Topics in Pediatrics

Herbert H. Pomerance Barry B. Bercu
Editors

Topics in Pediatrics

A Festschrift for Lewis A. Barness

Forewords by Allen W. Root and John S. Curran

With 113 Figures in 115 Parts

Springer-Verlag
New York Berlin Heidelberg
London Paris Tokyo Hong Kong

Herbert H. Pomerance, MD
Professor of Pediatrics
University of South Florida College of Medicine
Tampa, Florida 33612, USA;
Professor Emeritus
Department of Pediatrics
West Virginia University College of Medicine
Morgantown, West Virginia, USA

Barry B. Bercu, MD
Professor of Pediatrics
University of South Florida College of Medicine
Tampa, Florida 33612, USA

Library of Congress Cataloging-in-Publication Data
Topics in pediatrics : a festschrift for Lewis A. Barness / Herbert H. Pomerance, Barry B. Bercu, editors ; forewords by Allen W. Root and John S. Curran.
p. cm.
Includes bibliographical references.
ISBN-13: 978-1-4612-7925-9 e-ISBN-13: 978-1-4612-3230-8
DOI: 10.1007/978-1-4612-3230-8

1. Pediatrics. 2. Barness, Lewis A. I. Barness, Lewis A. II. Pomerance, Herbert H., 1918- . III. Bercu, Barry B.
[DNLM: 1. Pediatrics. WS 100 T6745]
RJ71.T67 1990
618.92–dc20
DNLM/DLC
for Library of Congress 89-21807

Softcover reprint of the hardcover 1st edition 1990

Typeset by Publishers Service, Bozeman, Montana.

9 8 7 6 5 4 3 2 1

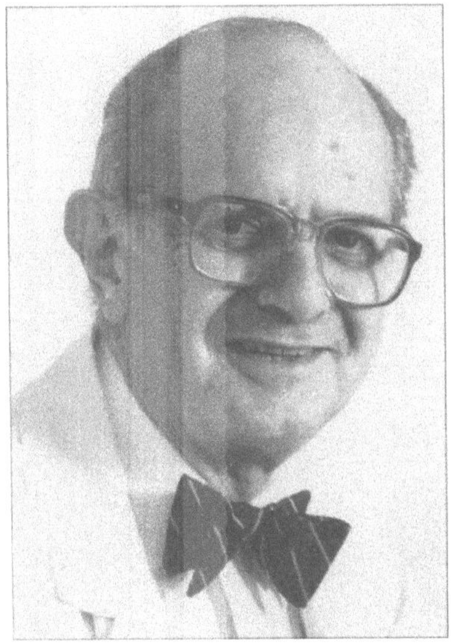

To Lewis A. Barness, MD, one of the few remaining great clinicians, whose love for children, for his peers and students, and for advancing knowledge through research, and whose dedication to improving the human condition, have made him a "legend in his own time."

Photograph by Don Pillai.

Foreword

ALLEN W. ROOT

On November 11 and 12, 1988, a "Festschrift" was held to honor "our Chief," Lewis A. Barness. Who is our Chief, and why was such an occasion held? I will not attempt to describe him in terms of his scientific and scholarly accomplishments, which have spanned more than four decades. Rather, I will describe the characteristics of an individual whose concern for humanity has made him the quintessential role model for countless students, residents, and graduate pediatricians around the world. The Chief's concern is manifested by his love for children and his tireless efforts on their behalf, as well as his genuine affection for his colleagues, all of whom are also his friends.

During the 2-day celebration, many of these friends had an opportunity to make comments which I believe capture portions of the essence of this remarkable human being:

> Many of us are better persons because of our association with the "Chief. . . ." Many of us have chosen pediatrics as a career as an unspoken act of tribute to him. . . . We love you and we thank you for making the world a better place to spend some time. (F. Oski)

> Lew fulfilled all our dreams . . . We all wish we could have done half so well. (R. Klein)

> [Your] ever-present evidence of concern for your fellow man . . . it is the quality of caring. (T. Oliver)

> Lew has achieved what all of us would have aspired to accomplish. . . . [He] is a masterful doctor, incredible teacher, inspirer of generations of young men and women.... (R. Kaye)

> Lew always knew the right question to ask. (D. Cornfeld)

> The best teacher . . . with modesty, human warmth, and understanding and honesty. . . . [He instilled an] optimistic spirit to explore new territories. (T. Scully)

> [Lew] created an atmosphere for learning that was vibrant. (W. Tunnessen)

> [Lew taught] four lessons – to enjoy children, to work hard, to be honest with yourself and with others, to have fun. . . . We all owe a debt of gratitude to Lew. (M. Kaback)

> [Lew has] the ability to crystallize thought [and to] open the vistas of the importance of pediatrics and child health and of child health advocacy. (J. Curran)

[Lew] continuously challenged us to ask the challenging question, . . . [taught] us how to learn and how to live. (D. Barrett)

Lew has been a mentor, a colleague, a friend to so many. He has been described as the "pediatrician's pediatrician." He is all of these and so much more. His legacy will be that of improved care and greater concern for children. It is for these reasons and many more that cannot be expressed in words that we gathered to honor Lew Barness.

Foreword

John S. Curran

Many years ago, Thomas Carlyle wrote: "All that man has done, said, thought, or been; they are written in the pages of books. They are the chosen possessions of mankind." These words, written just a century ago, embody the purpose for this volume acknowledging a few of the contributions that Lewis A. Barness, MD, has given to his students as a teacher, mentor, guide, and adviser through their own academic development to be numbered among the leaders of pediatric medicine today.

The professional development of the man we honor has touched many institutions and people. This path spans graduation from Harvard Medical School, to the only battalion surgeon that lost and was billed for an ambulance in the Philippines in World War II, to Boston Children's Hospital and the Massachusetts Institute of Technology, to association with Paul Gyorgy at the University of Pennsylvania, and the establishment of his lifelong interest in newborn nutrition and the fact that "breast is best." After 19 years at the University of Pennsylvania, he accepted a new challenge to found and nurture the Department of Pediatrics at the then brand-new University of South Florida College of Medicine in Tampa. As recipient of awards for distinguished teaching at both medical schools, the Borden Award and the Joseph B. Goldberger Award in Clinical Nutrition, he has demonstrated his ability to stimulate not only trainees and students but also his peers. Much of the reemphasis upon the importance of human milk and its components in human nutrition must be attributed to his leadership of the Committee on Nutrition of the American Academy of Pediatrics from 1974 to 1981.

This "Festschrift" has been a joyous occasion to honor the contributions of Lewis Barness, teacher, scholar, and friend. Not only is Lew Barness honored for his life and contributions to children's care, but there is also a commitment to make permanent in the pages of mankind some of the areas of interest and achievement of his students and friends. The variety of contributions is much like the interests of the "Chief" himself: they range from the newborn to the red and white cells, immune function, genetics and teratology, nutrition, and metabolic diseases to areas as current as medical education, health care delivery, ethics, human rights, and pediatric economics. Such is the measure of the Chief, his interest in children's affairs is protean, even though much of his interest has been in proteins: their optimal quality and quantity in human nutrition.

The Chief has never sat and will never sit on his laurels; there are too many questions to be asked and answers to be sought. The role of nucleotides in immune function and gut growth and the optimal fat blend for the human neonate are two of his current interests.

The Socratic method of his teaching will be remembered by every one of his students along with his water pistol and his deadly accuracy for the wayward or recalcitrant student. From the shuffle of his footsteps between both basic science and clinical labs, to the Snickers bars for lunch, to the irrepressible good humor, counsel and advice, we all salute him for his contributions to children and the development of his academic "children" who present these papers in honor and tribute to the Chief.

Preface

When we first accepted the task of creating a "Festschrift" for Lew Barness, we looked on it as a *labor of love*. Little did we realize that we would also need a love of labor, all of it most worthwhile for our dear friend.

One of the bigger problems we faced was that of explaining to others the meaning of the word Festschrift. Both of us knew the word, and its content. To aid us in explaining it, we felt it would be appropriate to consult a German-English dictionary. To our dismay, the word does not appear in the best one. Its parts do:

"*Fest*, n., festival; holiday; feast; fete; banquet." "*Schrift*, f., writing, hand; letters; script; text; book, publication; paper, review." Together, we have "a festive writing," and this definition has served us well.

To honor such a man as Lew Barness, we had to find everyone who occupied a place in his life. We tried. We obtained lists from Enid, Frank, Grant, and others. Mostly we prayed that we were not overlooking anyone, though we are sure we did, and we apologize to those we missed. Our list grew to almost 700 people, all of whom were invited to the celebration. Each was invited to write a letter, as per the definition above, to be bound into a book. Lew has this beautiful volume.

The "Fest" would not have been a festival without a banquet. The event filled a ballroom with 390 relatives, friends, colleagues, and students, all of whom were anxious to show their esteem. Modern technology permitted a videotaped record of the ceremonies, and Lew has this also.

The "Schrift" would not have been complete without "writings," and 26 colleagues responded with papers, some very scientific, some more practical, some rather philosophic. Two days were spent in their presentation. To culminate this, still in keeping with the definition, there came "publication," and we feel privileged to have been able to edit this volume, dedicated to Lew and produced with the love of all, including the publisher.

Herbert H. Pomerance
Barry B. Bercu

Encomium

This "Festschrift" is less to honor, and more to demonstrate our affection for, a man who has given so much of himself to each one of the contributors to this collection. We are all better persons because of our association with Lewis Abraham Barness, fondly known to many as "the Chief."

The Chief was born on July 31, 1921, and spent his childhood in Bucks County, Pennsylvania. He was graduated from Harvard College in 1941 and from the Harvard Medical School in 1944. While at Harvard College, he played on the Harvard baseball team and later joined the Abraham Lincoln Battalion in Spain. Following his graduation from medical school, he took what was then a prestigious internship at Philadelphia General Hospital, before entering the United States Army as a Captain in the Medical Corps.

After completing his Army service, he spent a year as a Research Fellow in Pediatrics at Boston Children's Hospital and the Massachusetts Institute of Technology. Following this year of preparation, he served as intern, assistant resident, and Fellow in Pediatrics at Boston Children's Hospital, completing these experiences in 1950. In 1951, he was appointed as an Associate in Pediatrics at the University of Pennsylvania School of Medicine, ultimately rising to the rank of Professor of Pediatrics in 1964. While at the University of Pennsylvania, he served as Chief of the Department of Pediatrics at Philadelphia General Hospital and at the Hospital of the University of Pennsylvania.

The Chief left the University of Pennsylvania in 1972 to create the post of Professor and Chairman of Pediatrics, at the University of South Florida College of Medicine. In 1986, he was also appointed Professor of Public Health.

The Chief is a modest man with many accomplishments. Among the most notable honors are his receipt of the Christian R. and Mary F. Lindback Foundation Award for Distinguished Teaching at the University of Pennsylvania in 1963; his election to membership in the honor society Alpha Omege Alpha in 1966; the award of an honorary Master of Arts degree at the University of Pennsylvania in 1971; the receipt of the Borden Award in 1972; the award of the Rudolph and Anita Noer Distinguished Professor Award at the University of South Florida in 1980; and receipt of the Joseph B. Goldberger Award in Clinical Nutrition in 1984.

Over the years, he has given a succession of honor lectureships at various universities. These include the Waldo Nelson Lecture at Temple University in 1971; the John P. Scott Lecture at the Children's Hospital of Philadelphia in 1981; the James Etteldorf Lecture at the University of Tennessee in 1984; the Frank A. Oski Lecture at SUNY Upstate Medical Center in 1985; the Sauer Lecture at Northwestern University in 1986; and the Packard Lecture to the Philadelphia Pediatric Society in 1986.

He holds memberships in the Society for Pediatric Research, the American Pediatric Society, the American Academy of Pediatrics, the American Association for the Advancement of Science, the American Institute of Nutrition, the American College of Nutrition, the American Society of Parenteral and Enteral Nutrition, and the American Academy of Certified Medical Nutritionists. He has managed to give maximum effort to each.

Indeed, he served as President of the American Pediatric Society in 1985 and 1986 and, seemingly, as the perpetual Recorder of the American Pediatric Society, from 1964 to 1974. He was Chairman of the Committee on Nutrition of the American Academy of Pediatrics from 1974 to 1981, a period of the Committee's greatest productivity and influence. He currently serves on the Editorial Board of *Nutrition Reviews*, the *Journal of Clinical Medicine and Nutrition*, and *Contemporary Pediatrics*. He is an Assistant Editor of *Pediatric Gastroenterology and Nutrition* and the Editor of *Advances in Pediatrics*.

His bibliographic citations begin with the now classic article entitled "The Utilization of Glycogen by Flies During Flight and Some Aspects of the Physiological Aging of *Drosophila*." The list now includes some 250 additional papers. He did much of the definitive work on the determination of the protein requirements of the low-birth-weight infant and was the first to demonstrate the relationship between vitamin B_{12} deficiency and methylmalonic aciduria. With one of us (G.A.M.), he helped to elucidate the nature of the congenital defects in organic acid metabolism in methylmalonic acidemia.

He is the author of the popular book entitled *A Manual of Pediatric Physical Diagnosis* and is coeditor of the textbook titled *A Core Textbook in Pediatrics*.

These accomplishments tell you nothing about the man for whom we all have a special fondness. A central portion of his life has always been his family, his devotion to his parents and his children (Carol, Laurie, and Joseph), his love for his first wife, Elaine, now deceased, and his romantic affection for his present wife, Enid Gilbert-Barness.

This recital has failed to mention the fact that the Chief has been regarded as the best teacher by his medical students and house staff, every year and in every place he has been. Many of us chose pediatrics as a career as an unspoken act of tribute to him.

No mention of Dr Barness could be complete without commenting on his perpetual optimism, his skill in helping people reach their potential, his intense intellectual curiosity, his ability to inspire those around him to seek answers to the problems that confront us, his modesty, his very poor jokes, and his equally bad taste in clothes. His clip-on bow ties and his water pistol are as much a part of him as the smell of tobacco, his "humble mumble," his diagnostic acumen, and his store of information and misinformation.

For all this and more, we love him and we thank him for making the world a better place for children and for all of us to spend some time.

FRANK A. OSKI
GRANT MORROW III

A Sonnet for Lew on the Occasion of His "Festschrift"

Man honours man in sundry various ways
By titles, prizes, and the earthly dime
But greater far than anyone who pays,
Are they who brought their company and time.
And so they honoured Lew Barness these days
Came to salute this man, modest and mild
Teacher, who touched their lives in many ways
Researcher, of metabolism of child.
Just as we love our parents' smile or mien
So students relish Lew, his teaching fun,
His stories with their final flaccid line,
Recall the showers from his water gun.
His students and his friends thus honoured Lew
"Friend of the child," one of a special few.

JOHN EMERY, MB, CHB, MD

Contents

Contributors

DOUGLAS J. BARRETT, MD, Associate Professor of Pediatrics, University of Florida College of Medicine, Gainesville, Florida, USA.

ROBERT L. BRENT, MD, PhD, DSc., Distinguished University Professor, Louis and Bess Stein Professor of Pediatrics, Chairman, Pediatric Department, Thomas Jefferson University, Philadelphia, Pennsylvania; Director, Division of Developmental Biology, Alfred I. duPont Institute, Wilmington, Delaware, USA.

DANIEL CHIU, PHD, Associate Research Biochemist, Children's Hospital Research Institute, Oakland, California, USA.

CHARLES D. COOK, MD, Professor of Pediatrics, University of Rochester School of Medicine and Dentistry, Rochester, New York, USA.

DAVID CORNFELD, MD, MSc, Professor of Pediatrics, University of Pennsylvania School of Medicine, Philadelphia, Pennsylvania, USA.

JUAN CUETO, BS, University of Miami School of Medicine, Miami, Florida, USA.

JOHN S. CURRAN, MD, Professor and Interim Chairman of Pediatrics, University of South Florida College of Medicine, Tampa, Florida, USA.

MARIA DELIVORIA-PAPADOPOULOS, MD, Professor of Pediatrics and Physiology, University of Pennsylvania School of Medicine, Philadelphia, Pennsylvania, USA.

FRANK B. DIAMOND JR, MD, Associate Professor of Pediatrics, University of South Florida College of Medicine, Tampa, Florida, USA.

JOHN L. EMERY, MB, CHB, MD, Professor Emeritus, Department of Pediatrics, University of Sheffield, Sheffield, England.

DANIEL A. GALVIS, BS, Graduate Student in Experimental Pathology, University of Southern California School of Medicine, Los Angeles, California, USA.

PARVIN GANJEI, MD, University of Miami School of Medicine, Miami, Florida, USA.

MARY M. GILBERT, MD, Assistant in Ophthalmology, Massachusetts Eye and Ear Infirmary, Clinical Instructor in Ophthalmology, Harvard University School of Medicine, Boston, Massachusetts, USA.

ENID GILBERT-BARNESS, MD, Professor of Pathology and Pediatrics, University of Wisconsin School of Medicine, Madison, Wisconsin, USA.

MUTAZ B. HABAL, MD, Director, Tampa Bay Craniofacial Center, Inc., Adjunct Professor of Material Science and Clinical Professor of Surgery, University of Florida, Research Professor, University of South Florida, Tampa, Florida, USA.

M. ELIZABETH HARTNETT, MD, Clinical Fellow in Ophthalmology, Massachusetts Eye and Ear Infirmary, Surgical Fellow, Eye Research Institute, Retina Foundation, Boston, Massachusetts, USA.

M. DARIA HAUST, MD, FRCP(C), Professor of Pathology, Pediatrics, and Obstetrics and Gynecology, University of Western Ontario, London, Ontario, Canada.

TATSUO HIROSE, MD, Associate Surgeon in Ophthalmology, Massachusetts Eye and Ear Infirmary, Associate Clinical Professor in Ophthalmology, Harvard Medical School, Associate Scientist, Eye Research Institute, Retina Foundation, Boston, Massachusetts, USA.

ROBERT KAYE, MD, Professor and Interim Chairman, Department of Pediatrics, Medical College of Pennsylvania, Philadelphia, Pennsylvania, USA.

ROBERT Z. KLEIN, MD, Professor of Pediatrics, Department of Maternal and Child Health, Dartmouth University Medical School, Hanover, New Hampshire, USA.

C. EVERETT KOOP, MD, The Surgeon General, United States Public Health Service, Department of Health and Human Services, Rockville, Maryland, USA.

JOSEPH H. KRUG, MD, Assistant in Ophthalmology, Massachusetts Eye and Ear Infirmary, Instructor in Ophthalmology, Harvard Medical School, USA.

FRANS KUYPERS, PHD, Assistant Research Biochemist, Children's Hospital Research Institute, Oakland, California, USA.

BENJAMIN H. LANDING, MD, Professor of Pathology and Pediatrics, University of Southern California School of Medicine, Los Angeles, California, USA.

CHARLES C. LOBECK, MD, Professor of Pediatrics, University of Wisconsin Medical School, Madison, Wisconsin, USA.

BERTRAM LUBIN, MD, Director of Medical Research, Children's Hospital of Oakland, Oakland, California, USA.

CELESTE M. MADDEN, MD, Assistant Professor of Pediatrics, State University of New York, Upstate Medical Center, Syracuse, New York, USA.

JOHN I. MALONE, MD, Professor of Pediatrics, University of South Florida College of Medicine, Tampa, Florida, USA.

MARIE C. MCCORMICK, MD, ScD, Associate Professor of Pediatrics, Harvard School of Medicine, Boston, Massachusetts, USA.

GRANT MORROW III, MD, Professor and Chairman, Department of Pediatrics, Ohio State University College of Medicine; Medical Director, Columbus Children's Hospital, Columbus, Ohio, USA.

MEHRDAD NADJI, MD, University of Miami School of Medicine, Miami, Florida, USA.

FRANK A. OSKI, MD, Given Professor and Chairman, Department of Pediatrics, Johns Hopkins University School of Medicine, Baltimore, Maryland, USA.

DONALD A. PIOUS, MD, Professor of Pediatrics and Immunology, Adjunct Professor of Genetics, University of Washington School of Medicine, Seattle, Washington, USA.

THOMAS M. RICHARDSON, MD, Assistant Surgeon in Ophthalmology, Massachusetts Eye and Ear Infirmary, Assistant Clinical Professor of Ophthalmology, Harvard Medical School, Boston, Massachusetts, USA.

ALLEN W. ROOT, MD, Professor of Pediatrics and Biochemistry, University of South Florida College of Medicine, Tampa, Florida, USA.

ARLAN L. ROSENBLOOM, MD, Professor of Pediatrics, University of Florida College of Medicine, Gainesville, Florida, USA.

DESMOND A. SCHATZ, MD, Assistant Professor of Pediatrics, University of Florida College of Medicine, Gainesville, Florida, USA.

THOMAS J. SCULLY, MD, Professor of Pediatrics, Associate Dean for Student Affairs, University of Nevada School of Medicine, Reno, Nevada, USA.

MASOUD SHAMSZADEH, MD, Clinical Assistant Professor of Pathology, University of Southern California School of Medicine, Los Angeles, California, USA.

DOROTHY I. SHULMAN, MD, Assistant Professor of Pediatrics, University of South Florida College of Medicine, Tampa, Florida, USA.

FRANK SINATRA, MD, Associate Professor of Pediatrics, University of Southern California School of Medicine, Los Angeles, California, USA.

JOHN W. SLEASMAN, MD, Assistant Professor of Pediatrics, University of Florida College of Medicine, Gainesville, Florida, USA.

BARBARA E. STRASSBERG, MD, Associate in Clinical Pediatrics, College of Physicians and Surgeons, Columbia University, New York; Associate Physician, Presbyterian Hospital of the City of New York, Riverdale, New York, USA.

WALTER W. TUNNESSEN, JR, MD, Associate Professor of Pediatrics and Dermatology, Johns Hopkins University School of Medicine, Baltimore, Maryland, USA.

CARMEN PATRICIA VALDES-DAPENA, MD, Resident in Family Medicine, Underwood Hospital, Underwood, New Jersey, USA.

MARIE VALDES-DAPENA, MD, Professor of Pathology and Pediatrics, University of Miami School of Medicine, Miami, Florida, USA.

ELLIOTT VICHINSKY, MD, Associate Director, Hematology/Oncology Department, Children's Hospital of Oakland, Oakland, California, USA.

THEADIS R. WELLS, HT (ASCP), Senior Research Technologist, Pathology Research Unit, Children's Hospital of Los Angeles, Los Angeles, California, USA.

1
Complications of Diabetes in Children: When Does the Clock Start Running?

JOHN I. MALONE

Pediatricians are frequently accused of not being properly concerned about the complications of diabetes in children. This statement is commonly made by physicians who inherit the care of the young adults who have complications secondary to diabetes with onset during childhood. Since these complications rarely become manifest during childhood or adolescence, it is alleged that pediatricians fail to understand the importance of good diabetic control for their prevention. The "complications" considered in this context are diabetic retinopathy, nephropathy, neuropathy, macrovascular disease leading to coronary artery disease, and peripheral vascular insufficiency which results in lower limb amputations. These problems tend to become clinically evident a number of years after the initial diagnosis of diabetes mellitus.

It is rare to recognize diabetic retinopathy before diabetes has been present for at least 5 years. Diabetic nephropathy is first recognized when the patient develops hypertension or protein in the urine. This generally requires 10 years of clinically recognized diabetes mellitus. If one considers that the prepubertal age for peak incidence of new cases of insulin-dependent diabetes mellitus (IDDM) is 5 to 6 years of age, it is easy to understand why pediatricians are rarely involved in managing the complications of IDDM. If one includes adolescents in pediatric practice (not a universal practice), it is found that the greatest number of youth have the onset of IDDM with the onset of puberty. Therefore, the associated complications will have their earliest recognition 5 to 10 years later.

It is important, however, before focusing on the complications of long-standing IDDM to recognize that certain *acute and subacute problems* are associated with IDDM which are of great importance for the affected child as well as the pediatrician (Table 1.1). These problems are (1) hypoglycemia (which occurs in all individuals who are insulin dependent); (2) diabetic ketoacidosis (the most common cause for diabetes-related hospitalizations in children between birth and 18 years of age); (3) growth failure (a common occurrence in association with

---

From the Section of Metabolic Diseases, Department of Pediatrics, University of South Florida College of Medicine, Tampa, Florida.
Presented in honor of Lewis A. Barness, MD, November 12, 1988.

TABLE 1.1. Acute and subacute complications of IDDM.

Hypoglycemia
Diabetic ketoacidosis
Growth failure
Psychosocial dysfunction

diabetes with onset prior to puberty); and (4) psychosocial dysfunction (immaturity and over dependence upon authority figures evolving from daily concern about the correct amount of food, exercise, and insulin in emotionally developing children). Each of these problems associated with IDDM has its onset at the time of clinical recognition of hyperglycemia and the initiation of insulin therapy.

Acute Complications

Hypoglycemia

Hypoglycemia occurs in all insulin-dependent patients. It is generally mild and easily managed by the consumption of extra food. It may be more severe and produce a spectrum of symptoms ranging from personality changes to loss of consciousness and seizures. The more severe stages of hypoglycemia are thought to cause some brain damage and may result in focal neurologic deficits such as paralysis. Deaths due to hypoglycemia continue to be reported in association with IDDM. Efforts to improve diabetic control with intensified insulin therapy as reported by the Diabetes Control and Complications Trial have resulted in a fivefold increase in the frequency of severe hypoglycemia (loss of consciousness and/or seizures).[1]

Diabetic Ketoacidosis

Diabetic ketoacidosis is the most common cause for hospitalization in children under the age of 18 years with diabetes.[2] This is a problem that is most commonly associated with failure of insulin administration. It occurs with greatest frequency in the adolescent who has assumed total responsibility for all insulin administration. It can occur, however, in younger children who are dependent upon adults who also may forget to administer the insulin.

Growth Failure

Growth failure is a common problem in children who have onset of diabetes prior to puberty. Poor metabolic control is associated with reduced levels of somatomedin-C[3] (insulinlike growth factor-1) as well as urinary loss of calcium and phosphorus[4] essential for bone growth and development. Insulin in and of itself has a growth-promoting function. Thus, physiologic quantities of insulin

TABLE 1.2. Chronic complications of IDDM.

Cardiac
Retinopathy
Cataracts
Neuropathy
Nephropathy

are required for normal growth and development and cannot be appropriately supplied by our current methods of delivering insulin to growing children.

Psychosocial Dysfunction

The standard parenting practice utilized to allow the normal progression from a dependent child to an independent adult is severely affected by the presence of a chronic disease requiring daily medical treatment. Diabetes is a chronic disorder requiring the injection of insulin one to three times a day as well as frequent needle punctures to collect blood samples for glucose monitoring. This is an activity that is emotionally distasteful and one that interferes with the normal progression of self-care duties that are initially the responsibility of the parents and should progress to the domain of the adolescent or young adult. The trial and error involved in this natural progression is not ideal for achieving the goal of "good metabolic control" and adds to the frustration that develops between the youths and their parents. Thus, adolescents with poor self-image and self-destructive activities are somewhat common in this patient population.

Each of these issues (hypoglycemia, ketoacidosis, growth failure, psychosocial dysfunction) is an important and difficult problem faced by the pediatrician. These problems begin with the onset of clinical diabetes and the initiation of insulin therapy. Many times rigid control of the blood glucose seems to lose importance in comparison with resolution of the above issues.

Chronic Complications

The chronic complications of diabetes start to produce obvious physical morbidity and reduced life expectancy approximately 5 years after the clinical onset of diabetes (Table 1.2). They become more evident after duration of diabetes for 10 years (Fig. 1.1). Since most children develop IDDM between 5 and 6 and between 10 and 12 years, it is easy to understand why preadolescent children appear to be spared the toxic effects of hyperglycemia. Drash reported an analysis of diabetic children followed at Children's Hospital of Pittsburgh.[5] He concluded that the prepubertal duration of diabetes had a "minimal influence" on the later risk of diabetic complications. In support of that clinical observation, Williamson and associates[6] have shown in streptozotocin diabetic rats that increased collagen cross-linking and increased vascular permeability associated with hyperglycemia

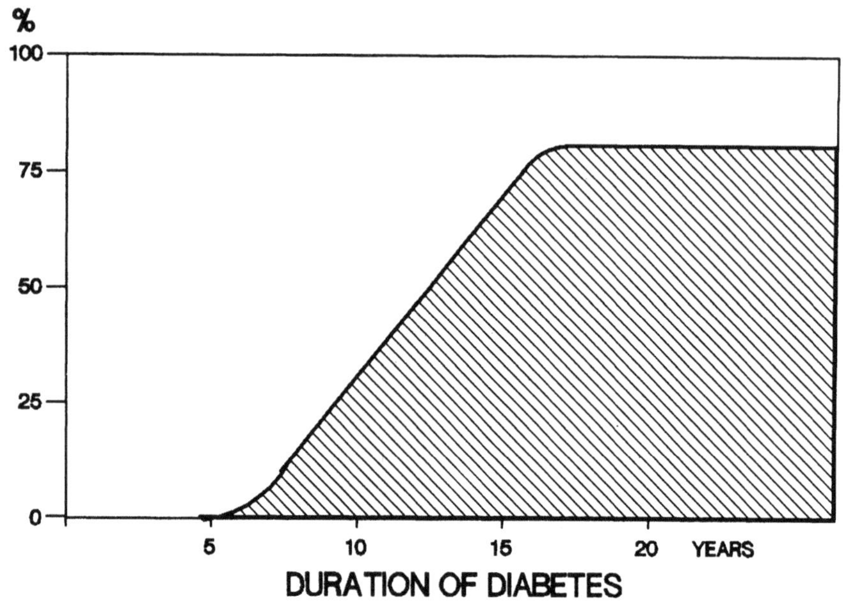

FIGURE 1.1. Prevalence of retinopathy (%) by duration of clinical diabetes (0 to 20+ years).

can be prevented by castration. They were also able to show that castration significantly reduced the activity of the polyol pathway which has been implicated as a metabolic cause of the long-term complications of diabetes mellitus (Table 1.3). These observations support the concept that children with diabetes may be protected from vascular complications prior to the onset of puberty.

Parents and pediatricians, with greater responsibility for the care of infants and young children, take comfort from the belief that diabetic complications do not occur during childhood. When faced with the impossible task of achieving good

TABLE 1.3. Albumen permeation and sorbitol content.

	N	New vessels	Sorbitol (mM/g wet wt)
Control			
Intact	8	1.99 ± 0.22	7.1 ± 1.9
Castrated	8	1.89 ± 0.24	5.7 ± 1.1
Diabetic			
Intact	9	3.11 ± 0.14[a]	14.7 ± 4.4[a]
Castrated	6	1.89 ± 0.14	9.1 ± 1.4

[a] Different from control.
Source: Williamson et al.[6]

TABLE 1.4. Microvascular abnormalities in girls with diabetes 7 to 18 years.[a]

Stage	Age (years) 7-9	10-11	12-13	14-15	16-18
0	5	12	23	9	7
1	7	31	23	11	5
2	1	10	6	2	4
3	1	1	1	8	2
% Positive	64	78	57	70	61
% 2, 3	14	20	13	33	33

[a] Microvascular abnormalities are noted at age indicated.

diabetic control in those children, there is great hope that elevated blood glucose values during childhood may not have the same detrimental effect as they do in later life.

Until the late 1970s, most of the medical community accepted the idea that the microvascular complications of diabetes really did not become manifest during childhood. Close examination of the retina of children with diabetes using fluorescein angiography, however, proved that microvascular abnormalities do occur in children with diabetes of less than 5 years' duration and prior to the onset of puberty[7] (Tables 1.4, 1.5). Moreover, investigators from three different institutions reported that improving metabolic control in a group of preadolescent children caused a rapid progression of retinopathy as the result of improved metabolic control[8] (Table 1.6).

Diabetic nephropathy is much more difficult to document than retinopathy because of the relative inaccessibility of the kidneys. The first clinical sign of nephropathy is the onset of hypertension and/or proteinuria. It is believed that structural changes occur in kidneys 10 to 15 years before the recognition of clinical proteinuria. The work of Silverstein and associates[9] indicates that histologic renal disease begins before puberty (Table 1.7). Individuals in this study with diabetes 10 years' duration or more had histologic changes consistent with diabetic nephropathy, plus proteinuria at 15 and 16 years of age, suggesting that the early

TABLE 1.5. Microvascular abnormalities in boys with diabetes 7 to 18 years.[a]

Stage	Age (years) 7-9	10-11	12-13	14-15	16-18
0	10	9	12	12	4
1	12	17	15	20	9
2	5	7	1	3	3
3	0	2	1	1	2
% Positive	49	74	59	67	78
% 2, 3	14	26	7	11	28

[a] Microvascular abnormalities are noted at age indicated.

TABLE 1.6. Microvascular disease before puberty.

	Female	Male	Male	Male
Bone age	11 years	ND	13.5	6
Pubertal stage	I	I	II	I
Retinopathy	Yes	Yes	Yes	Yes

Source: Daneman et al.[8]

structural defects of diabetic renal disease existed before puberty in those individuals. Other teenage individuals in this study had histologic evidence of diabetic nephropathy after 7 years of IDDM without clinical evidence of proteinuria. This circumstantial evidence suggests that histologic changes were present in the kidneys of the young postpubertal individuals 7 to 10 years earlier, when prepubertal.

Peripheral neuropathy is the most common complication of diabetes. Peripheral nerve dysfunction was well documented in a survey of children 3 to 8 years old with IDDM when compared to age-matched controls[10] (Table 1.8). The reduced nerve conduction velocities reported are believed to be the direct result of the hyperglycemia of IDDM and were found in prepubertal children.

Premature coronary artery disease is a significant complication and is the leading cause of death in diabetes. Hypercholesterolemia is a significant risk factor associated with premature coronary artery disease. Hypercholesterolemia occurs more commonly in children who have diabetes than in unaffected children of the same age[11] (Table 1.9). It is believed that this is directly related to the hyperglycemia associated with diabetes. The Bogalusa survey[12] reported that 4% of children less than 18 years of age had cholesterol values greater than 200 mg/dl. Six percent of our prepubertal females and 24% of our prepubertal males

TABLE 1.7. Nephropathy and IDDM in children.

Age (years)	Duration (years)	Proteinurea[a] (g/24 h)	Bx changes
16	11	3.5	4+
19	07	<0.24	2+
16	10	1.0	4+
16	14	3.5	4+
16	11	3.5	4+
20	06	<0.24	4+
23	10	1.0	3+
18	13	3.5	4+
15	13	1.0	4+
19	16	1.0	4+
20	07	<0.24	3+
21	11	3.5	4+

[a] Morphologic changes occur 10–15 years before proteinurea.
Source: Silverstein et al.[9]

TABLE 1.8. Childhood diabetic neuropathy (nerve conduction velocity m/sec), ages 3 to 8 years.

	Control	IDDM	P<
N	26	16	
Ulnar	65.4 ± 8.5	59.1 ± 5.2	0.01
N	25	16	
Median	58.3 ± 5.4	58.6 ± 9.5	NS
N	26	15	
Peroneal	57.5 ± 6.9	49.2 ± 6.5	0.001

Source: Gamstorp.[10]

had cholesterol levels greater than 200 mg/dl. This suggests that the hyperglycemia of IDDM is associated with increase of the coronary artery risk factor (cholesterol) in prepubertal children.

It appears that the microvascular/macrovascular complications of diabetes, which require 5 to 10 years to become manifest, have onset of the basic pathologic process closely timed to the initial onset of hyperglycemia. Since the prepubertal period is limited in duration and these vascular abnormalities require 5 to 10 years to evolve, this provides a false sense of security and safety. It may be more appropriate to accept the idea that the pathologic process causing tissue damage in diabetes begins with the onset of clinical hyperglycemia but the process is accentuated by the hormonal changes that occur with the onset of puberty. Growth hormone appears to be the most likely affector in this regard. Growth hormone is a major contributor to proliferative retinopathy. Growth hormone levels have also been shown to be elevated in association with IDDM. The observation that sex steroids accentuate growth hormone release to specific stimuli indicates a possible mechanism for an increase in microvascular abnormalities in association with puberty.

TABLE 1.9. Diabetes and hypercholesterolemia in children.

Males				
Cholesterol	Age < 10 years	Age 10–16	Age > 16	Duration
<200 mg/dl	75%	78%	60%	4 ± 2 years
200–240	12%	11%	30%	8 ± 2 years
>240	12%	11%	10%	4 ± 4 years
Females				
Cholesterol	Age < 8 years	Age 8–14	Age > 14	Duration
<200 mg/dl	94%	86%	50%	5 ± 3 years
200–240	06%	14%	31%	6 ± 3 years
>240	00%	00%	19%	6 ± 2 years

Thus, we cannot be reassured that there is a period of safety from hyperglycemia for prepubertal children. We must instead continue to look for more effective ways of treating diabetes in all children to restore normal metabolism since it is clear that the clock starts running for the complications of diabetes in children with the onset of hyperglycemia.

References

1. Lorenze R, Siebert C, Cleary P, Santiago J, Heyse S: Epidemiology of severe hypoglycemia in the DCCT. *Diabetes* 37:3A, 1988.
2. Crofford, O: *Report of the National Commission on Diabetes to the Congress of the United States*, Vol 3, part 2, DHEW Publication No (NIH) 76-1018, 1976.
3. Rudolf MCJ, Sherwin RS, Markowitz R, et al: Effect of intensive insulin treatment on linear growth in young diabetic patients. *J Pediatr* 101:333–339, 1982.
4. Malone JI, Lowitt S, Duncan JA, Shah SC, Vargas A, Root AW: Hypercalciuria, hyperphosphaturia in growth retardation in children with diabetes mellitus. *Pediatrics* 78:298–304, 1986.
5. Drash AL: Overview of complications in children with diabetes. Council on Diabetes in Youth American Diabetes Association annual meeting. New Orleans, June 1988.
6. Williamson JR, Rowold E, Chang K, et al: Sex steroid dependency of diabetes-induced changes in polyol metabolism, vascular permeability, in collagen cross-linking. *Diabetes* 35:20–27, 1986.
7. Malone JI, Grizzard WS, Epinoza LR, Achenbach KE, VanCader TC: Risk factor for diabetic retinopathy in youth. *Pediatrics* 73:756–761, 1984.
8. Daneman D, Drash AL, Lobes LA, Becker DJ, Baker LM, Travis LB: Progress retinopathy with improved control in diabetic dwarfism (Mauriac's syndrome). *Diabetes Care* 4:360–365, 1981.
9. Silverstein JH, Fennell R, Donnelly W, et al: Correlates of biopsied-studied nephropathy in young patients with insulin dependent diabetes mellitus. *J Pediatr* 106: 196–201, 1985.
10. Gamstorp I: Conduction velocity of peripheral motor nerves in mental retardation, diabetes and various neurologic diseases in childhood. *Acta Paediatr Scand* 53:408–416, 1964.
11. Malone JI, Shocken D: Diabetes and hypercholesterolemia in children. (Abstract) *Clin Res* 36:61A, 1988.
12. Freedman DS, Shear CL, Srinivasan SR: Tracking of serum lipids and lipoproteins in children over an eight year period: The Bogalusa study. *Prev Med* 14:203–216, 1985.

2
Life-Threatening Cerebral Edema in Diabetes: A Preventable Complication?

ARLAN L. ROSENBLOOM

Life-threatening cerebral edema (CE) is a disastrous complication that occurs almost exclusively in patients under 25 years of age. Although exceptional in any single physician's experience, several series suggest that it accounts for a substantial portion of diabetic ketoacidemia (DKA) associated deaths in childhood.

Over a 5-year period in Birmingham, England, three deaths occurred among 35 cases of DKA in the 10- to 19-year age group, and all were due to CE.[1] At the Joslin Clinic, from 1964 to 1966, there were 52 cases of DKA in an unknown age range with four deaths, of which two were the famous CE cases reported by Young and Bradley in 1967.[2] In a 35-year review of deaths in people under 20 with diabetes, the Pittsburgh Childen's Hospital group noted 17 DKA-associated deaths at onset of the diabetes, of which seven (41%) could be attributed to cerebral edema; and 19 deaths after diagnosis, of which four (21%) were due to CE.[3] Thus, at least 31% of DKA-associated deaths and 20% of all deaths in this age group could be attributed to cerebral edema. Travis[4] has seen two deaths and one case of severe neurological impairment due to cerebral edema in 24 years and 384 episodes of DKA.

This review is of 57 cases originally thought to be cerebral edema, 33 from the published literature[1,2,5-23] and 24 from information personally accumulated from various sources over the past decade. The questions addressed by this review are (1) whether there are any consistent circumstances that presage cerebral edema, (2) whether other intracranial disasters that clinically resemble cerebral edema are frequent, since they would influence choice of therapy, and (3) whether intervention to decrease intracranial pressure is effective. Finally, we will review etiological considerations in light of the clinical experience.

From the Department of Pediatrics, University of Florida College of Medicine, Gainesville, Florida.
Presented in honor of Lewis A. Barness, MD, November 12, 1988.

Are there Circumstances That Presage Cerebral Edema?

The rate of decrease of blood glucose, or the level of blood glucose attained, has been proposed as a mechanism for CE based on studies in rabbits made acutely hyperglycemic. In the 53 cases for which this could be analyzed, only three had a rate of blood glucose drop >100 mg/dl/h, and all three of these individuals were in the survivor group, two of them with little or no disability. Five individuals had blood glucose levels <200 mg/dl preceding neurologic collapse, and none had levels <100 mg/dl at that time.

Insulin may be a factor in the exchange of fluid and electrolyte across brain cell membranes, making the insulin dosage a consideration distinct from effects on glycemia. However, the advent of low-dose insulin therapy has not appeared to eliminate this problem, with six (about one third) of the cases in the low-dose era of the past 8 years being treated in this fashion.

Initial hyponatremia or subsequent fall in serum sodium concentration, due to either an inadequate sodium replacement or dysfunctional ADH response, has also been implicated. Calculated sodium concentrations at admission, in the 48 patients for whom these data are available, range from 130 to 179 mEq/dl. In 11 cases, the premorbid values were <130 mEq/dl and generally unrelated to the amount of sodium administered, which ranged in rate from 100 to 1,800 $mEq/m^2/24$ h.

Hypo- or hyperkalemia could be factors in the demise of these youngsters. There was only one instance of documented hypokalemia, and this was recognized and corrected in the hours before neurological collapse. The administration of bicarbonate has also been implicated. This review fails to demonstrate a consistent or even frequent use of bicarbonate.

The rate of fluid administration was calculated on the basis of current recommendations assuming 10% dehydration, with initial hydration in the first hour of 20/cc/kg body weight, and the remainder of the replacement and maintenance over the subsequent 23 hours.[24] A percentage of this ideal replacement regimen was calculated for 53 of the reports, excluding two from the literature in which the fluid administration data were not provided and two who had all of their hydration orally without recording of the volume. Rates varied from 30% to 450% of ideal, and there was an even split between those receiving <110% of estimated ideal and those receiving more than this amount. There was no difference in outcome with normal or overhydrated individuals. The two individuals completely hydrated by mouth died.

The review suggests other factors that may be important. Thirty-two of the 57 patients had new-onset diabetes, a proportion that seems greater than the general ketoacidosis experience. There were 10 subjects under 3 years of age and all were new-onset, as were all 14 under 5 years of age. The distribution of ages is disproportionate to the age incidence of diabetes in childhood, suggesting greater risk for the younger patient.

The oldest people in this group were a 23-year-old and a 28-year-old. Otherwise, they were all under 20 years of age, a circumstance that is all the more interesting when one considers the studies of Clements et al[25] showing increased CSF pressure as well as mild neurologic signs of cerebral edema in adults being treated for DKA, and the studies of Fein et al[26] showing ventricular compression by echoencephalography in similar patients. Why don't these adults develop life-threatening cerebral edema?

How Common Are Other Intracranial Disasters That Clinically Resemble Cerebral Edema?

Cerebral edema is, of course, the result of a variety of potential insults, including infection, toxins, trauma, and hypoxia. Intracranial disasters other than cerebral edema may occur during DKA and its treatment. Some suggestion of the heterogeneity of intracranial problems in DKA has been provided by the availability of CT scans over the past decade.

Just over half of the 29 patients having CT in this series showed diffuse cerebral edema on acute studies. Four had localized edema at the base of the brain; in one case this was suggestive of subarachnoid hemorrhage. Two had clear-cut subarachnoid hemorrhage, and one had basal artery thrombosis. Five were initially read as normal, but two of these who had follow-up scans were found to have had infarction in various loci of the brain. Two individuals did not have acute scans, but, following recovery, scans showed necrosis or infarcts.

Postmortem studies in 20 individuals who did not have scans were consistent with cerebral edema and in most cases brainstem herniation. However, one individual, a 3-month-old child admitted in coma, did not have diffuse edema but multiple thrombi, presumably due to a hypercoagulable state.[12] One reported case with cerebral edema noted at postmortem had encephalitis as part of his new-onset diabetes.[16] A 6-year-old son of a father with insulin-dependent diabetes was not in DKA on admission with a blood sugar of 855 mg/dl and a CO_2 of 20, but developed headaches half an hour after his first dose of insulin, followed by vomiting, and died with respiratory arrest 12h following the institution of IV fluids at an inadequate rate of 30% of anticipated need.

It would appear that some 10% to 15% of clinically typical cerebral edema will be due to thrombosis, infection, or hemorrhage.

What Are the Results of Treatment to Decrease Intracranial Pressure?

All 57 patients have been analyzed including those with diagnoses other than cerebral edema, since it is likely that treatment will need to be undertaken in an emergency before obtaining diagnostic verification. There have been eight survivors *without residua* of whom six were treated early, before the development of respiratory arrest, one treated after respiratory arrest, and one never treated. None had developed respiratory arrest.

The classification *disabled* refers to those individuals who have such problems as hypopituitarism, partial paralysis, a seizure disorder, or mild to moderate learning disability, but who nonetheless are capable of achieving independence. Six individuals treated early survived disabled.

Severely disabled refers to inability to achieve independence but not in a vegetative state, including total blindness with retardation and hypopituitarism or quadraplegia. One untreated one late-treated, and one early-treated patient fell into this category. Two treated early survived in the *vegetative* state, as did one not treated at all. Finally, *death* occurred in 17 out of 20 who were not treated, 13 out of 15 who were treated late, but only 7 out of 22 who were treated early.

These data differ markedly from the general impression that cerebral edema is universally fatal. Furthermore, they support the importance of careful neurologic monitoring during treatment of DKA to permit early intervention when unmistakable neurologic signs develop, such as bradycardia, blood pressure changes, incontinence, pupillary abnormalities, agitation, and headache. In all but one case, in which colloid solution was given very late, treatment was with mannitol and usually with hyperventilation and dexamethasone.

Etiologic Considerations

Numerous hypotheses have been put forth to explain the development of cerebral edema, and we have already dismissed these in all but the most blatant situations of overhydration or the use of very hypotonic fluids.

Suspecting that slowly metatolized polyols might be implicated in the development of cerebral edema, Clements et al[27] noted 20 years ago that if the blood glucose of a healthy anesthesized dog was raised to 400 to 600 mg/dl by intravenous glucose, the intracisternal fluid pressure fell as expected. But when the infusion was stopped after 4 h and rehydration was done with isotonic saline, the intracranial pressure consistently rose to pathologic levels. They could not attribute this to fluid overload or to water intoxication, and the brain showed obvious cerebral edema with increased concentrations of glucose and sorbitol. However, subsequent studies failed to implicate more than a partial osmolar contribution from sorbitol.[28] Identified were idiogenic osmols, culprits referred to by Finberg[29] in his studies of hyperosmolar dehydration in infants and children. There is an interesting parallel between the dilemmas of cerebral edema in children with DKA and that in infants and children with hypertonic dehydration. Finberg noted that sodium infusion in animals, simulating the hypernatremic state of children with high serum sodium levels, results in a sodium influx into brain cells but an exodus of taurine and glutamine with no net differential of osmols. Apparently, intracellular metabolism is generating the "idiogenic" osmols. There is certainly no contribution of hyperglycemia or polyols to the problem if nondiabetic hypertonic dehydration of infants and children.

In five unselected patients, aged 28 to 40 years, studied by Clements et al,[25] continuous monitoring of CSF pressure revealed consistent rises during treatment. In every case, this was associated with the development of drowsiness and in one, slurred speech 3 h after the start of treatment, followed by semistupor. In another, incoherence and agitation developed 4 h after treatment was instituted. All of these patients had been alert on admission. As with the dogs, this development did not appear to be related to overhydration.

Another interesting observation is that of Ditzel and colleagues,[30] who studied venous blood PO_2 and found it elevated during DKA, suggesting a failure of uptake in the peripheral tissues. They viewed this as histotoxic hypoxia, rather than a reflection of diminished tissue perfusion from hypovolemia. They pointed out that the effect of decreased tissue perfusion is a reduction in venous oxygen content, rather than an increase.

Fein et al[26] found decreased arterial PO_2 and alveolar arterial oxygen gradients during standard treatment of 18 patients with DKA aged 13 to 42 years. The PaO_2 was highest before treatment, decreased rapidly by 4 h, and more slowly thereafter. In only two of these 18 individuals did this create levels of oxygen saturation below 90%.

This group also did echoencephalography in 11 of these patients and found that 9 of them had substantial compression of the lateral ventricles, indicative of cerebral edema. It is noteworthy that, despite profound dehydration in these patients, there was no evidence of brain shrinkage in the pretreatment phase; this suggests the generation of idiogenic osmols to protect the brain from dehydration in this situation. Although these authors attributed their findings to the use of crystalloid volume loading, there is no comparison to the use of colloid or varying concentrations of crystalloid. In CT studies of six children, Krane and colleagues[31] similarly found ventricular compression and narrowing of the subarachnoid spaces.

While these studies of increased CSF pressure and some degree of cerebral edema as a regular feature of treatment of DKA are intriguing, they only befuddle us more in our attempts to understand why some patients have a disastrous expression of this phenomenon and why it occurs exclusively in children despite demonstrable experimental changes in adults.

Can We Prevent Life-Threatening Cerebral Edema?

The answer to this question is a highly qualified "maybe." On the basis of this review, we are able to make recommendations for reducing the risk of cerebral edema and, when it develops, to reduce the risk of fatality or severe brain damage. The first line of defense is the early recognition of diabetes, particularly in infants and young children, who appear unusually susceptible to intracerebral problems with diabetes just as they are with other fluid and electrolyte problems. Prevention of ketoacidosis in newly diagnosed patients, as well as established patients, is obviously going to be associated with decreased risks for intracerebral problems. In this context, we need to rethink the amount of vomiting and ketosis that is permissible in the home setting before these youngsters are brought to the hospital.

In a substantial number of patients there is usually a premonitory period when the development of cerebral edema can be suspected on the basis of headache, incontinence, dramatic change in arousal or behavior, pupillary changes, blood pressure changes, bradycardia, and hypothermia. Treatment with mannitol and hyperventilation, before the development of respiratory arrest, has appeared to be successful in several instances. Since early recognition requires careful monitoring, either an intensive-care setting or a closely supervised ward is necessary.

Certainly judicious treatment of DKA is important to prevent rapid osmolar shifts, hemodynamic compromise, and hypoxia. The minority of patients reviewed were clearly overhydrated, and this may have contributed to their course. Nonetheless, there was no relationship between the degree of overhydration and outcome or between the amount of sodium administered and the degree of fall in serum sodium concentration. The debate about whether we should be giving physiological concentrations of sodium in this condition, versus half normal saline, is no more resolved in DKA than it is in hypernatremic dehydration of infants and children.[32]

References

1. Fitzgerald MG, O'Sullivan DJ, Malins JM: Fatal diabetic ketosis. *Br Med J* 1:247–250, 1961.
2. Young E, Bradley RF: Cerebral edema with irreversible coma in severe diabetic ketoacidosis. *N Engl J Med* 12:665–669, 1967.
3. Scibili J, Finegold D, Dorman J, et al: Why do children with diabetes die? *Acta Endocrinol (Copenhagen)* Suppl 279:326–333, 1986.
4. Travis LB: Diabetic ketoacidosis. In Travis LB, Brouhard BH, Schreiner B-J, eds: *Diabetes Mellitus in Children and Adolescents.* Philadelphia: Saunders, 1987, p 159.
5. Taubin H, Matz R: Cerebral edema, diabetes insipidus, and sudden death during the treatment of diabetic ketoacidosis. *Diabetes* 17:108–109, 1968.
6. Hayes TM, Woods CJ: Unexpected death during treatment of uncomplicated diabetic ketoacidosis. *Br Med J* 4:32–33, 1968.
7. Warren P, Villaluz ES, Rosenberg H: Diabetic ketoacidosis with fatal cerebral edema. *Pediatrics* 43:620–622, 1969.
8. Manigand G, Auzepy F, Jan FL, et al: La mort par oedeme cerebral au cours de l'acido-cetose diabetique grave. *Presse Med* 77:790–792, 1969.
9. Metzger AL, Rubenstein AH: Reversible cerebral oedema complicating diabetic ketoacidosis. *Br Med J* 3:746–747, 1970.
10. Speirs AL, Stewart D, Adams H, et al: Fatal increase of intracranial pressure during management of diabetic ketosis. *Lancet* 2:879, 1971.
11. Warne GL: Fatal cerebral oedema with insulitis in diabetic ketoacidosis. *Med J Aust* 2:934–937, 1973.
12. Timperley WR, Preston FE, Ward JD: Cerebral intravascular coagulation in diabetic ketoacidosis. *Lancet* 1:952–956, 1974.
13. Menage JJ, Casenave C, Pelletier J, et al: Coma acido-cetosique avec diabete insipide d'evolution fatale par oedeme cerebral. *Sem Hop Paris* 52:948–952, 1976.
14. Duck SC, Weldon VV, Pagliara AS, et al: Cerebral edema complicating therapy for diabetic ketoacidosis. *Diabetes* 25:111–115, 1976.

15. Lufkin EG, Reagan TJ, Doan DH, et al: Acute cerebral dysfunction in diabetic ketoacidosis: Survival followed by panhypopituitarism. *Metabolism* 26:363–369, 1977.
16. Yoon J-W, Austin M, Onodera T, Notkins AL: Virus-induced diabetes mellitus. *N Engl J Med* 300:1173–1179, 1979.
17. Rosenbloom AL, Riley WJ, Weber FT, et al: Cerebral edema complicating diabetic ketoacidosis in childhood. *J Pediatr* 96:357–361, 1980.
18. Jos J, Hubert P, Mselati JC, et al: Oedeme cerebral aigu compliquant le traitement de l'acido-cetose diabetique de l'enfant. *Arch Fr Pediatr* 39:375–377, 1982.
19. Franklin B, Liu J, Ginsberg-Fellner F: Cerebral edema and ophthalmoplegia reversed by mannitol in a new case of insulin-dependent diabetes mellitus. *Pediatrics* 69:87–90, 1982.
20. Hayes PC, Newton RW: Reversible internal hydrocephalus complicating diabetic keto-acidosis. *Scot Med J* 29:195–197, 1984.
21. Garre M, Boles JM, Garo B, et al: Cerebral oedema in diabetic ketoacidosis: Do we use too much insulin? *Lancet* 1:220, 1986.
22. Keller RJ, Wolfsdorf JI: Isolated growth hormone deficiency after cerebral edema complicating diabetic ketoacidosis. *N Engl J Med* 316:857–859, 1987.
23. Kanter RK, Oliphant M, Zimmerman JJ, et al: Arterial thrombosis causing cerebral edema in association with diabetic ketoacidosis. *Crit Care Med* 15:175–176, 1987.
24. Schatz DA, Rosenbloom AL: Diabetic ketoacidosis: Management tactics in young patients. *J Crit Illness* 3:31–45, 1988.
25. Clements RS Jr, Blumenthal SA, Morrison AD, et al: Increased cerebrospinal-fluid pressure during treatment of diabetic ketosis. *Lancet* 2:657–661, 1971.
26. Fein IA, Rackow EC, Sprung CL, et al: Relation of colloid osmotic pressure to arterial hypoxemia and cerebral edema during crystalloid volume loading of patients with diabetic ketoacidosis. *Ann Intern Med* 96:570–574, 1982.
27. Clements RS Jr, Prockop LD, Winegrad AI: Acute cerebral edema during the treatment of hyperglycaemia: An experimental model. *Lancet* 2:384–386, 1968.
28. Guisado R, Arieff AI: Neurologic manifestations of diabetic comas: Correlation with biochemical alterations in the brain. *Metabolism* 24:665–679, 1975.
29. Finberg L, Luttrell C, Redd H: Pathogenesis of lesions in the nervous system in hypernatremic states. II. Experimental studies of gross and anatomic changes and alterations of chemical composition of the tissues. *Pediatrics* 23:46–53, 1959.
30. Ditzel J, Andersen H, Daugaard N: Tissue oxygenation in uncontrolled diabetes mellitus. *Lancet* 2:818, 1972.
31. Krane EJ, Rockoff MA, Wallman JK, et al: Subclinical brain swelling in children during treatment of diabetic ketoacidosis. *N Engl J Med* 312:1147–1151, 1985.
32. Finberg L: Dehydration and osmolality. *Am J Dis Child* 135:997–998, 1981.

3
Premature Pubarche: An Analysis of 102 Patients

ALLEN W. ROOT, FRANK B. DIAMOND, JR., BARRY B. BERCU, DOROTHY I. SHULMAN

Introduction

Premature pubarche is the clinical appearance of coarse sexual pubic hair before 8 years of age in the female and 10 years in the male, in the absence of signs of the gonadarche (thelarche in girls, testicular enlargement in boys).[1] Other signs of androgen excess in these children include the development of axillary hair or adult axillary odor, acne, and accelerated growth. In relationship to chronologic age, premature pubarche is associated with increased serum concentrations of dehydroepiandrosterone (DHEA) and/or its sulfate (DHAS) as well as androstenedione, testosterone, and dihydrotestosterone in many subjects.[2]

Normal adrenarche is accompanied by increased adrenocortical activity of 3β hydroxysteroid dehydrogenase and 17–20 lyase (P450-c17) enzymes, possibly due to an autoregulatory mechanism associated with the increased mass of the growing adrenal.[3,4] Height age and skeletal maturation are modestly advanced for chronologic age, and some but not all children with premature pubarche are overweight for height. This developmental pattern has been considered a benign pubertal variant, with subsequent normal linear growth, sexual maturation, and fertility.[5,6] However, this concept has been challenged by reports of children with variant or mild forms of congenital adrenal hyperplasia (CAH) or with the carrier status for this disorder.[7-9]

In order to define further the clinical and biochemical characteristics of children with premature pubarche we have reviewed our data concerning 102 patients with this diagnosis evaluated in the pediatric endocrinology unit of the University of South Florida College of Medicine over a 15-year period.

From the Section of Endocrinology, Department of Pediatrics, University of South Florida College of Medicine, Tampa, Florida.
Presented by Dr Root in honor of Lewis A. Barness, MD, November 11, 1988.

TABLE 3.1. Clinical characteristics of children with premature pubarche.

	Race	N	HA/CA	WA/HA	BA/CA
Female	Total	81	1.06 ± 0.17^a	1.10 ± 0.24	1.17 ± 0.24
	White	41	1.06 ± 0.18	1.12 ± 0.25	1.15 ± 0.21
	Black	25	1.06 ± 0.14	1.05 ± 0.23	1.24 ± 0.31
Male	Total	21	0.98 ± 0.18	1.13 ± 0.34	1.13 ± 0.21
	White	11	1.06 ± 0.19	1.23 ± 0.43	1.15 ± 0.26
	Black	9	0.89 ± 0.12	1.04 ± 0.17	1.07 ± 0.10

[a] Mean $\pm$ 1 SD.
Abbreviations: HA, height age; CA, chronologic age; WA, weight age; BA, bone age.

Materials and Methods

The charts of 102 children with premature pubarche who were less than 8 (girls) or 10 (boys) years of age when initially evaluated between 1973 and 1988 were reviewed. The clinical, hormonal, and radiographic data were abstracted. Bone ages were interpreted with the Greulich and Pyle atlas[10] by a pediatric radiologist not familiar with the patients. Serum concentrations of 17-hydroxypregnenolone, DHAS, DHEA, 17-hydroxyprogesterone (17OHP), androstenedione, and testosterone were measured by radioimmunoassay by previously reported methods.[11] Interassay coefficients of variations for these assays ranged between 10% and 24%. The adrenal androgen secretory response to adrenocorticotropin (ACTH) was assessed in 18 patients by the administration of synthetic 1-24 ACTH (0.25 mg by IV bolus) with determination of steroid concentrations prior to and 60 min after ACTH injection.

Results

Eighty percent of the patients were girls, and 31% of the females and 43% of the males were black (Table 3.1). The majority of girls with premature pubarche were evaluated between 5 and 8 years of age (Fig. 3.1), while boys presented between 4 and 10 years of age (Fig. 3.2). Eight of 13 children with premature pubarche less than 4 years of age when first examined were black. Thirty-one percent of the black girls with premature pubarche were less than 4 years of age at presentation, while 13 percent of white females were 4 years of age or younger.

Signs of androgen excess (axillary odor) began as early as 1 to 2 years. The children with premature pubarche were slightly taller and heavier and had advanced skeletal maturation in comparison with age-matched peers (Table 3.1). That adrenal androgens can advance skeletal maturation is evident in the growth pattern depicted in Figure 3.3. In the boy whose growth pattern is shown in Figure 3.3, linear growth rate was exceeded by the rate of skeletal maturation;

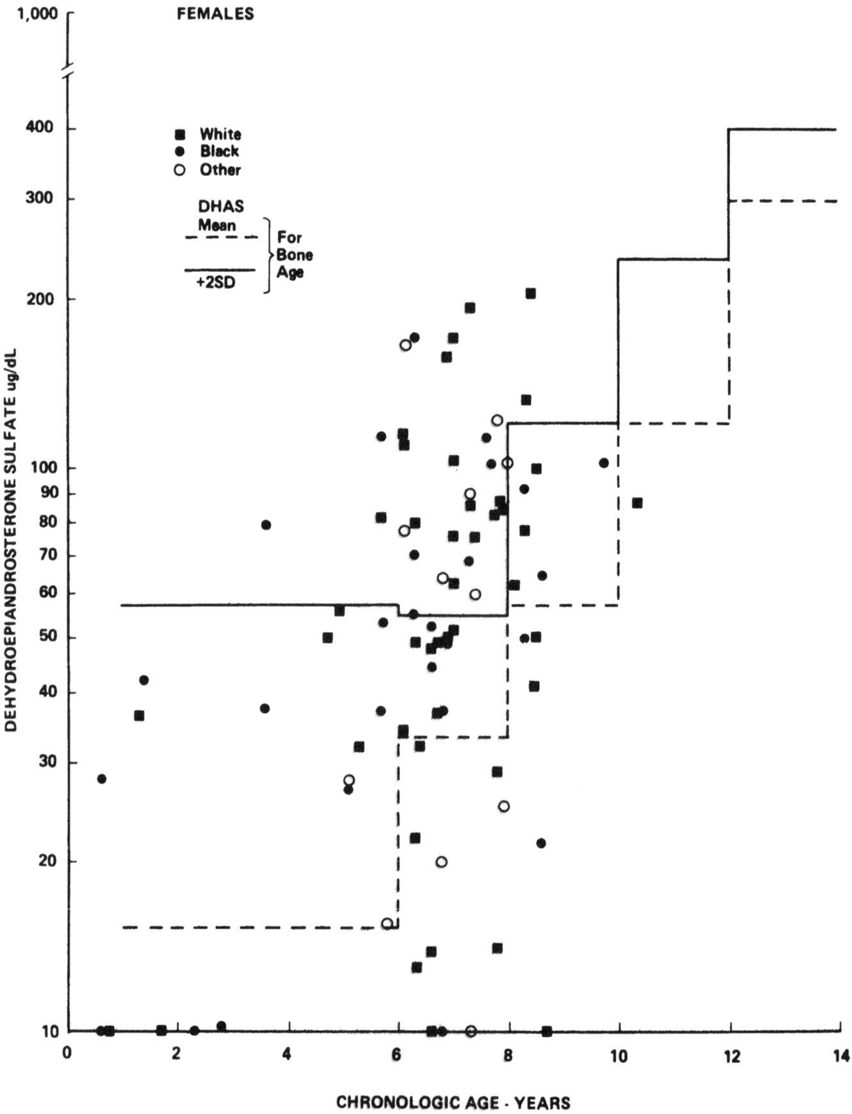

FIGURE 3.1. Serum concentrations of DHAS in girls with premature pubarche at initial evaluation.

since no other underlying abnormality was identified, the rapid skeletal development was attributed to his adrenal androgens.

Although serum concentrations of DHAS in girls with premature pubarche (Fig. 3.1) tended to be above the mean control value, they were usually within the normal range except between 6 and 8 years, when 25 of 48 DHAS levels

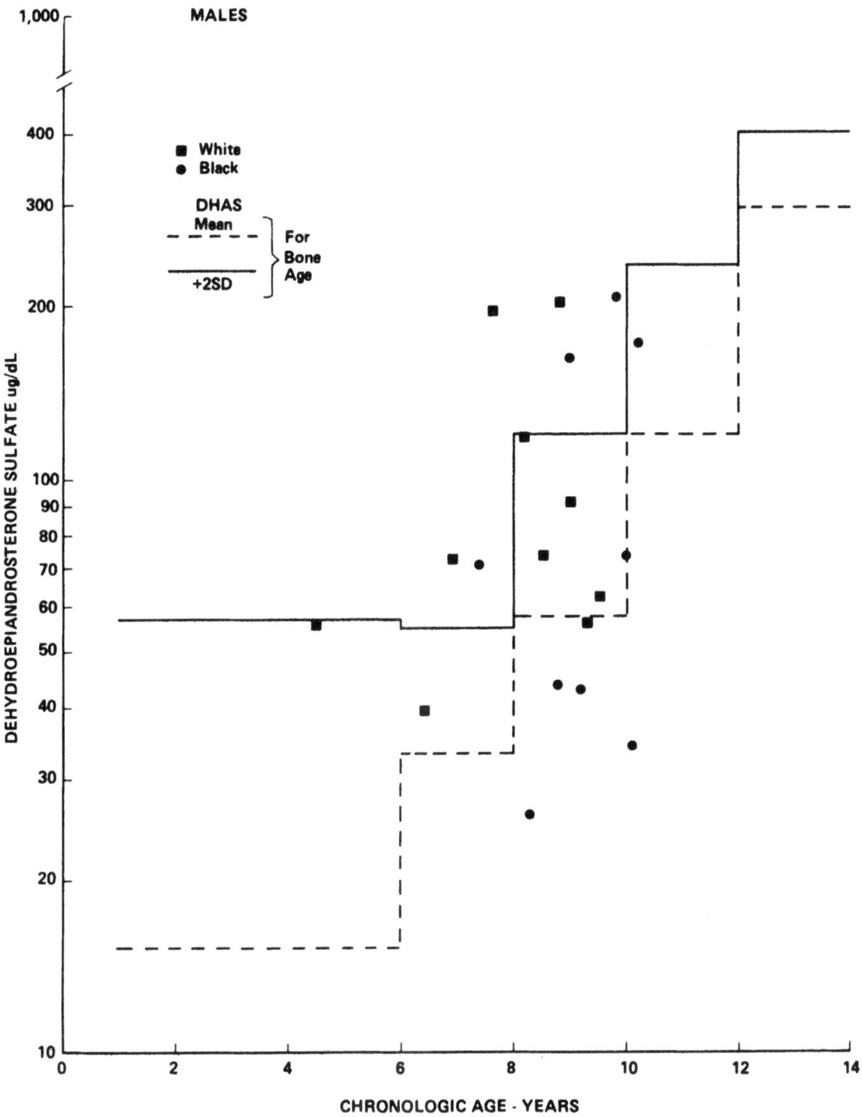

FIGURE 3.2. Serum concentrations of DHAS in boys with premature pubarche at initial evaluation.

were more than 2 SD above mean DHAS value. Between 6 and 8 years the mean (± SEM) DHAS concentrations of girls with premature pubarche were significantly higher than the control mean value (68.4 ± 9.0 and 70.1 ± 13.2 for white and black affected girls, respectively, versus 30.4 ± 7.6 μg/dL). The wide range of DHAS values (including specimens in which the DHAS concentration was

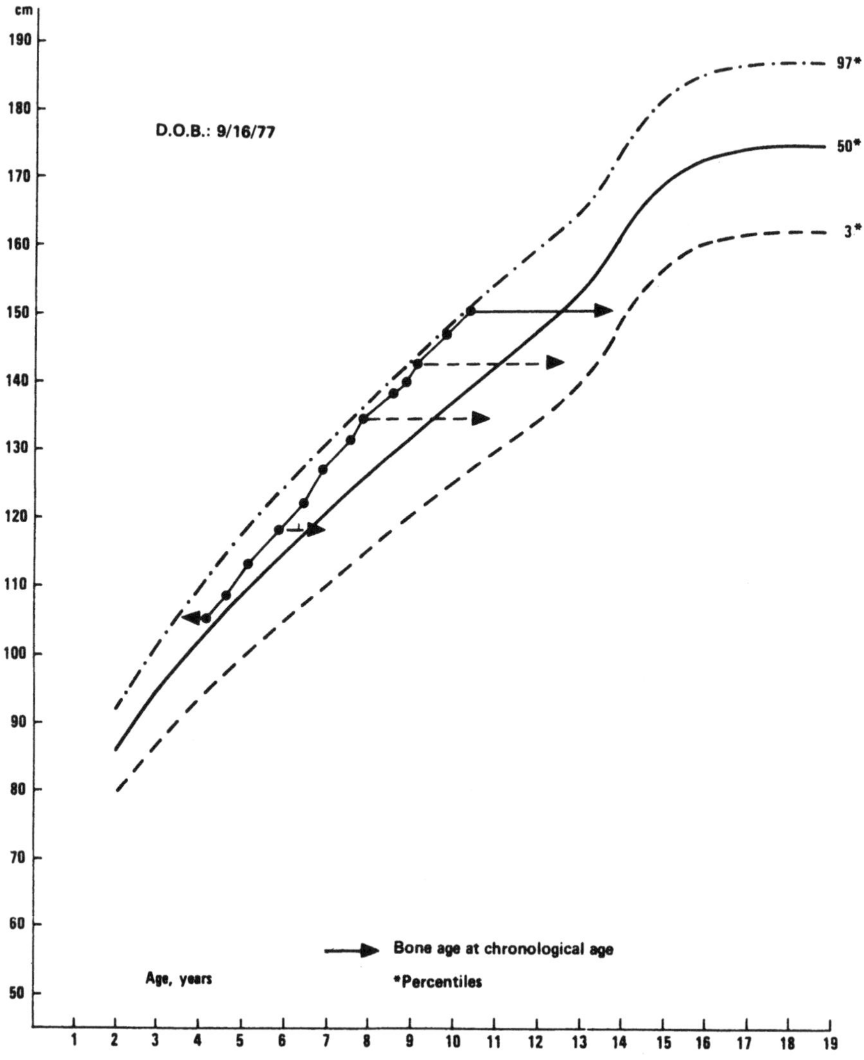

FIGURE 3.3. Actual and projected growth pattern of a boy with premature adrenarche who demonstrated marked acceleration of skeletal maturation with no other underlying abnormality.

below assay sensitivity) is apparent, suggesting that androgens other than DHAS probably contribute to the clinical manifestations of this entity. In three of four boys with premature pubarche (Fig. 3.2), serum DHAS values were more than 2 SD above the mean between 6 and 8 years, but in only 3 of 12 were levels high between 8 and 10 years of age. Follow-up of children with premature pubarche for up to 6 years has revealed no inordinately rapid progression in sexual matura-

TABLE 3.2. Incremental increase in serum concentrations of 17-hydroxyprogesterone (ng/dl) after administration of 0.25 mg 1–24 ACTH IV.

	N	Mean	SD	Range
Control	19	124	58	52–239
Heterozygotes for CAH	16[a]	339	170	88–722
Premature adrenarche	16[b]	238	143	92–650

[a] Group composed of parents of children with documented 21-hydroxylase-deficient CAH.
[b] Data derived from the 16 patients with premature adrenarche excluding data from two children with nonclassical congenital adrenal hyperplasia (see text).

tion or clinical evidence of androgen excess, but it should be emphasized that most of the patients are still young.

To determine the frequency of the heterozygous carrier state for, or the incidence of, 21-hydroxylase deficiency in our population of children with premature pubarche, ACTH tests were performed in 18 children (three of them black) (Table 3.2). Three patients (two girls, one boy, all white) had increments in serum concentrations of 17-OHP (405, 430, and 650 ng/dL) that were above the control range (239 ng/dl), suggesting the carrier state for 21-hydroxylase deficiency. In two white girls the increments of 17-OHP (2691, 3922 ng/dL) were compatible with the nonclassical form of congenital adrenal hyperplasia.[12] In this population there were no children with significantly exaggerated secretion of 17-hydroxypregnenolone or DHEA after ACTH administration.

Discussion

The control of normal adrenarche is unclear, and the pathophysiology of premature adrenarche is therefore unknown. Premature adrenarche is accompanied by increased serum concentrations of DHEA, DHAS, and other androgens to values that may be lower than or comparable to those in normal older children with Tanner stage II pubic hair growth.[2,6] Serial studies by other investigators have demonstrated persistently elevated androgen values which increase appropriately for chronologic age and skeletal maturation,[2] findings similar to ours. Premature adrenarche appears to be less common in boys than in girls. Affected boys are often obese and may have evidence of central nervous system dysfunction.

Whether there is a race-dependent variation in DHAS concentrations is unknown. Kaplowitz et al[13] reported upper normal DHAS values of 26 μg/dl and 57.3 μg/dl in normal black females less or more than 6 years of age, respectively. The DHAS data of Katz et al[14] for American black youth are similar to ours derived from a mixed population. In healthy African boys and girls, DHAS concentrations remain quite low (<20 μg/dl) until 12 years of age.[15] Kaplowitz et al[13] have reported a preponderance of black females (19/22) among children with premature adrenarche, while Oberfield and Levine [16] reported that in a population of 34 children with premature adrenarche, 14 were black and 20 Hispanic. Ten of 31 patients studied by Morris et al[17] were black. Among our children, 31% of the girls and 43% of the boys were black. In our general pediatric endocrine population, 8% of the patients are black. It is unclear if these data indicate geographical variability (Virginia, New York, Massachusetts, and Florida, respectively) or a true increase in incidence of premature pubarche in the black population in America.

The concept that premature adrenarche is a benign process in all children has been challenged by reports of children with premature pubarche in whom ACTH-stimulated serum concentrations of 17-OHP are greatly elevated.[7] These children have a nonclassical or variant form of mild 21-hydroxylase-deficient congenital adrenal hyperplasia (CAH), often associated with the HLA haplotype B14–DR1.[12] Temeck et al[7] evaluated the steroid secretory response to ACTH in 23 children with premature pubarche. In 13 children the 17-OHP levels were similar to those of normal children with Tanner stage III pubic hair development. In seven subjects (29%) the 17-OHP responses were within the range of nonclassical 21-hydroxylase-deficient subjects. Basal 17-OHP levels in the nonclassical CAH subjects overlapped with those of normal Tanner pubic hair stage II to III children and heterozygote subjects, implying that a random value is inadequate to identify patients with nonclassical CAH and clinical premature pubarche. Rappaport et al[18] reported that 2 of 30 girls with premature pubarche had 17-OHP secretory responses to ACTH consistent with nonclassical 21 hydroxylase deficiency, but neither Oberfield and Levine[16] nor Morris et al[17] observed this abnormality in 65 patients with premature pubarche whom they evaluated. Ten percent of the patients in our limited study had greatly exaggerated 17-OHP secretory response to ACTH, compatible with nonclassical congenital adrenal hyperplasia.

In the study of Temeck et al,[7] 1 of 13 patients with idiopathic premature adrenarche and 2 of 21 in the general population with Tanner stage II to III pubic hair growth had 17-OHP secretory responses compatible with the heterozygous carrier state for CAH. Although these investigators did not find a link between the heterozygous state for 21-hydroxylase deficiency and premature pubarche, Granoff et al[8] reported that 9 of 10 girls with premature adrenarche had 17-OHP secretory responses to ACTH within the range for heterozygotes for this enzyme deficit. Knorr et al[9] stated that 31 of 75 children with premature pubarche had a heterozygote 17-OHP response to ACTH. Three of 18 children in our study had 17-OHP secretory responses to ACTH suggestive of the carrier state for 21-hydroxylase deficiency.

In their study of 23 children with premature pubarche, Temeck et al[7] also identified three children (13%—one male) with a suspected defect in activity of 3β-hydroxysteroid dehydrogenase-(3β-HSD) activity identified by an exaggerated 17-hydroxypregnenolone secretory response after ACTH administration compared to a population of normal subjects with Tanner stage II to III pubic hair development. We identified no such patients in our studies. However, Rappaport et al[18] and Oberfield and Levine[16] reported incidences of 3β-HSD deficiency of 26% and

12%, respectively, in children with premature pubarche. Whether these are indeed subjects with a pathologic defect in 3β-HSD activity or ones with "exaggerated" but otherwise appropriate adrenarchal changes in adrenal function[3] will require further study and long-term follow-up of many more such patients.

Although premature pubarche/adrenarche is considered a benign variant of puberty, long-term hormonal studies of the reproductive endocrine system and of fertility in such patients have not been reported. Such data are essential.

Acknowledgments. The authors thank Judy Zamanillo for her nursing skills; Gregory Duckett, Margaret Sweetland, Ching Shi Hu, and Lorraine Forson for their technical assistance; and Etta Tucker for her secretarial competence.

References

1. Diamond FB Jr, Root AW: Delayed sexual maturation and sexual precocity. In Conn RB (ed): *Current Diagnosis*. Philadelphia: Saunders, 1985, pp 1252–1264.
2. Korth-Schutz S, Levine LS, New MI: Serum androgens in normal prepubertal and pubertal children and in children with precocious adrenarche. *J Clin Endocrinol Metab* 42:117–124, 1976.
3. Rich BH, Rosenfield RL, Lucky AW, Helke JC, Otto P: Adrenarche: Changing adrenal response to adrenocorticotropin. *J Clin Endocrinol Metab* 52:1129–1136, 1981.
4. Dickerman Z, Grant DR, Fairman C, Winter JSD: Intraadrenal steroid concentrations in man: Zonal differences and developmental changes. *J Clin Endocrinol Metab* 59:1031–1036, 1984.
5. Sigurjonsdottir TJ, Hales AB: Premature pubarche. *Clin Pediatr* 7:29–33, 1968.
6. Voutilainen R, Perheentupa J, Apter D: Benign premature adrenarche: Clinical features and serum steroid levels. *Acta Paediatr Scand* 172:707–711, 1983.
7. Temeck JW, Pang S, Nelson C, New MI: Genetic defects of steroidogenesis in premature pubarche. *J Clin Endocrinol Metab* 64:609–617, 1987.
8. Granoff AB, Chasalow FI, Blethen SL: 17-Hydroxyprogesterone responses to adrenocorticotropin in children with premature adrenarche. *J Clin Endocrinol Metab* 60:409–415, 1985.
9. Knorr D, Bidlingmaier F, Holler W, Kuhnle U, Meiler B, Nachman A: Is heterozygosity for the steroid 21-hydroxylase deficiency responsible for hirsutism, premature pubarche, early puberty and precocious puberty in children? *Acta Endocrinol* Suppl 279:284–289, 1986.
10. Greulich WW, Pyle SI: *Radiographic Atlas of Skeletal Development of the Hand and Wrist*, 2d Ed. Palo Alto, CA: Stanford University Press, 1959.
11. Reiter EO, Root AW: Effect of an infusion of Gn-RH upon levels of sex hormones in prepubertal and pubertal girls: Evidence for relative ovarian insensitivity. *Steroids* 30:61–69, 1977.
12. Speiser PW, New MI: Genotype and hormonal phenotype in nonclassical 21-hydroxylase deficiency. *J Clin Endocrinol Metab* 64:86–91, 1987.
13. Kaplowitz PB, Cockrell JL, Young RB: Premature adrenarche. Clinical and diagnostic features. *Clin Pediatr* 25:28–34, 1986.

14. Katz SH, Hediger ML, Zamel BS, Parks JS: Blood pressure, body fat, and dehydroepiandrosterone sulfate variation in normal adolescence. *Hypertension* 8:277–284, 1986.
15. Mavoungou D, Gass R, Emane MN, Cooper RW, Roth-Meyer C: Plasma dehydroepiandrosterone, its sulfate, testosterone and FSH during puberty of African children in Gabon. *J Steroid Biochem* 24:645–651, 1986.
16. Oberfield SE, Levine LS: Precocious adrenarche in NYC black and hispanic children. *Endrocrinology* 122:211A, 1988.
17. Morris AH, Reiter EO, Geffner ME, Lippe BM, Itami RM, Mayes D: Absence of non-classical congenital adrenal hyperplasia in patients with precocious adrenarche. *J Clin Endocrinol Metab* 69:709–715, 1989.
18. Rappaport R, Goldstein S, Skuza K, Robey C, Hess A, Chou J: Adrenal steroidogenic defects in children and adolescents with disordered puberty. *Endocrinology* 122: 211A, 1988.

4
In Utero Protection of the Brain of the Hypothyroid Infant

ROBERT Z. KLEIN

The prime question when Dussault[1] initiated neonatal hypothyroidism screening 14 years ago was how much if any of the brain damage leading to intellectual retardation in infantile hypothyroidism was postnatal. The fact that the IQs and school achievements of the patients of the New England Congenital Hypothyroidism Collaborative are indistinguishable from those of their siblings and peers proves that nearly all of this brain damage in sporadic infantile hypothyroidism is postnatal.[2-4] Figure 4.1 shows the latest Stanford-Binet IQs for 121 patients at 3 to 5 years. The means for patients and controls were both 105 $\pm$ 15 (SD). The stippled background represents a normal Gaussian distribution derived from these means and standard deviations. It is obvious that the distribution of the patients' IQs is normal. Figure 4.2 is similarly constructed and shows the WISC-R IQ at 6 years for 57 patients. The mean IQ of the patients was 109 $\pm$ 13, and that of the controls was 110 $\pm$ 13.

It had been suggested that hypothyroid children had specific learning disabilities since even those with normal IQs were unable to progress in school.[5-8] There were no concurrent controls in these studies, and where individual IQ data were available, those who did poorly in school had significantly lower IQs than the remainder of the patients (McFaul et al[7]). All but two of the patients with learning problems in this study had IQs below 95, 1 SD below the normal mean in most recent studies.[4,9]

The New England Hypothyroidism Collaborative compared the performance of its hypothyroid patients with those of their siblings and peers in school.[10] The IQs were derived from a WISC-R abbreviated to five items and were correlated with Peabody Individual Achievement Test scores standardized for age for 60 patients and for 119 controls (88 classmates of the same age and sex as the patients and 31 siblings of the patients) after a minimum of kindergarten and 3 additional years in school. Nine patients and their classmates had finished the

---

From the New England Congenital Hypothyroidism Collaborative and the Department of Maternal and Child Health, Dartmouth University Medical School, Hanover, New Hampshire.
Presented in honor of Lewis A. Barness, MD, November 11, 1988.

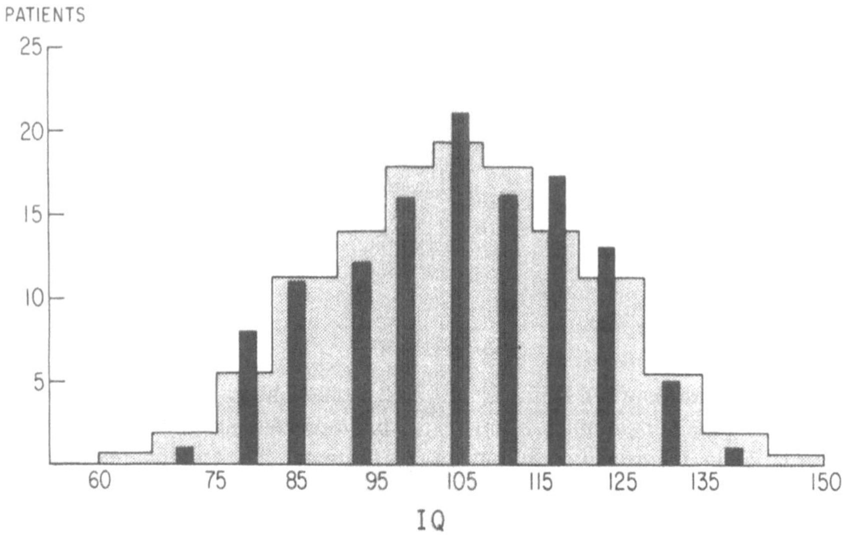

FIGURE 4.1. Distribution of latest Standord-Binet IQ scores for 121 patients 3 to 5 years of age. Mean IQ for patients was 105 ± 15 (SD) and was 105 ± 15 for controls as well. Stippled background represents calculated normal distribution for 121 individuals with this mean and standard deviation.

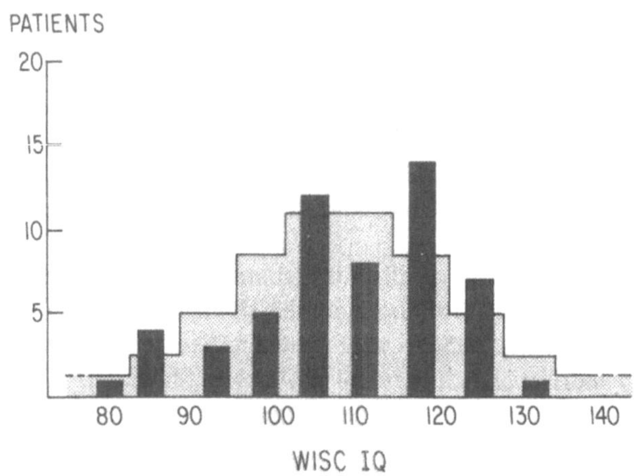

FIGURE 4.2. Distribution of WISC-R IQ scores at age 6 years for 57 patients. Control mean was 110 ± 13, patient mean was 109 ± 13. Graph is plotted as in Figure 4.1.

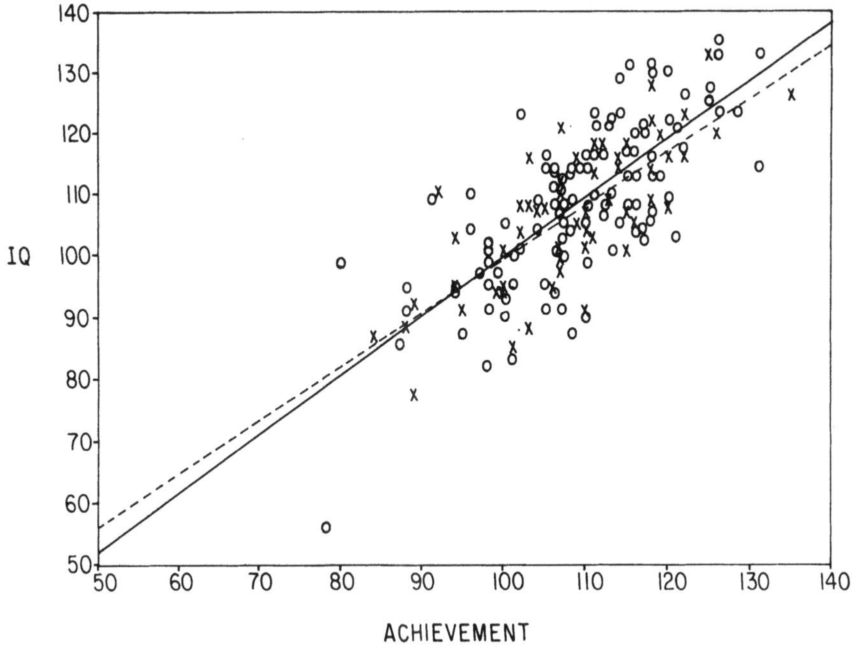

FIGURE 4.3. Relationship of IQ to Peabody Individual Achievement Test scores standardized for age for 60 patients (X and ---) and 119 controls (O and —). Regression equations are y = 92x + 8.1 for controls and y = .87x + 12.1 for patients.

fourth grade, and 51 patients and their classmate controls had finished the third grade. Four siblings had finished the fifth grade, 10 the fourth, and 17 the third grade. Figure 4.3 shows the regression lines and the individual distribution for patients and controls using IQ as the independent variable and school achievement test scores as the dependent variable. The lines are identical.

There were also no differences in mean global IQs, 107 ± 1.5 (SEM) for the patients vs 109 ± 1.2 for the controls, or in school achievement test scores. Table 4.1 shows the school progress through the third grade of 68 patients, 81 of their siblings, 83 classmates of the same sex and age as the patients, and 80

TABLE 4.1. School progress through the third grade.

	Hypothyroid Patients (N=68)	Siblings (N=81)	Controls (N=163)
No problems	70.6%	69.2%	70.1%
Repeated a grade (K to 3)	13.3%	18.5%	16.9%
Special education	7.4%	8.6%	4.1%
Tutoring	8.8%	3.7%	9.8%

There are no statistically significant differences among the three groups.

siblings of the classmates. The same percentage of patients as of controls progressed without difficulty through the first three grades. There were no statistically significant differences in the incidences of the various types of school problems.

What was originally a secondary question now becomes the primary one. What protects the fetal brain in utero? Second, why are endemic cretins not protected? Although direct proof in humans may prove impossible for practical reasons, it seems most likely that maternal thyroid hormone protects the fetal brain even though conventional wisdom is that transplacental passage is inadequate.

In the past it has been suggested that there was some factor in utero that substituted for thyroid hormones. No such factor has been identified, and even if one had been, it would not explain the failure of protection in endemic cretinism per se.

I once suggested that the infant with sporadic infantile hypothyroidism might be protected against thyroid deficiency in utero by late and slow development of deficiency since there is demonstrable loss of thyroid function postnatally.[11] This became unlikely when two of our patients (one with goitrous hypothyroidism and one with a nondemonstrable gland) were found retrospectively to have had thyroid dysfunction at 16 and 17 weeks of gestation. Kourides found elevated amniotic fluid TSH concentrations in fluid obtained at these times.[12] Whether this represented relatively compensated thyroid disease or significant thyroid deficiency at that time cannot be determined.

What is the evidence that transplacental passage of maternal thyroid hormone might protect the fetal brain? It was demonstrated in 1956[13] that in humans the passage of T4 and T3 from mother to fetus at term was slow. In this study radioiodinated thyroid hormone was administered to six mothers, 2 to 8 h prior to delivery, to one mother 18 h before delivery, and to two mothers whose children were not born until 3 and 7 days after injection of ^{131}I-thyroxine.[13] The specific activity in cord blood was 2.3% to 7.9% of the specific activity in maternal blood at delivery in those infants born 2 to 8 h postinjection. It was 13% in the child born at 18 h postinjection. In the children born at 3 and 7 days, however, it was 32% and 48%, respectively. When radiolabeled triiodothyronine was administered similarly instead of thyroxine to mothers whose children were born 8 to 16 h later, the cord blood specific activity was 10% to 21% that of the mother's blood.

A later study showed that, at delivery 2 to 8 h post oral administration, cord serum activity was 5% of the simultaneous maternal serum activity for T4 and 25% for T3. When inorganic ^{131}I was similarly administered, cord blood activity was 30% to 100% that of maternal blood.[14] Fairly consistent suppression of newborn T4 concentration could be achieved by Raiti et al by the administration of the huge dose of 300 μg of T3 to mothers for 6 weeks preceding delivery.[15] As has been pointed out, there is no evidence that placental passage of thyroid hormones is inadequate early in pregnancy.[11] That at least some thyroid hormone does pass the human placenta from the mother to the fetus early in pregnancy has been demonstrated by the finding of reverse T3 in amniotic fluid before the time when the fetal thyroid is active.[16]

Morreale de Escobar and co-workers have shown[17,18] that, in rats, the fetal brain contains significant amounts of thyroid hormones long before the fetal thyroid produces any. If the dam is thyroidectomized, fetal brain contains no demonstrable thyroid hormones before day 17 of gestation, when the fetal thyroid becomes active. Normal fetal brain triiodothyronine concentration is maintained when both dam and fetuses are made hypothyroid with thiouracil derivatives if thyroxine is given to the dam.[19] The dose of thyroxine was sufficient to maintain normal serum and tissue T4 concentrations in the mother, but T4 concentration was only about 50% of normal in fetal serum and tissues. It was, however, preferentially taken up and deiodinated by the brain of the fetus. Brain 5′ deiodinase is increased in the hypothyroid rat fetus.[20] T3 concentrations are low in fetal plasma and lungs in this experimental situation.

Obviously, there is no proof of preferential uptake in the brain of the human fetus. Since the newborn with hypothyroidism usually shows minimal or no other signs of tissue deficiency except in bone maturation, one would have to postulate further that other tissues besides the brain must have some preferential ability to deiodinate T4 to T3 for their own use or to take up serum T3. Teleologically one might infer from the disproportionately elevated reverse T3 concentration in the fetus, the low concentration, the rapid increase in T3 and T4, and the fall in reverse T3 at birth that the fetus needs much lower circulating concentrations of active thyroid hormones than does the infant. The postnatal increase of T4 concentrations into the normal range before treatment in 27% of hypothyroid infants with ectopic thyroid tissue in the New England series suggests the same. Both these findings, however, would be equally compatible with the theory that the mothers supply some other factor to their fetuses that substitutes for thyroid hormones.

If the theory that transplacental passage of maternal thyroid hormone is adequate to support the hypothyroid fetus is true, it would also help explain some long unanswered questions about endemic cretinism. The worst central nervous system problems occurred in those who by the time of birth had received enough iodine to be euthyroid, and these problems were not relieved by postnatal treatment.[21] Some postulated that since the deaf-mutism, spastic gaits, and other neurologic problems existed without postnatal hypothyroidism and similar problems were rarely if ever seen in sporadic hypothyroidism, these CNS effects were the direct result of iodine deficiency and not hypothyroidism. The occurrence of similar deaf-mutism in patients in nonendemic areas with tissue resistance to thyroxine suggested the opposite.[22] It has been suggested that the mothers with endemic hypothyroidism could not supply their fetuses with enough thyroxine to protect them in the first 12 weeks of gestation (i.e., before the time when the normal fetal thyroid gland secretes hormone but during the time when these CNS injuries were thought to occur) and so their offspring had deaf-mutism, spastic paraplegias, etc.[11] This would be supported by the findings of Morreale de Escobar's group. Similarly, the fetus with tissue resistance to thyroxine would not be protected in the first 12 weeks of gestation no matter how much thyroxine passed the placenta from the mother. In endemic cretins, the combination of maternal and fetal thyroid deficiency after the fetal thyroid should have been producing hormone may also have contributed to later cognitive retardation.

The second line of evidence comes from clinical studies of infants with transient hypothyroidism whose mothers are hypothyroid. Ordinarily, children with transient hypothyroidism of various causes are not intellectually retarded.[11] However, Goldsmith et al[23] reported a family in which grandmother and mother had autoimmune thyroid disease. The grandmother had a goiter but was euthyroid. The mother became hypothyroid sometime between the age of 6 years, when she had an inflammatory process in the neck, and adolescence. She maintained persistently high antimicrosomal and antithyroglobulin antibodies. Her treatment was inadequate much if not all the time. She had six children with autoimmune transient hypothyroidism. All four survivors were markedly mentally retarded although they were treated with thyroxine from the day of birth. Treatment was probably not adequate some of the time because of the family situation. Indeed, some of the children had clinical signs of hypothyroidism early in life before their thyroids had fully recovered. A similar family was reported by Matsuura et al.[24] The children were reported as having normal intelligence without treatment even though the mother had been hypothyroid in one of the pregnancies. This contradiction was only recently cleared up. Continued observation of the child revealed that the original observation had been wrong and the product of the pregnancy during which the mother was hypothyroid was indeed mentally retarded. This stimulated Matsuura to study 22 mother-child pairs where the mother had autoimmune thyroiditis.[25] Two of the mothers were hypothyroid during pregnancy. The children of all 22 mothers were followed with psychometric tests. The offspring of the two mothers who were hypothyroid during pregnancy had lower than normal IQs; these were also significantly lower than the children of the other 20 mothers who had adequate replacement thyroxine during pregnancy or were never hypothyroid.

Francis and Riley[26] reported another mother with a goiter and hypothyroidism who had persistent circulating immunoglobulin which blocked the binding of TSH to thyroid cells and inhibited TSH stimulation of cyclic AMP in thyroid tissue. She was clinically hypothyroid in her first pregnancy, and the child was developmentally retarded with poor attention span and motor function. The mother's replacement theory was adequate during the next two pregnancies, and the infants were considered to be normal though no measurements of cognition were reported for any of the children. Brown et al[27] have shown that these blocking antibodies correlate with transient hypothyroidism in the offspring better than do titers of antithyroglobulin and antimicrosomal antibodies.

As part of a series of investigations, Man and Serunian[28] studied the children of 210 mothers who were euthyroid in pregnancy, of 15 found to have BEI concentrations in the hypothyroid range but adequately treated, and of 21 whose subnormal BEI concentrations were not adequately corrected. The incidence of hypothyroidism in the overall study was 3% as diagnosed by two or more low BEI concentrations, one low BEI with clinical signs of hypothyroidism, previous history of hypothyroidism, or reproductive difficulties. The children of the mothers with hypothyroidism had significantly lower IQs than those of the children of the other two groups of mothers when tested at 4 and 7 years of age. Whether the hypothyroid mothers also had autoimmune thyroiditis and their children had transient hypothyroidism is unknown. The incidence of autoimmune thyroiditis in women of childbearing age is reported to be 5% to 15%, but only a small proportion of them are actually hypothyroid.[29] In any event, this study further suggests that maternal thyroxine may protect fetal CNS development.

Finally, there is a significant postnatal decrease in serum T4 concentration in patients with infantile hypothyroidism who have no demonstrable thyroid tissue on scanning. The mean T4 of 33 such children on neonatal screening in the New England program was 2.9 ± 0.21 (SE) μg/dl, and this fell to 1.9 ± 0.31 at an average of 3 weeks later.[3] Such a decrease was not seen in 62 patients with demonstrable thyroid tissue on scanning. It is conceivable but most unlikely that all the patients with atrophic glands had such a rapid postnatal involution. On the other hand, it is obvious that the amount of maternal hormone crossing the placenta is inadequate to maintain serum T4 concentrations in the normal range for newborns or older children.

Thus, the preponderance of evidence suggests but does not prove that transplacental passage of maternal thyroid hormones protects the fetus against the inadequacies of its own thyroid. Unfortunately, one simple study that might prove the theory is unethical. It would involve preventing fetal damage to endemic cretins by treating their mothers with thyroid hormone. Since adequate amounts of prophylactic iodide are known to do just this, the study cannot be done.

Until the theory is disproved, however, there are certain practical measures that should be taken to prevent fetal brain damage. All women with autoimmune thyroid disease, hypothyroidism, or any condition that might lead to hypothyroidism should be carefully monitored and treated with complete replacement doses of thyroxine to ensure maintenance of the high-normal T4 concentrations of pregnancy. If the current incidence of hypothyroidism in pregnant women is of the order of magnitude of that found by Man and Serunian,[28] thyroid screening should be instituted for all pregnant women. Thyroid hormone administration to pregnant women being treated for hyperthyroidism was used 25 years ago by Herbst and Selenkow although evidence for its efficacy was never reported.[30] Selenkow et al[31] later extended the indications for provision of thyroid replacement therapy essentially to all circumstances in which hypothyroidism might occur in pregnancy. The risk of thyroxine administration in all these circumstances is truly minuscule compared to any possible risk of fetal brain damage.

References

1. Dussault JH, Coulombe P, Laberge C, et al: Preliminary report on a mass screening program for neonatal hypothyroidism. *J Pediatr* 86:670, 1975.
2. New England Congenital Hypothyroidism Collaborative: Effects of neonatal screening for hypothyroidism: Prevention of mental retardation by treatment before clinical manifestations. *Lancet* 2:1095–1098, 1981.

3. New England Congenital Hypothyroidism Collaborative: Characteristics of infantile hypothyroidism discovered on neonatal screening. *J Pediatr* 104:539–544, 1984.
4. New England Congenital Hypothyroidism Collaborative: Neonatal hypothyroidism screening: Status of patients at 6 years of age. *J Pediatr* 107:915–919, 1985.
5. Von Harnack GA, Wallis H: Zur psychopathologie der hypothyreose in kindesalter. *Monatsschr Kinderheilkd* 108:373–376, 1960.
6. Zabransky S, Richter R, Hanefeld F, et al: Zur prognose der angeborenen hypothyreose. *Monatsschr Kinderheilkd* 123:475–476, 1975.
7. MacFaul R, Dorner S, Brett EM, et al: Neurological abnormalities in patients treated for hypothyroidism from early life. *Arch Dis Child* 53:611–619, 1978.
8. Wolter R, Noel P, DeCock P, et al: Neuropsychological study in treated thyroid dysgenesis. *Acta Pediatr Scand* Suppl 277:41–46, 1980.
9. Brand C: Bryter still and bryter. *Nature* 328:110, 1987.
10. New England Congenital Hypothyroidism Collaborative: Neonatal thyroid screening: Now we are nine. In Delange F (ed): *Research in Congenital Hypothyroidism*. New York: Plenum Press, 1988 (in press).
11. Klein RZ: Infantile hypothyroidism then and now: The results of neonatal screening. *Curr Probl Pediatr* 15:1–58, 1985.
12. Kourides IA: Personal communication, 1984.
13. Grumbach MM, Werner SC: Transfer of thyroid hormones across the placenta at term. *J Clin Endocrinol Metab* 16:1392–1395, 1956.
14. Kearns E, Hutson W: Tagged isomers and analogues of thyroxine (their transmission across human placenta and other studies). *J Nuclear Med* 4:453–461, 1963.
15. Raiti S, Holzman GB, Scott RL, Blizzard RM: Evidence for the placental transfer of triiodothyronine in human beings. *N Engl J Med* 277:456–459, 1967.
16. Klein AH, Murphy BEP, Artal R, et al: Amniotic fluid thyroid hormone concentration during pregnancy. *Am J Obstet Gynecol* 126:626–631, 1980.
17. Obregon MJ, Mallol J, Pastor R, Morreale de Escobar G, et al: L-thyroxine and 3,5,3′,-triiodo-L-thyronine in rat embryos before the onset of fetal thyroid function. *Endocrinology* 114:305–307, 1984.
18. Morreale de Escobar G, Pastor R, Obregon MJ, Escobar del Rey F: Effects of maternal hypothyroidism on the weight and thyroid content of rat embryonic tissues before and after the onset of fetal thyroid function. *Endocrinology* 117:1890–1900, 1985.
19. Morreale de Escobar G, Obregon MJ, Ruiz de Ona C, Escobar del Rey F: Transfer of thyroxine from the mother to the rat fetus near term: effects on brain 3,5,3′-triiodothyronine deficiency. *Endocrinology* 122:521–531, 1988.
20. Ruiz de Ona C, Obregon MJ, Escobar del Rey F, Morreale de Escobar G: Developmental changes in rat brain 5′-deiodinase and thyroid hormones during the fetal period: The effects of fetal hypothyroidism and maternal thyroid hormones. *Pediatr Res* 24:588–594, 1988.
21. Koenig MP. Endemic goiter and endemic cretinism. In Gardner LI (ed): *Endocrine and Genetic Disease of Childhood and Adolescence*. Philadelphia: Saunders, 1975, pp 260–269.
22. Refetoff S, DeGroot LJ, DeWind LT: Studies of a sibship with apparent hereditary resistance to the intracellular action of thyroid hormone. *Metabolism* 21:723–756, 1972.
23. Goldsmith RE, McAdams AJ, Larsen PR, et al: Familial autoimmune thyroiditis: Maternal fetal relationship and the role of generalized autoimmunity. *J Clin Endocrinol Metab* 37:265–275, 1973.

24. Matsuura N, Yamada Y, Nohara Y, et al: Familial neonatal transient hypothyroidism due to maternal TSH-binding inhibitor immunoglobulins. *N Engl J Med* 303:738–741, 1980.
25. Matsuura N: Neonatal transient hypothyroidism. In Delange F (ed): *Research in Congenital Hypothyroidism*. New York: Plenum Press, 1988 (in press).
26. Francis G, Riley W: Congenital familial hypothyroidism secondary to transplacental thyrotropin-blocking autoantibody. *Am J Dis Child* 141:1081–1083, 1987.
27. Brown RS, Keating P, Mitchell E: Maternal thyroid- blocking immunoglobulins in congenital hypothyroidism. In Delange F (ed): *Research in Congenital Hypothyroidism*. New York: Plenum Pres, 1988 (in press).
28. Man EB, Serunian SA: Thyroid function in human pregnancy. IX. Development of retardation of 7-year-old progeny of hypothyroxinemic women. *Am J Obstet Gynecol* 125:949–957, 1976.
29. Davies T, Cobin R: Thyroid disease in pregnancy and post-partum period. *Mt Sinai J Med* 52:59–77, 1985.
30. Herbst AL, Selenkow HA: Combined antithyroid-thyroid therapy of hyperthyroidism in pregnancy. *Obstet Gynecol* 21:543–550, 1963.
31. Selenkow HA, Birnbaum MD, Hollander CS: Thyroid function and dysfunction during pregnancy. *Clin Obstet Gynecol* 16:66–108, 1973.

5
The Role of Oxidation in Diseases of the Human Erythrocyte

BERTRAM LUBIN, FRANS KUYPERS, ELLIOTT VICHINSKY, DANIEL CHIU

Introduction

Considerable evidence exists that red blood cells (RBC) are oxidatively damaged in vivo.[1-10] Since these cells have limited ability to repair such damage, the cumulative injury resulting from oxidation can contribute to cell death. In red cells characterized by congenital or acquired structural defects, susceptibility to oxidant injury is often increased.[2] However, the extent to which oxidant injury contributes to shortened survival of these RBC is not clearly determined. We will discuss factors that render the red cell susceptible to oxidant injury, review several clinical disorders in which red cell oxidant injury has been reported, and provide a rationale for designing therapies to prevent oxidative damage.

Biologically important oxidants that have the potential to initiate or participate in oxidative reactions to RBC lipids and proteins include superoxide anion (O_2^-), hydroxy radical ($OH^\cdot$), lipid hydroperoxides (R-OOH), singlet oxygen ($^1O_2$), and hydrogen peroxide (H_2O_2). Red cell lipids and proteins may be the target of these oxidants. Oxidation of lipids usually involves unsaturated fatty acyl groups, although cholesterol may also be oxidized.[11] Oxidized phospholipid fatty acyl chains are removed from the glycerol backbone by phospholipase A_2 and then reduced by glutathione peroxidase.[12] Proper reacylation of these lysophospholipids is required to repair the membrane phospholipids. If this repair process is impaired, red cell phospholipid composition may be altered. Protein oxidation usually involves an attack on sulfhydryl groups. Unlike lipid repair, structurally altered proteins are either removed by proteolysis or rendered nonfunctional or dysfunctional as a consequence of the oxidative event. The resulting effects of these changes in lipids and/or proteins are likely to affect red cell structure and function.

Several factors that increase the red cells' susceptibility to oxidative damage are listed in Table 5.1.[6] The high oxygen content of the red cell places it in an

---

From the Children's Hospital Oakland Research Institute, Oakland, California (B.L., F.K., E.V., D.C.) and the Center for Advanced Medical Technology, San Francisco, California (D.C.).
Presented by Dr. Lubin in honor of Lewis A. Barness, MD, November 11, 1988.

TABLE 5.1. Factors that render the red cell susceptible to oxidant injury.

High content of O_2
Autooxidation of hemoglobin
Iron content (free iron, heme, denatured hemoglobin)
Polyunsaturated fatty acids and
Sulhydryl containing proteins
Membrane structural changes during passage through the microcirculator
Constant exposure to external oxidants
Antioxidant capacity
Superoxide dismutase
Vitamin E level
Reduced glutathione

environment conducive to oxidative reactions. The instability of hemoglobin, characterized by its spontaneous oxidation to methemoglobin, generates a constant source of superoxide anion. In certain pathologic conditions where hemoglobin auto-oxidation is accelerated, denatured hemoglobin, called hemichrone, binds to the membrane.[13-24] The iron in this denatured hemoglobin can be an extremely potent initiator of oxidative processes through a chemical reaction called the Fenton reaction.[25,26] Red cells undergo considerable shape change as they traverse the microcirculation. The stress placed on the membrane during shape change, particularly in pathologic red cells, may alter membrane organization and increase susceptibility of lipid and protein domains to oxidant injury. Red cells are constantly exposed to oxidant challenge generated during normal metabolic processes, from drugs or their metabolites and from granulocytes that have been activated as part of an inflammatory response.[27,28] Considering all of these factors, it is surprising that the red cell does so well in withstanding oxidant insult.

Hemolytic Anemia in Vitamin E-Deficient Premature Infants

One of the earliest clinical descriptions of a disorder in which oxidation contributed to shortened red cell survival was the hemolytic anemia associated with vitamin E deficiency in premature infants.[29] This condition is associated with hemolysis, thrombocytosis, and edema in premature infants fed formulas containing an elevated ratio of polyunsaturated fatty acids (PUFA) to vitamin E.[29,30]

Correction of hemolysis and other clinical features resulted when vitamin E supplementation was provided to these infants. In vitro studies of vitamin E-deficient red cells revealed that lipid peroxidation preceded the onset of hemolysis.[29] Additional studies demonstrated that proteins as well as lipids were oxidized and that a number of cellular properties such as volume regulation, cation permeability, and cell deformability were altered.[30]

Studies on vitamin E-deficient red cells provided the stimulus to pursue the role of oxidation in the pathophysiology of other hemolytic anemias. As in the

TABLE 5.2. Several clinical red cell disorders in which increased susceptibility to oxidative damage has been reported.

A.	Membrane
	Vitamin E deficiency
	Congenital hemolytic anemia
	Spherocytosis
	Pyropoikilocytosis
	Elliptocytosis
	Infection mediated
B.	Enzyme
	GGPD deficiency
	GSH peroxidase deficiency
	GSH synthetase deficiency
	Pyruvate kinase deficiency
C.	Hemoglobin
	Thalassemia
	Unstable hemoglobin
	Sickle cell anemia

red cell from the premature infant, an imbalance between oxidant stress and antioxidant defense renders the red cell susceptible to oxidative injury. Congenital red cell disorders in which an increased susceptibility to oxidant injury has been reported are listed in Table 5.2.

A number of hemolytic anemias due to membrane defects[31-34] have RBC with increased susceptibility to oxidant injury. We hypothesize that the disruption in membrane integrity resulting from the congenital defect (usually in skeletal proteins) alters the organization of protein sulfhydryl groups or phospholipid side chains within the membrane. Thus they are not protected from oxidant injury by virtue of an intact membrane structure. Attempts to prevent oxidant damage, to inhibit further membrane insult, and to stabilize the defective membrane structure using antioxidants have received little attention.

Red cell enzyme deficiencies, particularly those associated with pathways involved in maintaining adequate levels of reduced glutathione, are clinically associated with increased hemolysis following exposure to an oxidant.[6] Studies on G6PD- deficient red cells have demonstrated both in vivo and in vitro abnormalities consistent with oxidative damage.[4,5] Since a source of reduced glutathione is required to neutralize oxidants within red cells, inability to regenerate reduced glutathione from oxidized glutathione removes the red cell's major cytoplasmic antioxidant pathway. As a consequence, these oxidants attack protein and lipid components of the cell membrane. The alteration in lipids and proteins that has been reported in the Mediterranean variants of G6PD deficiency are sufficient to contribute to the hemolytic anemia associated with these disorders.[4,5] Other defects in the hexose monophosphate shunt, such as glutathione reductase and glutathione peroxidase deficiency, are similarly affected.[6] Studies of red cells from patients with enzyme deficiencies in the glycolytic pathways have also demonstrated abnormal susceptibility to oxidant injury. In these disorders, perhaps the inability to maintain adequate NAD/NADH ratios to stabilize certain cellular metabolic processes may contribute to their susceptibility to oxidants.[2]

Vitamin E supplementation in patients with Mediterranean variants of G6PD deficiency has yielded variable results.[35-38] In affected children and adults, a slight increase in hemoglobin and a decrease in reticulocyte count have been reported; however, the significance of these changes in regard to the patient's overall clinical status remains to be established. Other studies have failed to demonstrate a change in hematologic parameters following therapy with vitamin E.[37,38] Failure to respond to vitamin E supplementation does not exclude an oxidant mechanism in the pathogenesis of hemolysis or the possibility that other antioxidants or combinations of antioxidants might not have therapeutic value.

Qualitative or quantitative disorders of hemoglobin synthesis offer an interesting model to study oxidant-induced cellular injury. The thalassemias, where an imbalance in globin change synthesis is associated with excess globin chains, either alpha in the case of beta thalassemia, or beta in the case of alpha thalassemia, demonstrate evidence for membrane oxidation.[3,6,10,39,40] The excess hemoglobin chains, which bind to the inside of the cell membrane, may dissociate into heme and globin, form an aggregate called Heinz bodies, or oxidize into a hemichrome. The heme moieties and free iron are particularly important in regard to oxidant injury.[20-24] This iron, when in proximity to polyunsaturated fatty acids or sulfhydryl-containing proteins, readily initiates oxidant damage. Ascorbic acid, within the cytoplasm of the cell or its membrane, may enhance or reduce the oxidant potential of this iron.[41] Membrane-permeable agents, which chelate iron and block its ability to generate free radicals, may be useful as antioxidants in these conditions.[42]

Red cells containing unstable hemoglobins are also susceptible to oxidant injury. These disorders are clinically characterized by hemolysis following exposure to oxidant drugs or during infection, where oxidants are generated by stimulated granulocytes.[43] The unstable hemoglobin, once oxidized to methemoglobin, rapidly denatures generating Heinz bodies, hemichromes, hemin, and probably free iron. In Hb Koln, in vivo evidence of oxidant injury, correlates with extent of hemolysis.[44,45]

The sickle erythrocyte has several unique features in regard to its susceptibility to oxidant injury. Although sickle cell disease is due to an inherited defect in hemoglobin (B_6 valine $\rightarrow$ glutamic acid), the interaction between this structurally abnormal hemoglobin and the cell membrane results in a number of molecular events consistent with oxidant injury. The extent to which these secondary oxidant-induced alterations contribute to the pathophysiology of sickle cell disease remains to be determined.[6,8,9,46,47] Stocks et al[2] initially reported that the sickle RBC releases excessive amounts of malondialdehyde (MDA) when exposed to hydrogen peroxide. Subsequently, we reported that the amount of MDA generated by deoxygenated (sickled) cells was markedly increased when compared to that generated by oxygenated (biconcave disc shape) sickle cells. This demonstrates that change of shape altered cell membrane susceptibility to oxidation

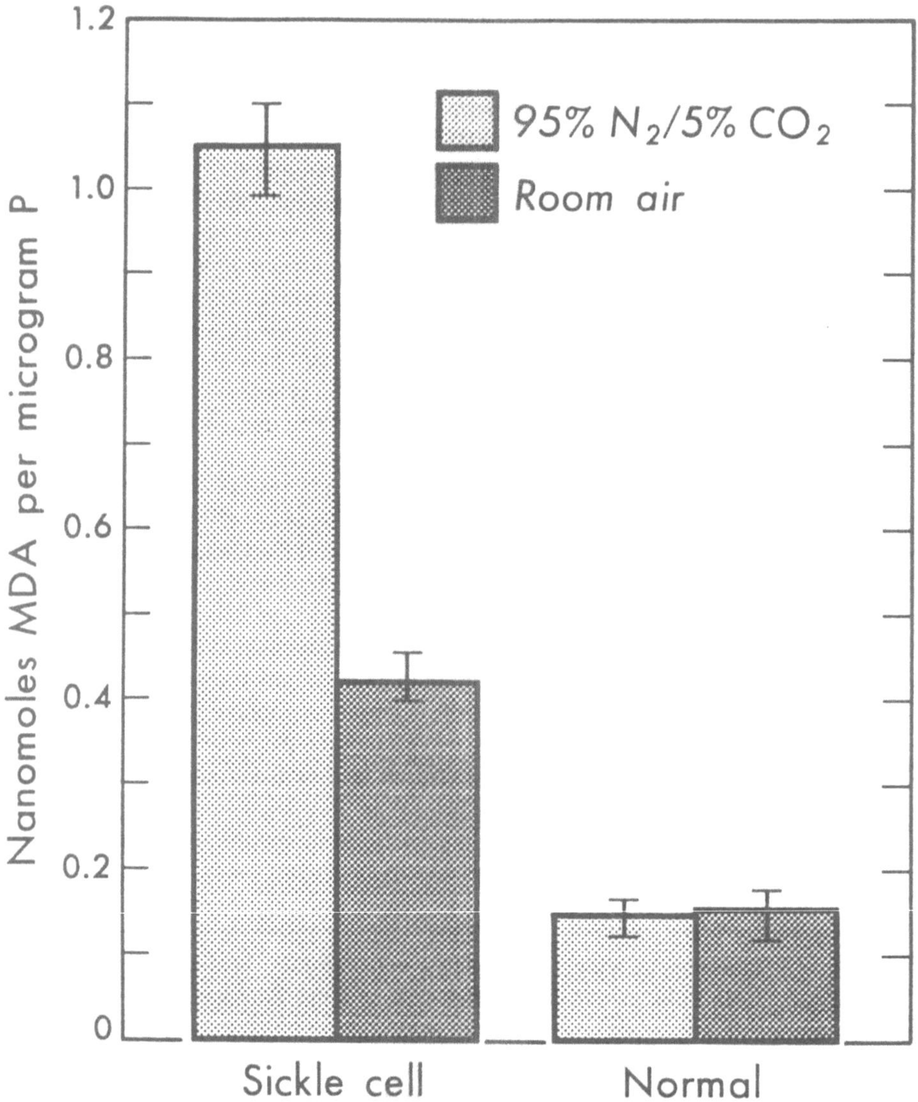

FIGURE 5.1. Effect of sickling on the susceptibility of sickle erythrocytes to lipid peroxidation. The MDA generated from normal and sickle erythrocytes following 2 h incubation under either room air or 95% N_2/5% CO_2 at 37°C was measured. The mean values as well as the ranges are shown. (From Chiu et al.[48])

(Fig. 5.1).[48] Prior addition of vitamin E to sickle red cells in vitro inhibited the MDA generation even under deoxygenated conditions.[49]

It is likely that several factors contribute to the susceptibility of sickle cells to oxidative damage. These are indicated in Table 5.3. Low vitamin E[49,50] and vitamin C[51,52] levels in sickle cell patients have been reported. The etiology of these

TABLE 5.3. Factors contributing to the susceptibility of sickle erythrocytes to peroxidative damage.

Low vitamin E and C
Sickle hemoglobin autooxidation
Membrane-associated hemoglobin
Dissociation of heme and intercalation into membrane lipids
Dissociation of iron from heme
Abnormal membrane phospholipid organization

deficiencies has not been determined. Because of the instability of sickle hemoglobin, sickle erythrocytes spontaneously generate significant quantities of superoxide, peroxide, and hydroxyl radical.[53] These radicals can serve as the initiator of oxidant reactions in the red cell membrane. Furthermore, membrane-associated heme and hemichrome as well as elevated free iron released from denatured sickle hemoglobin create a cellular environment where oxidant injury can occur.[22,23]

Several lines of evidence for in vivo oxidation have been demonstrated in lipid and protein domains of the sickle cell membrane. Cross-linked products of lipids and lipid/protein complexes resulting from reactions with MDA have been reported.[54] Evidence of membrane protein oxidation has included functional alterations in skeletal protein interactions (spectrin–actin–band 4.1)[55] and abnormalities in band 4.1.[9] Defects in several membrane-bound enzymes such as Ca/Mg ATPase[56] also appear to reflect oxidant injury.

The previously mentioned association of alteration in shape with MDA generation suggested that the perturbations in membrane structure accompanying the change in shape associated with sickling render the cell susceptible to injury by oxidants.[46] Phospholipids within the red cell membrane are asymmetrically organized within the bilayer, with sphingomyelin (Sph) and phosphatidylcholine (PC) in the outer leaflet, phosphatidylethanolamine (PE) predominantly in the inner leaflet, and all of the phosphatidylserine (PS) in the inner leaflet.[57] The aminophospholipids (PS and PE), which are rich in polyunsaturated fatty acids, are more susceptible to oxidation than the choline-containing phospholipids. We decided to determine if changes in membrane phospholipid organization accompanied the process of sickling and thereby contributed to the observed change in oxidant susceptibility. Using several probes to identify membrane lipid orientation, abnormalities were demonstrated in sickled erythrocytes.[48,58,59] As shown in Figure 5.2, when cells sickle, the amount of PE in the exterior leaflet of the bilayer increases and 10% to 20% of the PS can be detected in this leaflet. This destabilization of the normal architecture of the lipid bilayer (exposure of aminophospholipids containing PUFA) may contribute to the susceptibility of sickled cells to oxidant injury.

Possible alterations in molecular species of phospholipids induced by oxidation could also contribute to pathologic changes in sickle erythrocytes – in particular, changes in cell hydration. Using a phospholipid exchange protein to transfer phospholipids between red cells separated into dense and light fractions (using a

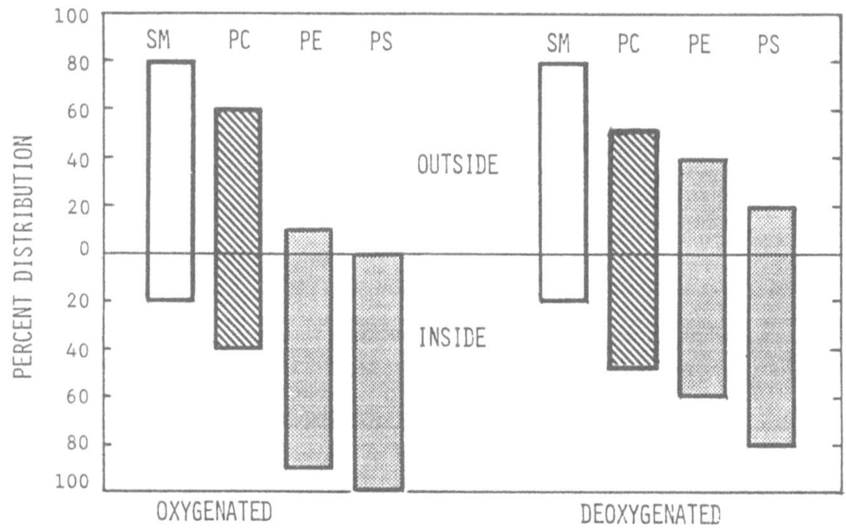

FIGURE 5.2. Proposed distribution of membrane phospholipids in sickle erythrocyte under oxygenated and deoxygenated conditions. (Reproduced from Lubin et al.[58] by copyright permission of the American Society for Clinical Investigation.)

density gradient), Kuypers et al[60] demonstrated rehydration of dense sickle cells (Fig. 5.3). This improvement in cell hydration occurred without a net change in phospholipid composition or change in membrane proteins. It is possible that the exchange protein replaced a critical mass of altered phospholipid (perhaps oxidized phospholipid) with native phospholipid, thereby facilitating the cell's potential to maintain hydration and regain its water content. Since an increase in mean cell hemoglobin concentration accelerates the rate of hemoglobin polymerization (if dehydration of dense cells is due, in part, to oxidized phospholipids), then oxidation of membrane lipids would be a factor that could potentiate the tendency of cells to sickle.

Recently, a sulfhydryl-containing protein has been identified in red cells that assists in maintaining the asymmetric distribution of membrane aminophospholipids.[61] This protein, called an aminophospholipid translocase or flipase, requires adenosine triphosphate to transport aminophospholipids from outer to inner membrane. Studies using electron spin-labeled phospholipid probes have shown that transport of aminophospholipids from the exterior leaflet to the interior leaflet of the membrane is impaired in sickle erythrocytes.[62] Data support the hypothesis that in the spiculed portion of the sickled red cell, where hemoglobin polymers protrude through the cytoskeleton and separate the lipid bilayer from membrane skeletal proteins, transbilayer mobility of phospholipids is increased.[63] We hypothesize that this is because the interactions between cytoskeletal proteins and lipids, which stabilize lipid organization, are weakened in the spicule. As a consequence, in the spicule of the sickled cell, phosphatidyl-

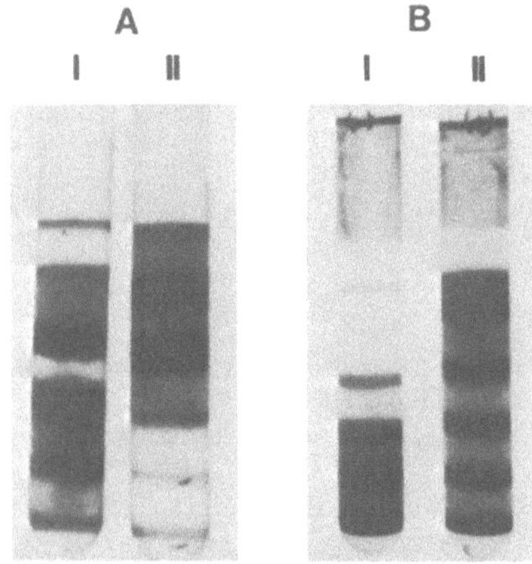

FIGURE 5.3. Density-dependent separation of sickle RBCs on a discontinuous stractan gradient after incubation for 8 h at 37°C in absence (I) or presence (II) of 1 µmol/L phosphatidylcholine transfer protein (PCTP). Note shift to lighter density in the PCTP-treated cells. (A) Nonseparated population of sickle RBCs; (B) dense sickle cells, harvested from a stractan gradient with a density greater than 1.1149 g/mL.

serine can distribute evenly over the lipid bilayer. Since lipids move laterally in the bilayer, PS molecules translocated from inner to outer membrane leaflet in these spicules will move to domains of the membrane where the cells are not spiculated. If the aminotranslocase were intact, these PS molecules would be transported back to the inner leaflet of the bilayer and remain in proximity to skeletal proteins such as spectrin and band 4.1.[64] If the aminotranslocase is oxidized, as appears to occur in sickle erythrocytes, the PS that is on the exterior in the spicules would remain in the outer leaflet even if it moved laterally in the membrane. The combination of dissociation of lipids from proteins in membrane spicules and oxidation of the aminophospholipid translocase could explain the translocation of phosphatidylserine noted in sickled red cells. This hypothesis, schematically represented in Figure 5.4, illustrates a unique effect of oxidative damage in sickle red cells. Since red cells with PS on their surface have procoagulant activity,[63] adhere to monocyte-macrophages,[65] and activate complement,[66] these alterations in PS organization may contribute to the pathophysiology of sickle cell disease.

Consequences of Membrane Oxidative Damage

The consequence of membrane oxidative damage in congenital hemolytic anemias may be profound. Changes in membrane deformability and permeability that accompany oxidant injury can alter cell viability and contribute to intravascular lysis. Low et al[67] reported that hemoglobin, which associates with band 3,

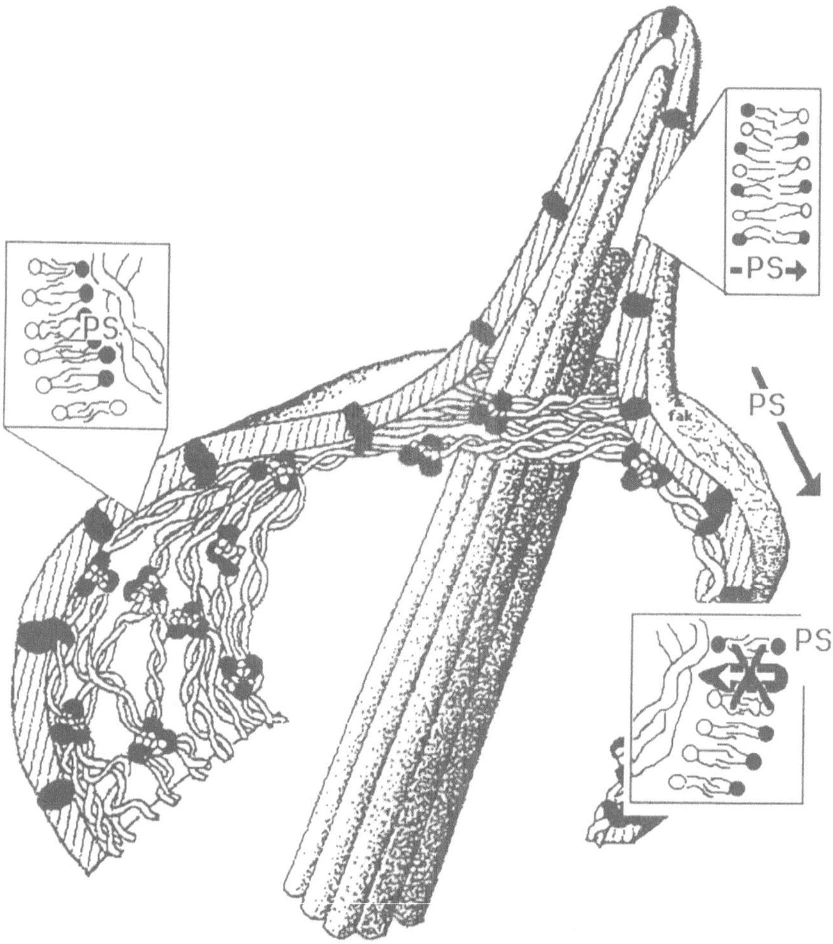

FIGURE 5.4. Proposed model for PS flow (both vertical and lateral) in oxidatively damaged sickled cells. Arrows indicate direction of PS flow. Loss of membrane phospholipid asymmetry occurs in the spicules which are devoid of red cell skeletal proteins. PS diffuses laterally in the exterior leaflet. Inhibition of the flipase results in retention of PS in the exterior leaflet.

causes aggregations of band 3, creating an antigenic structure on the red cell surface, which can serve as a site for macrophage recognition. Hebbel and Miller[68] showed that MDA, when added to RBC, alters membrane structure and serves as a site for macrophage recognition. Snyder et al[69] demonstrated that oxidation of normal RBC results in their recognition by macrophages as well as shortened in vivo survival.[70]

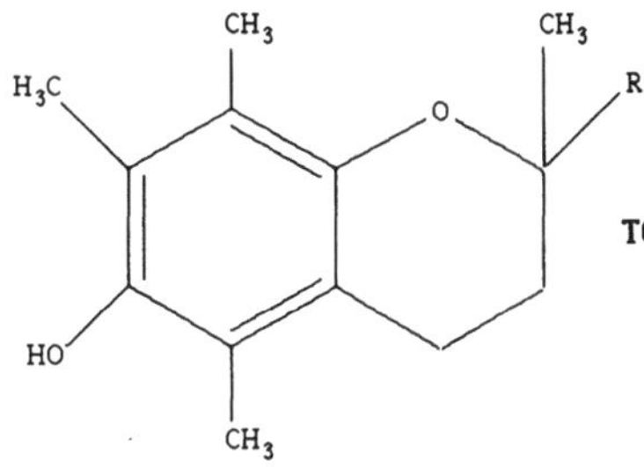

TOCOPHEROL (VITAMIN E)

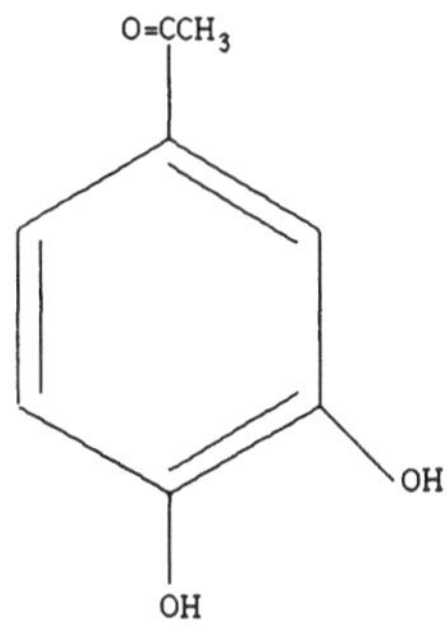

3,4 DIHYDROXYACETOPHENONE

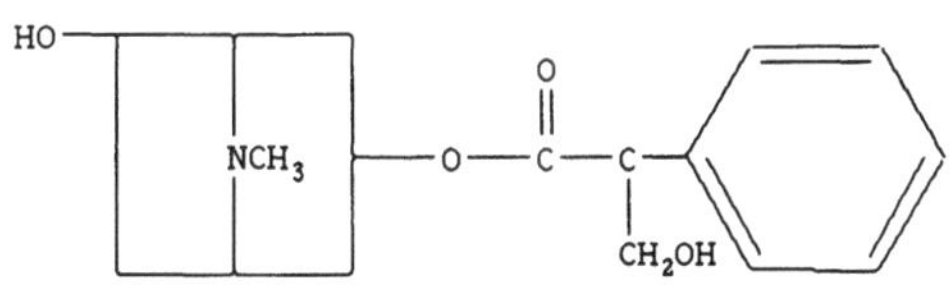

ANISODAMINE (6542)

FIGURE 5.5. Chemical structures of tocopherol (vitamin E) and the two purified ingredients from Chinese herbs, 3.4 dihydroxyacetophenonl and anisodamine.

Strategies to Prevent Red Cell Oxidative Damage

In contrast to the wealth of information regarding evidence for oxidant injury in the pathology of certain red cell disorders, strategies to prevent oxidant damage have demonstrated limited effect in vivo. Except for vitamin E deficiency in the premature infant, therapy with vitamin E has not resulted in dramatic improvement in most oxidant-susceptible red cell disorders. Although this may be due to an inadequate dose of vitamin E, it is also possible that vitamin E given alone provides protection against certain components of an oxidant insult but not against others. Furthermore, oxidative membrane damage may be compartmentalized to specific lipid or protein domains. Prevention of oxidant damage may require combinations of hydrophobic and hydrophilic antioxidants which protect different components of the cell. Chelating agents such as deferoximine or penicillamine should be evaluated, since iron bound to a chelating agent cannot initiate free-radical reactions.[42] Clinical studies employing water-soluble, membrane-permeable chelators, in combination with hydrophobic and hydrophilic antioxidants, would be of theoretical benefit.

Chinese herbal medicines have been found to contain a number of antioxidants. Studies on two of these agents in our laboratory, dihydroxyactophenone and anisodamine, have demonstrated protective effects on lipid peroxidation and hemoglobin oxidation.[70] The chemical structure of these two drugs in comparison to vitamin E is shown in Figure 5.5. The water-soluble nature of these antioxidants may be particularly useful in preventing protein oxidation.

In summary, we have reviewed evidence that supports the hypothesis that oxidative damage is important in the pathophysiology of congenital and acquired hemolytic anemias. Stimulated by the work of Oski and Barness[29] on the vitamin E-deficient premature infant, extensive effects of oxidant injury on red cells have been demonstrated. Although this article did not refer to the relationship between oxidant injury and cell aging, the oxidant-induced findings reported in pathologic red cells are consistent with premature red cell aging. Prevention of disease is one of the pediatrician's goals. Therefore, the burden is ours to find the "fountain of youth"—at least for the red cell.

Acknowledgments. This work was supported in part by the National Institutes of Health grants HL27059, HL 20985, HL 21016, HL 36255, HL 37593, and AM 32094.

References

1. Dodge JT, Cohen G, Kayden H, et al: Peroxidation hemolysis of red blood cells from patients with abeta lipoproteinemia (acanthocytosis). *J Clin Invest* 46:357–368, 1967.
2. Stocks J, Offerman EL, Modell CB, et al: The susceptibility to autoxidation of human red cell lipids in health and disease. *Br J Haematol* 23:713–724, 1972.
3. Rachmilewitz EA, Lubin BH, Shohet SB: Lipid membrane peroxidation in β thalassemia major. *Blood* 47:495–505, 1976.
4. Allen DW, Johnson GJ, Cadman S, et al: Membrane polypeptide aggregates in glucose-6-phosphate dehydrogenase-deficient and in vitro aged red blood cells. *J Lab Clin Med* 91:321–327, 1978.
5. Johnson GJ, Allen DW, Cadman S, et al: Red cell membrane polypeptide aggregates in glucose-6-phosphate dehydrogenase mutants with chronic hemolytic disease. *N Engl J Med* 301:522–527, 1979.
6. Chiu D, Lubin B, Shohet SB: Peroxidation reactions in red cell biology. In Pryor W (ed): *Free Radicals in Biology*, Vol V. New York; Academic Press, 1982, pp 115–160.
7. Jain SK, Yip R, Hoesch RM, et al: Evidence of peroxidative damage to the erythrocyte membrane in iron deficiency. *Am J Clin Nutr* 37:26–30, 1983.
8. Rank BH, Carlson J, Hebbel RP: Abnormal redox status of membrane-protein thiols in sickle erythrocytes. *J Clin Invest* 75:1531–1537, 1985.

9. Schwartz RS, Rybicki AC, Heath RH, et al: Protein 4.1 in sickle erythrocytes: Evidence for oxidative damage. *J Biol Chem* 262:15666–15672, 1987.
10. Prasartkaew S, Bunyaratvej A, Fucharoen S, et al: Oxidative stress and antioxidant enzymes in hemoglobin H disease. *BDOAS* 23(5A):193–198, 1988.
11. Girotti AW, Bachowski GJ, Jordan JE: Lipid peroxidation in erythrocyte membranes: Cholesterol product analysis in photosensitized and xanthine oxidase-catalyzed reactions. *Lipids* 22:401–408, 1987.
12. Van Kuijk FJGM, Sevanian A, Handelman GJ, et al: A new role for phospholipase A_2: Protection of membranes from lipid peroxidation damage. *TIBS* 12:31–34, 1987.
13. Jacob HS: Mechanisms of Heinz body formation and abnormal hemoglobin molecule. *Semin Hematol* 7:341–354, 1970.
14. Rachmilewitz EA: Denaturation of the normal and abnormal hemoglobin molecule. *Semin Hematol* 11:441–462, 1974.
15. Wetterstroem N, Brewer GJ, Warth JA, et al: Relationship of glutathione levels and Heinz body formation to irreversibly sickled cells in sickle cell anemia. *J Lab Clin Med* 103:589–596, 1984.
16. Waugh S, Low PS: Hemichrome binding to band 3: Nucleation of Heinz bodies on the erythrocyte membrane. *Biochemistry* 24:34–39, 1985.
17. Mannoji M, Sugihra T, Yawata Y: Heinz body formation in red cell membrane disorders: Its acceleration in membrane lipid abnormalities. *Scand J Haematol* 35: 257–263, 1985.
18. Reinhart WH, Sung LA, Chien S: Quantitative relationship between Heinz body formation and red blood cell deformability. *Blood* 68:1376–1383, 1986.
19. Waugh SM, Willardson BM, Labotka RJ, et al: Heinz bodies induce clustering of band 3, glycophorin and ankyrin in sickle cell erythrocytes. *J Clin Invest* 78:1155–1160, 1986.
20. Shaklai N, Shviro Y, Rabizadeh E, et al: Accumulation and drainage of hemin in the red cell membrane. *Biochim Biophys Acta* 821:355–366, 1985.
21. Janney SK, Joist JH, Fitch CD: Excess release of ferriheme in G6PD-deficient erythrocytes: Possible cause of hemolysis and resistance to malaria. *Blood* 67:331–333, 1986.
22. Kuross SA, Rank BH, Hebbel RP: Excess heme in sickle erythrocyte inside-out membranes: Possible role in thiol oxidation. *Blood* 71:876–882, 1988.
23. Liu SC, Zhai S, Palek J: Detection of hemin release during hemoglobin S denaturation. *Blood* 71:1755–1758, 1988.
24. Chiu D, Lubin B: Oxidative hemoglobin denaturation and RBC destruction: The effect of heme on red cell membranes. *Semin Hematol* 2:128–135, 1989 (in press).
25. Sadrzadeh SMH, Grat E, Panter SS, et al: Hemoglobin: A biologic Fenton reagent. *J Biol Chem* 259:14354–14356, 1984.
26. Puppo A, Halliwell B: Formation of hydroxyl radicals from peroxide in the presence of iron. *Biochem J* 249:185–190, 1988.
27. Weiss SJ: The role of superoxide destruction of erythrocyte targets by human neutrophils. *J Biol Chem* 255:9912–9917, 1980.
28. Claster S, Chiu DTY, Quintanilha A, Lubin B: Neutrophils mediate lipid peroxidation in human red cells. *Blood* 64:1079–1084, 1984.
29. Oski FA, Barness LA: Vitamin E deficiency: A previously unrecognized cause of hemolytic anemia in the premature infant. *Pediatrics* 70:211–220, 1967.
30. Ritchie JH, Fish MB, McMasters V, et al: Edema and hemolytic anemia in premature infants. *N Engl J Med* 279:1185–1190, 1968.

31. Becker PS, Lux SE: Hereditary spherocytosis and related disorders. *Clin Haematol* 14(1):15–43, 1985.
32. Palek J: Hereditary elliptocytosis and related disorders. *Clin Haematol* 14(1):45–87, 1985.
33. Lande WM, Mentzer WC: Haemolytic anemia associated with increased cation permeability. *Clin Haematol* 14(1):89–103, 1985.
34. Rybicki AC, Heath R, Wolf JL, et al: Deficiency of protein 4.2 in erythrocytes from a patient with a Coombs negative hemolytic anemia. *J Clin Invest* 81:893–901, 1988.
35. Corash H, Spielberg S, Bartsocas C, et al: Reduced chronic hemolysis during high-dose vitamin E administration in Mediterranean-type glucose-6-phosphate dehydrogenase deficiency. *N Engl J Med* 303:416–420, 1980.
36. Johnson GJ, Vatasserg GT, Finkel B, et al: High-dose vitamin E does not decrease the rate of chronic hemolysis in glucose-6-phosphate dehydrogenase deficiency. *N Engl J Med* 308:1014–1017, 1983.
37. Hafez M, Amar ES, Zedan M, et al: Improved erythrocyte survival with combined vitamin E and selenium therapy in children with glucose-6-phosphate dehydrogenase deficiency and mild hemolysis. *J Pediatr* 108:558–561, 1986.
38. Newman GJ, Newman TB, Bowie LJ, et al: An examination of the role of vitamin E in glucose-6-phosphate dehydrogenase deficiency. *Clin Biochem* 12:149–151, 1979.
39. Rachmilevitz EA, Kahane I: The red cell membrane in thalassemia. *Br J Haematol* 46:1–6, 1980.
40. Joshi W, Leb L, Piotrowski J, et al: Increased sensitivity of isolated alpha subunits of normal human hemoglobin to oxidative damage and crosslinkage with spectrin. *J Lab Clin Med* 102:46–52, 1983.
41. Canfield LM, Gollan JL, White AG, et al: Serum antioxidant activity in normal and abnormal subjects. *Ann Clin Biochem* 16(6):299–306, 1979.
42. Sullivan JL: Iron, plasma antioxidants, and the oxygen radical disease of prematurity. *Am J Dis Child* 142:1341–1344, 1988.
43. Platt OS, Falcone JF: Membrane protein lesions in erythrocytes with Heinz bodies. *J Clin Invest* 82:1051–1058, 1988.
44. Flynn TP, Allen DW, Johnson GJ, et al: Oxidant damage of the lipids and proteins of the erythrocyte membranes in unstable hemoglobin disease. *J Clin Invest* 71:1215–1223, 1983.
45. Allen DW, Burgoyne CF, Groat JD, et al: Comparison of hemoglobin Koln erythrocyte membrane with malondialdehyde-reacted normal erythrocyte membrane. *Blood* 64: 1263–1269, 1984.
46. Chiu D, Vichinsky E, Yee M, et al: Peroxidation, vitamin E and sickle cell anemia. *Ann NY Acad Sci* 393:323–335, 1982.
47. Rice-Evans C, Omorphos SC, Baysal E: Sickle cell membranes and oxidative damage. *Biochem J* 237:265–269, 1986.
48. Chiu D, Lubin B, Shohet SB: Erythrocyte membrane lipid reorganization during the sickling process. *Br J Haematol* 41:223–234, 1979.
49. Chiu D, Lubin B: Abnormal vitamin E and glutathione peroxidase levels in sickle cell anemia. *J Lab Clin Med* 94:542–548, 1979.
50. Natta C, Machlin L: Plasma levels of tocopherol in sickle cell anemia subjects. *Am J Clin Nutr* 32:1359–1362, 1979.
51. Ho T, Liu T, Vichinsky E, et al: Vitamin C levels in patients with sickle cell anemia. *Clin Res* 32:120, 1984 (abstract).

52. Jain SK, Williams DM: Reduced levels of plasma ascorbic acid (vitamin C) in sickle cell disease patients: Its possible role in the oxidant damage to sickle cell in vivo. *Clin Chim Acta* 149:257–261, 1985.
53. Hebbel RP, Eaton JW, Balasirgam M, et al: Spontaneous oxygen radical generation by sickle erythrocytes. *J Clin Invest* 70:1253–1259, 1982.
54. Jain SK, Shohet SB: A novel phospholipid in irreversibly sickled cells: Evidence for in vivo peroxidative membrane damage in sickle cell disease. *Blood* 63:362–367, 1984.
55. Platt OS, Falcone JF, Lux SE: Molecular defect in the sickle erythrocyte skeleton. *J Clin Invest* 75:266–271, 1985.
56. Dixon E, Winslow RM: The interaction between (Ca^{+2}-Mg^{+2})-ATPase and the soluble activator (calmodulin) in erythrocytes containing haemoglobin S. *Br J Haematol* 47:391–397, 1981.
57. Zwaal RFA, Roelofsen B, Comfurins P, et al: Organization of phospholipids in human red cell membranes as detected by the action of various purified phospholipases. *Biochim Biophys Acta* 406:83–86, 1975.
58. Lubin B, Chiu D, Bastacky J, et al: Abnormalities in membrane phospholipid organization in sickled erythrocytes. *J Clin Invest* 67:1643–1649, 1981.
59. Franck PFH, Chiu DTY, Op den Kamp JAF, et al: Accelerated transbilayer movement of phosphatidylcholine in sickled erythrocytes. *J Biol Chem* 258:8435–8442, 1983.
60. Kuypers FA, Chiu D, Mohandas N, et al: The molecular species composition of phosphatidylcholine affects cellular properties in normal and sickle erythrocytes. *Blood* 70:1111–1118, 1987.
61. Devaux PF: Phospholipid flipases. *FEBS Lett* 234:8–12, 1988.
62. Zachowski A, Craescu CT, Galacteros F, et al: Abnormality of phospholipid transverse diffusion in sickle erythrocytes. *J Clin Invest* 75:1713–1717, 1985.
63. Franck PFH, Beavers EM, Lubin BH: Uncoupling of the membrane skeleton from the lipid bilayer. *J Clin Invest* 75:183–190, 1985.
64. Rybicki AC, Heath R, Lubin B, et al: Human erythrocyte protein 4.1 is a phosphatidylserine binding protein. *J Clin Invest* 81:255–260, 1980.
65. Schwartz RS, Tanaka Y, Fidler IJ, et al: Increased adherence of sickled and phosphatidylserine-enriched human erythrocytes to cultured human peripheral blood monocytes. *J Clin Invest* 75:1965–1972, 1985.
66. Tomasko MA, Chudwin DS: Complement activation in sickle cell disease: A liposome model. *J Lab Clin Med* 112:248–253, 1988.
67. Low PS, Waugh SM, Zinke K, et al: The role of hemoglobin denaturation and band 3 clustering in red blood cell aging. *Science* 227:531–533, 1985.
68. Hebbel RP, Miller W: Phagocytosis of sickle erythrocytes: Immunologic and oxidative determinations of hemolytic anemia. *Blood* 64:733–741, 1984.
69. Snyder LM, Fortier NL, Trainor J, et al: Effect of hydrogen peroxide exposure on normal human erythrocyte deformability, morphology, surface characteristics, and spectrin-hemoglobin cross-linking. *J Clin Invest* 76:1971–1977, 1985.
70. McKenney J, Valeri CR, Mohandas N, et al: Decreased in vivo survival of oxidatively damaged red cells. *Blood* 72(5, Suppl 1):32a, 1988.
71. Chiu D, Pan HC, Kuypers FA, et al: Purified ingredients from chinese herbs protect human red cells against oxidant-induced damage. *Blood* 70(5) (Suppl 1):38, 1987 (abstract).

6
Combined Immunodeficiency Caused by a Transactive Regulatory Mutation: A New Mutational Class

Donald A. Pious

Our laboratory research has focused on the genes, gene regulation, protein structure, and function of HLA, the human major histocompatibility complex (MHC) of humans. In this paper I will focus on our work on HLA gene regulation and its defects as newly recognized causes of combined immunodeficiency. The HLA complex is a cluster of genes located on the short arm of chromosome six. HLA class II genes code for the heterodimeric cell surface glycoproteins HLA-DR, -DQ and -DP; both the heavy (A) and light (B) chain genes of class II molecules are in the MHC cluster. HLA class II molecules are expressed on B cells, activated T cells, macrophages, and some epithelial and other cells. In some cells, the levels of class II expression are coordinately increased by γ-interferon, IL-4, or tumor necrosis factor (TNF). Class II molecules function by binding peptides derived from degraded exogenous protein antigens; the generation by cells of immunogenic peptides from soluble exogenous proteins is known as antigen processing. The resulting peptide class II complex "presents antigen to" (ie, activates) specific helper or suppressor T cells by binding to a peptide- and HLA class II antigen-specific T cell receptor, expressed clonally. The ability of HLA molecules to bind given peptides is allele specific; the high degree of polymorphism in these genes therefore results in genetic differences in the capacity to mount immune responses to particular immunogens. In addition, certain HLA alleles are strong susceptibility factors for particular autoimmune diseases.

The research described in this paper can be thought of as a kind of "reverse genetics." In the usual sense of the terms, "direct genetics" proceeds from determining the phenotype produced by a mutation, to inferring the structure and action of the normal gene in which it occurred; reverse genetics, on the other hand, starts from the cloned gene and uses it to determine the primary structure of its gene product and to study its action in the cell. In our case we first defined a transactive factor required for transcription of all HLA class II genes by char-

---

From the Departments of Pediatrics, Immunology and Genetics, University of Washington, Seattle.
Presented in honor of Lewis A. Barness, MD, November 11, 1988.

acterizing a unique mutant we had isolated in cell culture. We then obtained evidence by genetic complementation that a mutation in this gene is responsible for a syndrome of primary combined immunodeficiency characterized by defective expression of HLA class II genes.

We initially devised a selective system for isolation of HLA mutants using antibodies to HLA specificities plus complement. With this selective system, we have isolated a large number of HLA mutants of different kinds from a cultured diploid, EB virus-transformed B lymphoid cell line, T5-1. T5-1 was cultured from a donor selected on the basis of heterozygosity for all six class I and II specificities; because HLA genes are expressed codominantly, it is easy to determine the genotype of any HLA loss mutant from such a cell line by simple serological assays. We have used the different kinds of mutants generated by mutagenesis and immunoselection: (1) for structure-function mapping of HLA molecules, using point mutants within the HLA structural genes and DNA sequencing together with functional assays; (2) for gene mapping on the short arm of chromosome 6, using heterozygous deletion mutants and recombinant gene probes; and (3) for exploring mechanisms that regulate expression of HLA genes, using mutants defective in HLA regulation. Most of the work described below stems from the characterization of one mutant, designated 6.1.6, which has given us our first insights into the complex mechanisms by which class II genes are regulated.

We[1] isolated 6.1.6 and other mutants using the frame-shift mutagen ICR 191 and an antibody specific for HLA-DR3. It was recognized that 6.1.6 was unique among the several hundred mutants isolated in that it appeared to have lost expression of all HLA Class II alleles from both haplotypes in a single step. One obvious possibility was that 6.1.6 had undergone deletions of the HLA regions of both chromosomes 6. However, no chromosome 6 deletions were detected in 6.1.6 by karyotypic analysis. Prior to the time that class II molecular probes became available, it was not possible to determine whether submicroscopic deletions were present in 6.1.6. However, statistical considerations made it unlikely that it could have undergone deletions of the class II regions of both chromosomes 6. Several lines of evidence subsequently confirmed that the class II genes were intact in 6.1.6 but were not being expressed.

Evidence that the class II genes in 6.1.6 were intact came first from somatic cell hybridization experiments in which 6.1.6 was fused to other B cell lines with class II specificities different from those of T5-1, the progenitor of 6.1.6.[2] The class II genes of 6.1.6 were reexpressed in these hybrids, indicating that in 6.1.6, the class II genes, although not expressed, were capable of being expressed. Additional evidence for the intactness of class II genes was obtained by Levine and Pious.[3] A minority population of partial revertants from 6.1.6 was isolated by fluorescence-activated cell sorting. On the basis of these findings, we postulated that the defect in 6.1.6 was in a factor required for class II expression and that the factor was "transactive"—that is, the factor missing in 6.1.6 could be supplied by its hybridization partner in the somatic cell hybrids.[2,3] We estimated that the rate of occurrence of 6.1.6-like mutations in T5-1 was very low and was consistent with a mutagen-induced "double hit" affecting both alleles of the transactive factor gene.

This appears to be the first report in which a mutation in a transactive gene regulator was proposed as the basis for loss of expression of a mammalian gene or genes. The multiplicity of HLA loci and their high degree of polymorphism made it possible to obtain and use a multiply heterozygous cell line in these studies. This was crucial initially in providing the markers to recognize that 6.1.6 might have a mutation in a transactive factor which coordinately regulates class II genes. For genes that are neither polymorphic nor members of multigene families, recognizing mutations in transactive factors will be more difficult, but not impossible.

At this juncture molecular probes for class II genes were needed to further investigate the nature and action of the postulated transactive factor deficient in 6.1.6. At that time a number of investigators (Erlich, Cetus Corp.; Mach, the University of Geneva; and Auffrey and Strominger, University of Harvard) had succeeded in isolating class II cDNAs and provided them to our laboratory. We used Northern blotting with probes for all the major expressed class II genes, and found that class II mRNAs were virtually absent in 6.1.6, indicating that the defect might be at the level of class II gene transcription or stability.[4] Using Southern blotting with restriction enzymes which distinguish between methylated and nonmethylated cytosines, we also found that in congenic pairs of cells that differed only in class II gene expression, such as progenitor T5-1 and mutant 6.1.6, and 6.1.6 and its revertants, a cytosine is methylated in class II genes that are expressed and is demethylated in class II genes that are not expressed.[5] This difference in the state of methylation of class II genes between T5-1 and 6.1.6 suggested that the transactive factor missing in 6.1.6 acted at a level involving class II genes themselves, eg, at the level of class II gene transcription rather than mRNA stability.

To obtain more definitive evidence about the site of action of the postulated class II transactive factor, we used the method of nuclear runoff transcription to measure the rates of transcription of class II genes in T5-1 and 6.1.6.[6] We found that there was essentially no detectable transcription of class II genes in 6.1.6. Taken together, these results thus defined genetically a transactive factor that is deficient in 6.1.6 and is required for transcription of HLA class II genes in B cells.

In collaboration with Salter and Cresswell, we subsequently used genetic complementation analysis to define a second transcriptional regulator of class II gene expression.[7] To determine whether two different recessive mutants defective in the same function have mutations in the same gene, somatic cell hybrids are made between the two. If the function is restored in the hybrids, the mutants are said to be "complementing" and the mutations are considered to be in different genes. If the function is not restored in the hybrids, the mutants are "noncomplementing," and the mutations are considered to be in the same gene. We asked whether the class II transactive transcriptional factor missing in two T leukemia cell lines that do not transcribe their class II genes was the same as that missing in 6.1.6. This was done by measuring class II expression in somatic cell hybrids made between 6.1.6 and the T leukemia lines and determining whether the class II genes from either or both genomes were expressed in the hybrids. We found that the class II genes from both genomes were expressed in these hybrids, indicating that the transcriptional factor missing in the T leukemia lines was different from that missing in 6.1.6. These results thus defined a second class II transactive transcriptional regulator. Additional complementation studies, described below, indicate that at a minimum there are three such class II transcriptional factors, and there may well be more.

At about the time our first report[1] on the 6.1.6 mutation appeared, Touraine et al[8] reported a child with severe combined immunodeficiency and reduced expression of HLA antigens on peripheral blood mononuclear cells. Over the succeeding years about 25 similar patients were described, mostly in Europe and among children of Turkish or North African origin. These patients probably do not constitute a single homogeneous group; they differ both clinically and in the relative effects of the mutations on HLA class I and II expression. The immune deficiency is frequently severe and is often fatal, as it is in some other, etiologically distinct forms of combined immunodeficiency. One instance of the disease in siblings has been reported, and the disorders are believed to result from recessive mutations. Although it was known at the time of Touraine's first report[8] that the ability of "antigen presenting cells" (APCs) to present soluble antigens required that the APCs express class II antigens, the exact nature of the role of class II molecules in presentation has only been recognized more recently. Hence, the causal relationship between the defect in HLA expression and combined immunodeficiency was initially not clear. Studies on the nature of the defect in these patients have been complicated in part by difficulties encountered in transforming peripheral blood B cells from these patients by EB virus for purposes of obtaining permanent cell lines. However, a few such cell lines from patients were eventually obtained.

It then became feasible to determine by complementation analysis whether the defects in the patients were in the same genes as are deficient in 6.1.6. RJ 2.2.5, a mutant phenotypically similar to 6.1.6 which had recently been immunoselected from a B cell line by Accolla,[9] was also available for study. These studies, done collaboratively with Accolla and Strominger,[10] showed that complementation for the defect in class II transcription did not occur in hybrids made between cells of one patient, TF, and mutant 6.1.6. However, complementation did occur in hybrids made[8] between cells from TF and mutant RJ 2.2.5 and between mutants RJ 2.2.5 and 6.1.6. These results suggest that the defects in the patient TF and in mutant 6.1.6 are in the same gene, whereas that in mutant RJ 2.2.5 is in a different gene. More recently, Hume and Lee[11] have studied two additional patients by complementation analysis with each other and with 6.1.6 and RJ 2.2.5. They found that hybrids made between cells of one of their patients and RJ 2.25 were noncomplementary, whereas hybrids made with all the other pairs from the four cell lines were complementary. These studies suggest that there are a minimum of three transactive regulators of class II gene transcription, mutations which lead to severe combined immunodeficiency. Not all combinations of cells from patients, class II nonexpressing T cells, and mutant cells have yet been included in the complementation matrix; further complementation studies and/or cloning the transactive factor genes (see below) are needed to determine whether these three genes define all the specific transactive factors regulating class II transcription.

A major goal now is to clone the genes for these transactive factors that regulate transcription of the HLA genes. After transactive genes are cloned, it would be possible to determine how they interact to regulate class II expression and how their expression is regulated. It might also provide a basis for gene therapy for these patients. As a first step toward cloning, attempts have been made to define the binding sites for the transactive factors in or around the class II genes, using various approaches. Because class II genes are for the most part regulated in coordinate fashion, one approach is simply to search for DNA sequence homologies among different class II genes immediately upstream from their transcriptional start sites, in the so-called "promoter" regions. The 5′ flanking regions of genes are the most common (but not the only) sites of interactions between DNA and regulatory proteins. In the 140 nucleotides immediately 5′ of the transcription start sites of the class II genes there are three stretches of homology of 8 to 15 nucleotides called W, X, and Y boxes.[12,13] These homologous sequences are prime candidates for sites of transactive transcriptional regulatory protein binding.

To further define the target DNA for the class II transactive factors, use has been made of so-called gel shift or gel retardation assays with defined class II DNA fragments and aqueous extracts of nuclei. It is possible in this way to identify nuclear proteins that bind specifically to the class II fragments as well as the DNA sequences to which they bind. Several labs have reported such binding sites in or around class II genes. The most interesting report in the context of combined immunodeficiency was by Reich et al.[14] They reported that a nuclear factor from cells of normal individuals which binds to the W and X box in gel shift assays was absent in cells from a patient with combined immunodeficiency and absent class II expression.

A third approach to defining the targets of the class II DNA transactive factors is to make gene constructs consisting of fragments of a class II gene or its flanking DNA fused to a "reporter" gene (a gene whose product is distinguishable from those made by the intended recipient cells), to transfect these gene constructs into class II expressing cells, and to determine the level of expression of the reporter gene as a measure of the promoter activity of the fragment. Using a set of such constructs, made with different lengths of DRA gene 5′ flanking region, the minimal promoter of the DRA gene has been defined as the segment from 131 bp 5′ to 31 bp 3′ of the transcription start site.[15-17] Shoval et al[17] found that expression of this fragment in transfected cells closely parallels that of the endogenous DRA gene: a construct with this fragment of the DRA gene is expressed at high levels in T5-1 and other B cell lines and in γ-interferon-induced HeLa, and at low or undetectable levels in 6.1.6, in uninduced HeLa cells, and in the class II nonexpressing T leukemia lines CEM and HSB. Expression of this gene construct made with a 162-bp DRA gene promoter thus parallels that of the endogenous class II genes in cells with different levels of class II transcription and modes of regulation. This 162-bp fragment thus appears to be the minimum DNA sequence containing the *cis* regulatory sites necessary for appropriate transcription of the

DRA gene. The pattern of expression of the DRA promoter constructs in T5-1 and 6.1.6 further suggests that the missing transactive protein in 6.1.6 is an X box binding protein. Additional studies will be necessary to confirm this.

These results may provide the basis for cloning the transactive factor genes. A strategy devised by Staudt et al[18] for cloning immunoglobulin regulatory proteins is currently being pursued by us and others, in attempts to clone genes for the class II regulatory proteins. Briefly, cDNA libraries from cells expressing high levels of class II genes are cloned into bacterial "expression vectors," that is, into bacteriophages, in such a way as to allow the cDNA inserts to be expressed as eukaryotic-bacterial fusion proteins in the bacterial host strain. The limit class II gene promoter or a fragment thereof is then used as a probe to screen by "Southwestern" blotting for lysogens expressing the transactive factor protein that specifically binds to the probe, as a means of identifying the appropriate cDNA insert. It has been possible in this way to identify cDNA clones coding for transactive transcriptional regulatory proteins that bind to the class II promoter fragment. A critical test that has not yet been carried out is to transfect full-length cDNA clones of this type in mammalian expression vectors into the mutant cells in order to show that expression of the transfected DNA corrects the defect in class II gene transcription in the mutant. Such a result would fulfill a genetic version of Koch's postulates and would constitute a most satisfying end point in the characterization of the first inherited defect in man recognized as caused by a mutation in a regulatory gene.

Acknowledgments. In addition to Lew Barness, who gave me a start in research, I would like to acknowledge and thank those in my lab who performed the work described: postdoctoral fellows Paul Gladstone, Eva Stimac, and Simcha Shoval; graduate students Fred Levine and Sherry Kempin; and my collaborators, Henry Erlich, Jack Strominger, Bernard Mach, Peter Cresswell, and Russell Salter.

References

1. Gladstone P, Pious D: Stable variants affecting a B cell alloantigen in human somatic cells. *Nature* 271;459–461, 1978.
2. Gladstone P, Pious D: Identification of a *trans*-acting function regulating HLA-DR expression in a DR-negative B cell variant. *Somatic Cell Genet* 6:285–298, 1980.
3. Levine F, Pious D: Revertants of the HLA class II regulatory mutant 6.1.6: Implications for the regulation of Ia gene expression. *J Immunol* 132:959–962, 1984.
4. Levine F, Mach B, Erlich H, Pious D: Transcriptional regulation of HLA class II and invariant chain genes. *J Immunol* 134:637–640, 1985.
5. Levine F, Pious D: Different roles for cytosine methylation in HLA class II gene expression. *Immunogenetics* 22:427–440, 1985.
6. Stimac E, Lyons S, Pious D: Transcription of HLA class II genes in the absence of B-cell-specific octamer-binding factor. *Mol Cell Biol* 8:3734–3739, 1988.
7. Salter R, Alexander J, Levine F, Pious D, Cresswell P: Evidence for two *trans*-active genes regulating HLA class II antigen expression. *J Immunol* 135:4235–4238, 1985.

8. Touraine J, Betael H, Souillet G, et al: Combined immunodeficiency disease associated with absence of cell surface HLA-A and -B antigens. *J Pediatr* 93:47–51, 1978.
9. Accolla R: Human B cell variants immunoselected against a single Ia antigen subset have lost expression of several Ia antigen subsets. *J Exp Med* 157:1053–1058, 1983.
10. Zhi Y, Accolla R, Pious D, Zegers B, Strominger J: Two distinct loci regulating class II gene expression are defective in human mutant and patient cell lines. *EMBO J* 7:1965–1972, 1988.
11. Hume C, Lee J: Congenital immunodeficiencies associated with absence of HLA class II antigens on lymphocytes result from distinct mutations in *trans*- acting factors. *Hum Immunol* (in press).
12. Saito H, Maki R, Clayton L, Tonegawa S: Complete primary structures of the E β chain and gene of the mouse major histocompatibility complex. *Proc Natl Acad Sci USA* 80:5520–5624, 1983.
13. Kelly A, Trowsdale J: Complete nucleotide sequence of a functional HLA-DRβ gene and the region between the DPβ1 and DPα1 genes: Comparison of the 5′ ends of the HLA class II genes. *Nucleic Acids Res* 13:1607–1621, 1985.
14. Reith W, Satola S, Sanchez C, et al: Congenital immunodeficiency with a regulatory defect in the MHL class II gene expression lacks a specific HLA-DR promoter binding protein. *Cell* 53:897–906, 1988.
15. Sherman P, Basta P, Ting J: Upstream sequences required for tissue specific expression of HLA-DRα gene. *Proc Natl Acad Sci USA* 84:4254–4258, 1987.
16. Tsang S, Nakanishi N, Peterlin B: B-cell-specific and interferon-gamma-inducible regulation of the HLA-DR alpha gene. *Proc Natl Acad Sci USA* 85:8598–8602, 1988.
17. Stimac E, Shoval S, Kempin S, Pious D: Manuscript in preparation.
18. Staudt L, Clerc R, Singh H, et al: Cloning of a lymphoid-specific cDNA encoding a protein binding the regulatory octamer DNA motif. *Science* 241:577–580, 1988.

7
Arterial Wall in Genetic Disorders: Selected Topics

M. DARIA HAUST

Introduction

With the exception of one area, the congenital malformations, the available information pertaining to the status of arteries in genetic diseases is meager, fragmented, and at times contradictory. Moreover, some of the normal arterial changes accompanying the development from infancy to adult life[1] have been misinterpreted in many reports as representing lesions.

There have been a few recent attempts at summarizing the existing knowledge on some aspects of the subject. These are neither up to date nor complete, notwithstanding the fact that most of these data appeared in the form of chapters in, or specialty textbooks.[2-10] It is therefore understandable that this presentation cannot serve as a complete overview of the subject.

The purposes of this communication are (1) to outline the modus in which arteries may be involved in genetic diseases; (2) to illustrate the mural changes of "normal" segments of arteries in three selected disorders; (3) to summarize in general terms some clinical consequences of arterial involvement; and (4) to discuss briefly the potential of the arterial wall as an important source of tissues for study of the as yet unknown bases of genetic diseases and other disorders.

Modus of Arterial Involvement in Genetic Diseases

In genetic diseases the arterial involvement ranges from alterations that may be apparent on gross examination as either changes of configuration and size or recognizable lesions affecting the wall to changes that may be appreciated upon light or electron microscopic examination only. Pathophysiologically, these alterations may be considered broadly in four categories.

From the Department of Pathology, Pediatrics, and Obstetrics and Gynecology, University of Western Ontario and the Children's Psychiatric Research Institute, London, Ontario, Canada.
Submitted in honor of Lewis A. Barness, MD, November 1988.

Congenital Malformations

Whereas a particular type may affect specific sets of arteries or segments thereof, it is important to emphasize that arterial malformations seldom, if ever, occur in genetic disorder as pathognomonic or isolated lesions. In some disorders they are often associated with other cardiovascular malformations and almost invariably are part of a multisystem involvement.

Chromosomal Disorders Often Associated with Congenital Arterial Malformations[4,5,9,11-16]

Of the known aberrations of autosomal chromosomes, all are associated with arterial malformations with one exception (Wolf's syndrome[4]). In the group of sex chromosome disorders, the Turner and Klinefelter syndromes show an increased incidence of such malformations. Some are characteristically present in a given disease – eg, aortic coarctation in the Turner syndrome, or pulmonary stenosis (as a part of tetralogy of Fallot) in the Klinefelter syndrome. However, whereas the former is a common association, the latter is not. No malformation is pathognomonic for a given syndrome.

Little is known about the microscopic features of malformed arteries, although studies in this area have been initiated.[17]

Monogenic Disorders (Autosomal and X-Linked [Recessive and Dominant])

Approximately 2% to 3% of all congenital cardiovascular malformations (of which 75% involve the arteries) occur in this disease group. When present they are characteristic but again, not pathognomonic.[2,3] For example, pulmonary arteriovenous fistulas are observed in the Osler-Rendu-Weber syndrome, patent ductus arteriosus in incontinentia pigmenti, and aortic coarctation in Sturge-Weber syndrome and neurofibromatosis.[2,3,5] Stenosis of pulmonary and/or renal artery may also be present in the latter. In some monogenic diseases, arterial changes do not represent true congenital malformations but are the consequence of the underlying a priori alterations of the arterial wall – eg, the aneurysms in the Marfan and Ehlers-Danlos syndromes.

The arterial structure at light and electron microscopic level have been studied in members of this disease group, and the interested reader is referred to the available chapter in a relatively recent textbook.[10] However, in many instances the reviewed literature relates to the obviously affected arteries, and the information about the more subtle changes of the arterial wall has seldom been cited.

Multifactorial Diseases (Interaction of Polygenic and Environmental Components)[2,3,18-21]

On the basis of clinical observations, some authors suggest that approximately 90% of all cardiovascular malformations are expressions of this disease group.[3,22-25] It is known that certain forms of arterial malformations have a definite sex preponderance[26,27] and that these diseases are less commonly encountered in female than in male infants. Approximately one third of patients with congenital cardiovascular malformations have several relatives with similar defects. Conversely, there is a two- to fivefold increase in risk of such malformations occurring in subjects whose first-degree relatives (parents, siblings) are affected. Nevertheless, cardiovascular malformations are not determined exclusively by genetic factors, as was shown by studies of monozygous twins (see above references).

Specific or Characteristic Arterial Lesions

In certain genetic diseases, the arterial lesions display features allowing for a considerable narrowing of the differential diagnoses or even diagnostic for a single disorder. For example, birefringent crystals of calcium oxalate are present in arterial walls in hyperoxaluria (oxalosis)[28-39]; bluish-black ochronotic pigment (oxidation and polymerization product of homogentisic acid) in ochronosis[40-51]; amyloid in certain forms of familial amyloidosis[52,53]; characteristic membranes and membrane-bound vesicles (or particles) in familial lecithin-cholesterol acyltransferase deficiency[54]; concentric, fibrous intimal lesions of coronary arteries in Hurler's syndrome[55]; nodular lesions involving the small-size arteries of several organs in neurofibromatosis[55]; and others.

In some genetic diseases with generalized involvement of connective tissues (eg, cutis laxa, osteogenesis imperfecta, and Marfan's and Ehlers-Danlos' syndromes) arterial changes and sequelae reflect the universality of the primary affected tissues. The arterial changes represent components of a "constellation" in a given disease rather than an isolated characteristic feature thereof. However, the manifestation of such arterial changes, eg, an aneurysm, may also be a feature of the same or different "constellation" in other disorders. Different diseases may show a predilection for different arteries. For example, the aorta is almost invariably affected in some types of the Ehlers-Danlos[56,57] and Marfan[8,10] syndromes but is usually not involved in other connective tissue disorders, such as pseudoxanthoma elasticum.[58] In the latter, the peripheral arteries (femoral, radial, ulnar) display the characteristic focal intimal and circumferential medial calcification of elastic fibers.

Similarly, in heredofamilial forms of amyloidosis, the amyloid is deposited in arterioles in Mediterranean fever or in the periarteriolar space in the Finnish type. In other types it may have a segmental (cerebral arteries in Iceland-type) or generalized (Denmark-type) distribution.[52,53,59] Segmental predilection may be expressed even in the same artery. For example, in Morquio's syndrome (genetic mucopolysaccharidosis IV), the intimal thickening of the pulmonary artery reportedly affects largely the trunk (as well as the coronary arteries).[60,61] The proximal segments of the coronary arteries in Friedreich's ataxia are normal, but the intima is markedly thickened in the intramural branches.[62] A similar distribution of lesions consisting of fibromuscular intimal proliferation, with luminal narrowing, has been reported to occur in the severe, X-linked recessive form of Duchenne muscular dystrophy.[63,64]

Arterial changes may be also generalized with no predilection for any one type or segment—for example in Menkes' syndrome (steely hair syndrome). These changes consist of patchy, widespread degeneration.[65-68] Generalized changes have also been described in a number of lysosomal diseases with accumulation of specific storage substances. For example, ceramide trihexoside accumulates in arterial cells in Fabry's disease,[69-73] and other substances characterizing various lysosomal disorders may also accumulate in arterial cells.[10] It should be stressed, however, that a generalization cannot be made because more than one substance may be accumulating in tissues in a given disease, and the "expression" in arterial mural cells may be quite variable. In the majority of diseases in the above ("lysosomal") category, specific localized identifiable lesions are not a feature, and these are thus not included in the category under discussion.

Finally, certain genetic diseases have an affinity for a specific arterial layer, or one mural component. Thus, in ochronosis the bluish-black pigment is deposited in all three layers, but the inner media is most severely affected[40-51]; intimal deposition (of storage substances) characterizes Hurler disease[10,55]; and in hyperoxaluria (oxalosis), the oxalate crystals involve the media of muscular and elastic arteries.[28-39]

Modification of Nongenetic Arterial Lesions

Little information exists on general tissue reactions of the arterial wall in genetic diseases, such as are encountered in inflammation, circulatory disturbances, various forms of regressive or degenerative changes, or arterial neoplasia. The existing knowledge is very meager, indeed, and largely limited to lesions of atherosclerosis.

Familial Hyperlipoproteinemias (FHLP)

Genetically, biochemically and clinically this group of diseases is heterogeneous. The FHLP have been classified into types I to V on the basis of levels of various classes of plasma lipids.[74-80] The underlying defects have not been identified to date in all.[74-82] The mode of inheritance is known in some: autosomal-recessive in type I; autosomal-dominant in the familial combined hyperlipidemia of type II. It is assumed autosomal to be dominant in type V and has not been established in others.[74-82] A number of subgroups have been emerging of late, and it is reasonable to anticipate that a new classification of the FHLP will be forthcoming soon. Pertinent to the present discussion, and of interest, is the fact that reports on the newly emerging subgroups seldom include data on the arterial status.

The FHLP were included in this presentation to illustrate that even in genetic diseases of the same broad category, the arterial wall may (types II to V) or may not (type I) modify the known—ie, atherosclerotic lesions. In the four types in which it does, the process is accelerated, but the pattern of the distribution of lesions is only altered in one: while it is predominantly abdominal in normal subjects, it affects the ascending aorta in type II.[10,55,77,83] The morphology of the lesion is modified in type III.[83]

Other Heritable Diseases and Atherosclerotic Lesions

To date, we have explored whether and how one form of early atherosclerotic lesions, the fatty streak, may be modified by the arterial wall itself in the following disorders: Wolman's disease; infantile form of GM_1-gangliosidosis; Hurler's syndrome; Ehlers-Danlos syndrome (EDS) type IV; and a newly described entity of generalized hypoplastic aorta whose features suggest a primary, presumed genetic, disorder of the arterial smooth muscle cells.[84] Subtle or considerable modifications of the fatty streaks were observed at the ultrastructural level in all the above diseases tested. The "superimposed" changes varied from one entity to another and appeared to be characteristic for a given disorder. Since the numbers of patients and lesions were small, the observations must await validation by study of a large series of arteries in each group. To avoid repetition, the reader is referred to the available reports.[55,85]

Changes in Arterial Wall Makeup

Since the altered metabolism in genetic diseases is inherent in all cells, it is to be expected that the arterial cells share such genetic "misinformation." Alterations at functional level do not have to exist despite the demonstrable metabolic changes. This is the case in other situations: eg, the circulating red blood cells in Gaucher's disease function adequately. Similarly, a morphologically detectable or definable arterial lesion may not be present, particularly in early life. Whether in some genetic disorders, an arterial lesion would become demonstrable if the affected children lived long enough cannot be ascertained.

In general, little effort has been made in the past to assess the arterial wall in these diseases, other than the lesion-containing segments. Thus the structural status of the lesion-free ("normal") arterial wall has not been studied systematically. Such explorations might provide clues concerning the nature of a given disease, or assist in unraveling other diseases—eg, atherosclerosis. The results of detailed studies of arterial structure may require a reassessment of clinical implications of certain disease entities. It has been recognized recently that one of the causes of morbidity and mortality in tuberous sclerosis (TS), a disorder with autosomal-dominant inheritance,[86-90] is the development and rupture of arterial aneurysms. It has been known for over three decades that, in TS, in addition to myocardial rhabdomyoma, "adenoma sebaceum", depigmentation of hair, cortical tubera and subependymal nodules in the brain, fibrous plaques in the soft tissues, cysts and hamartomas in the kidneys, and other changes, the angiomatous component of the renal hamartomas consists of abnormally structured vessels.[86-92] It became apparent only lately that other segments of the vasculature may also be altered,[93-100] suggesting that the arterial changes may be widespread.

The arterial changes in TS are associated with development of aneurysms of the thoracic or abdominal aorta[93-96,98,100] and the basilar artery,[97] and occlusive lesions in the iliac[96] and internal carotid[97] arteries. In one child,[100] in addition to aneurysms in the abdominal aorta and a major branch of one renal artery, occlusive lesions were found in proximal segments of the common iliac, main renal, and superior mesenteric and coronary arteries. On gross inspection of the intimal surface, "plaques" were observed in the arch and descending thoracic aorta. Microscopically, there were varying degrees of intimal lipid-free fibrocellular proliferations. Patchy degeneration and loss of elastic tissue, proliferation of collagen, and a striking thickening (with occasional obliteration) of vasa vasorum were also observed.[100] It has been suggested[100] that the nature of the fibrocellular proliferation is similar to that of arterial dysplasia.[101,102]

Our own studies showed, on microscopic examination, only aneurysmal dilatations in small branches of pulmonary arteries and focal intimal and/or medial changes of the aorta (Fig. 7.1) consistent with those reported by others.[100] Mural alterations resembling those of the aorta were also observed in a few muscular arteries of varying size. None had the striking appearance of walls of the intrarenal arteries (Fig. 7.2). As described in detail elsewhere,[55] the latter lacked almost invariably a definable structural organization, and the constituent smooth muscle cells had a peculiar stellate shape.

The experience with TS (identification of arterial aneurysms, the underlying mural changes and clinical sequelae) supports the contention that unraveling structural details of arterial walls is not an esoteric exercise, even in today's era of domination of medical science by biochemistry. Knowledge forthcoming from morphological studies may aid in the understanding of the basis of possible serious clinical consequences.

Three other genetic diseases were selected to illustrate that aortic segments, with an unremarkable intimal surface on gross inspection, showed a considerably altered mural structure on microscopic examination.

Infantile GM_1 gangliosidosis is one of three phenotypes of the GM_1 gangliosidosis, an autosomal-recessive disorder caused by a deficiency of acid β-galacto-

---

►

FIGURE 7.1. Aorta in tuberous sclerosis shows a thickened intima (upper half of photomicrograph) consisting of alternating cellular and fibrous layers. Focal areas of paucity of cells and fragmentation of elastic lamellae contain pools of ground substance (arrows). Hamalum, Phloxine, Saffron stains. Magnification ×280.

FIGURE 7.2. Intrarenal artery in tuberous sclerosis shows stellate-shaped cells. Note the variable thickness of the wall and lack of distinct layers. Masson's trichrome. Magnification ×300.

FIGURE 7.3. Conventionally processed aortic wall in infantile GM_1 gangliosidosis displays no obvious changes. Retrospectively, some medial cells may be vacuolated (arrows). Weigert-Hart elastica, Nuclear Fast Red, Metanil Yellow stains. Magnification ×320.

FIGURE 7.4. Plastic-embedded aortic wall in infantile GM_1 gangliosidosis shows the presence of numerous vacuoles in the mural smooth muscle cells. Toluidine Blue stain. Magnification ×1,200.

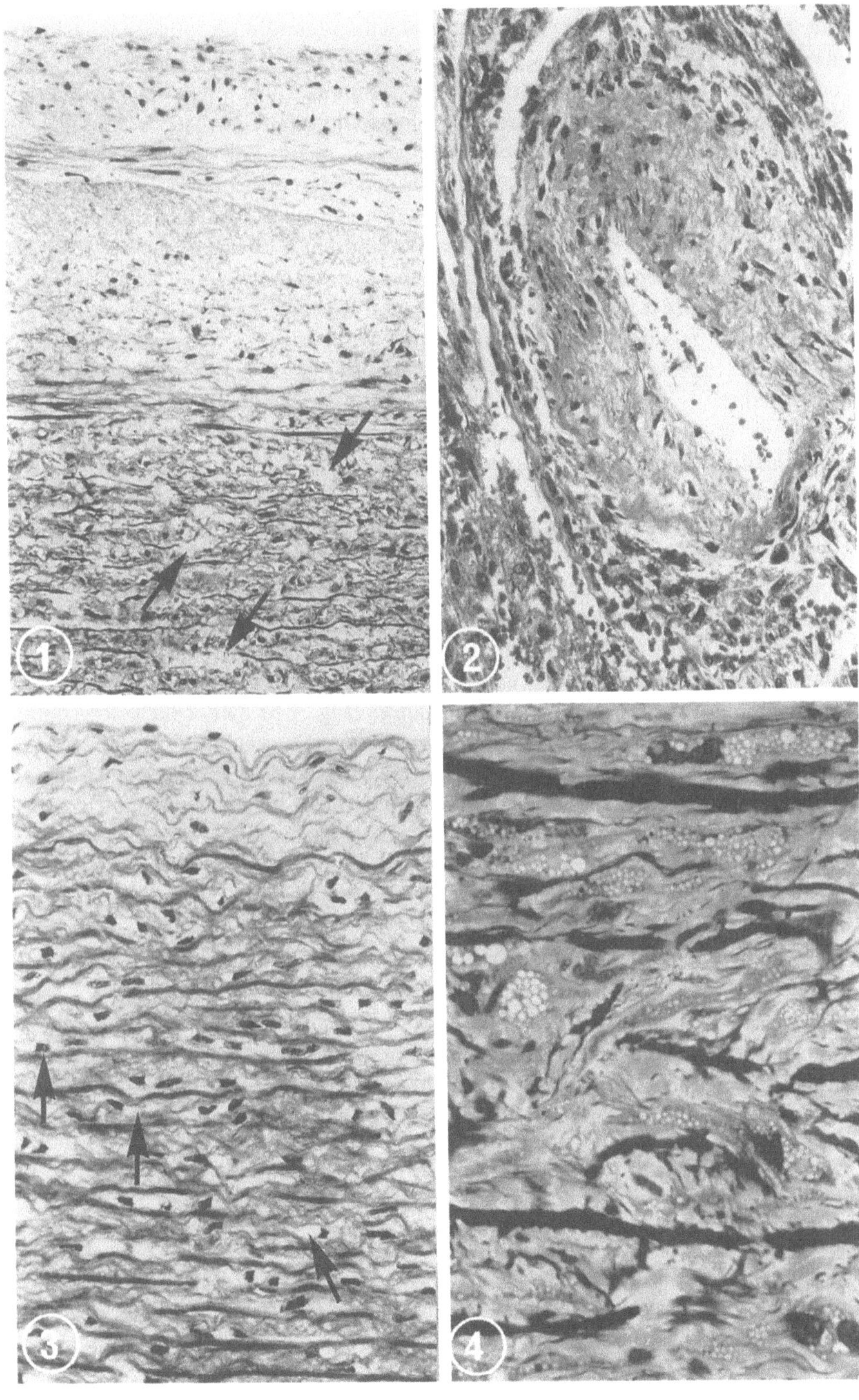
1
2
3
4

sidase.[103,104] In all, GM_1-ganglioside and its asialo derivative GM_{A1} are stored in the nervous system,[105,106] whereas galactose-containing oligosaccharides accumulate in the viscera.[103]

Children with the infantile form become symptomatic at a few months of age. They have coarse facial features, hepatosplenomegaly, dysostosis multiplex, peripheral edema, occasional ascites,[107] macular cherry-red spot (in ~ 50% of affected children), and retardation of mental and motor development. The patients usually die at the age of 2 years. Children with cardiac involvement reportedly die from heart failure[108,109]; they may possibly represent a variant of the disorder.

Little has been reported on the status of the vascular system in all forms of GM_1 gangliosidosis. In a few instances, endothelial vacuoles were observed in capillaries of skin, rectal mucosa, and some other tissues[107,109-112]; vacuolated vascular smooth muscle cells were mentioned in one report, but the vessel was not identified.[112]

In our studies neither gross nor microscopic examination of paraffin-embedded tissues (Fig. 7.3) showed changes of the aortic wall (exempting the usual fatty streaks of infancy and childhood). However, 1-μ-thick sections of plastic-embedded tissues processed for electron microscopy showed vacuolation of both the intimal and medial smooth muscle cells (SMCs), with the former being less affected than the latter. In the media, the SMCs were often considerably distended by a large number of vacuoles (Fig. 7.4).

Ultrastructurally (Figs. 7.5, 7.6), the vacuoles showed the presence of two distinct inclusion materials. The majority contained small amounts or traces of finely granuloreticular or floccular substances (Fig. 7.5). Other inclusions consisted of straight or twisted slender structures suggesting tubular configurations and their cross sections (Fig. 7.6). Nonspecific myelin figures were at times present in vacuoles. The floccular/reticulogranular material resembled substances such as mucopolysaccharides and possibly represents galactose-containing oligosaccharides.[103,113,114] The nature of the second type of vacuolar inclusions is unknown. It is tempting to assume that they are related to GM_1 gangliosides or their derivatives. These observations of the aortic SMCs are believed to be the first made at the ultrastructural level[55]; detailed studies of other features of the "normal" aortic wall in this disorder continue.

Hurler's syndrome is an autosomal-recessive disorder classified with genetic mucopolysaccharidoses.[115,116] While more than one variant exists, the most common is the classical form first described by Hurler and resulting from deficiency of the enzyme α-L-iduronidase. Visceral storage and urinary excretion of derma-

---

►

FIGURE 7.5. Electron microscopy. Aortic smooth muscle cells in GM_1 gangliosidosis show cytoplasmic vacuoles that are empty or that contain a small amount of finely floccular (top cell) or granular substance. The processes of two cells on the left are free of vacuoles. Magnification ×14,000.

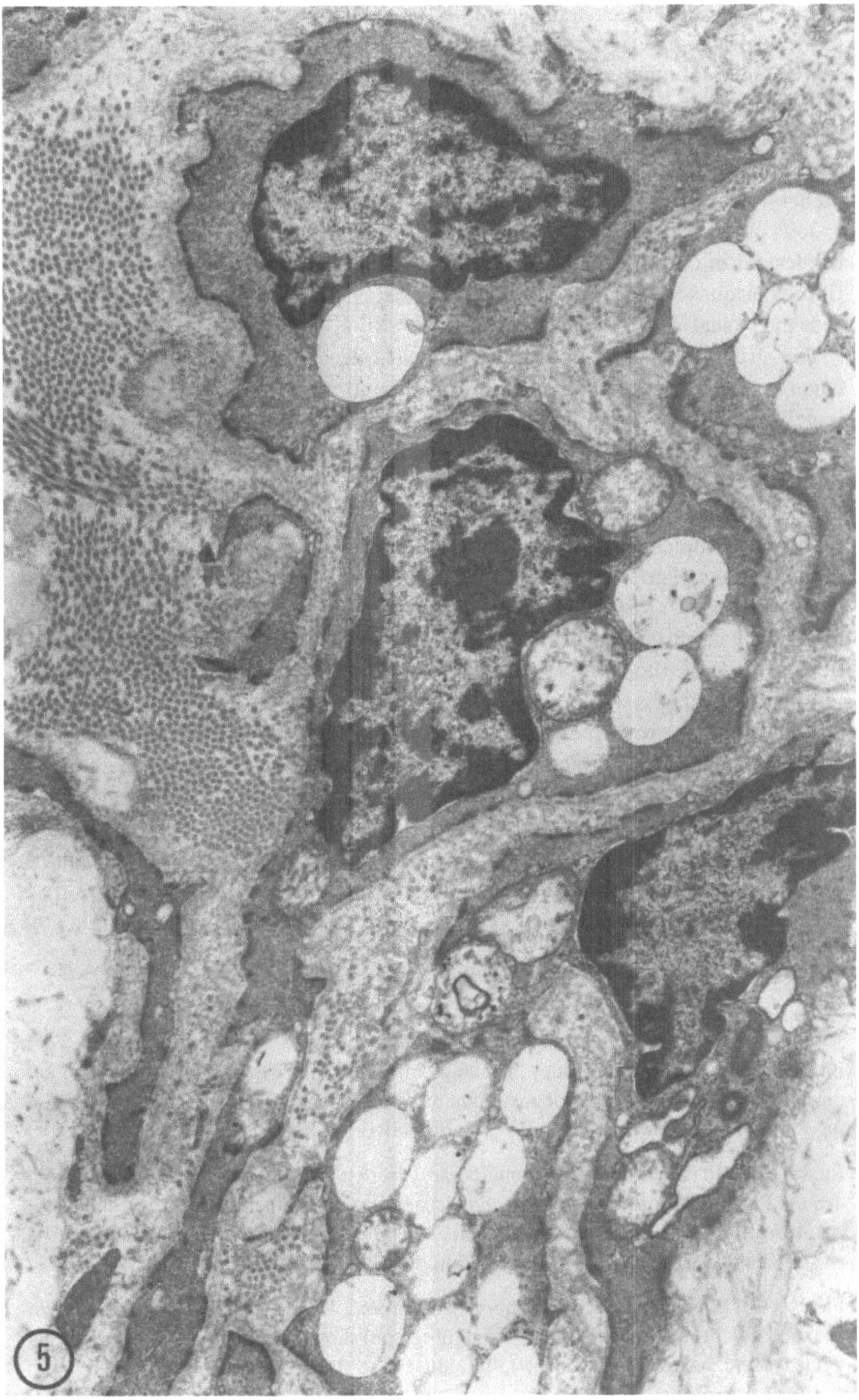
5

tan and heparan sulfates, and accumulation of gangliosides GM_2, GM_3, and GD_3 in the central and peripheral nervous system, characterize this disorder. The consequent clinical manifestations of coarse facial features, severe mental retardation, dysostosis multiplex, dwarfism, corneal opacities, hepatosplenomegaly, and lesions in the cardiovascular system and other tissues/organs have been described repeatedly.[116] It has been agreed that in general, cardiovascular involvement often causes morbidity and mortality in this disorder, and the characteristic lesions of the coronary arteries underlie this sequence of events. These concentric lesions of coronary arteries have been studied in some detail,[10,55] as were the fibrous plaques in the aorta and in other arteries. The latter are believed to represent the "usual" atherosclerotic lesions.[10]

The structural features of the aortic wall free of lesions on gross inspection have not been reported often or in detail, and available information is based largely on light microscopic examination. Relevant to our observations is the following statement made with reference to aorta: "Intimal thickening [is] due to proliferation of fibrous connective tissue and vacuolated cells" (from Ferrans and Boyce,[10] p 950; legend to Fig. 25.4C).

Our own studies indicate that the basic constituents and the overall structure of the aortic wall differ considerably from normal aorta and become accentuated with age (Figs. 7.7 to 7.11). These changes may be summarized briefly as follows. Early in life (first decade) it is apparent, even on light microscopic examination, that while the intima seems to be normal (ie, the physiological diffuse intimal thickening is within normal limits for age[1]), paucity and fragmentation of elastic lamellae prominently affect the media (Fig. 7.7). The intimal SMCs appear to be unremarkable, and questionable vacuoles may be seen in a few medial cells (Fig. 7.8). However, electron microscopy discloses that even in early life some intimal SMCs contain inclusions (Fig. 7.9). These consist of "bodies" of conglomerated membranes arranged parallel in a straight or curved fashion. Small, almost empty vacuoles are in close vicinity and on occasion contain a fine-granular or floccular substance. The inclusions occupy a small cytoplasmic area and are present in a few SMCs only.

►

FIGURE 7.6. Electron microscopy. Tissue as in Figure 7.5. The vacuoles in the smooth muscle cell contain short and long, straight or twisted slender fibrils (probably representing tubules) and their cross sections. Magnification ×23,000.

FIGURE 7.7. Plastic-embedded thoracic aorta from a young patient with Hurler's syndrome. Fragmentation and paucity of elastic lamellae, loss of cellular polarity, and loss of "stratification" are prominent in the media, but the intima (above the ill-defined internal elastic lamina; arrow) appears normal. Toluidine Blue stain. Magnification ×290.

FIGURE 7.8. Plastic-embedded coronary artery from a 15-year-old boy with Hurler's syndrome. Low intima (upper half of microphotograph) shows large smooth muscle cells distended with black inclusion (arrow). Toluidine Blue stain. Magnification ×320.

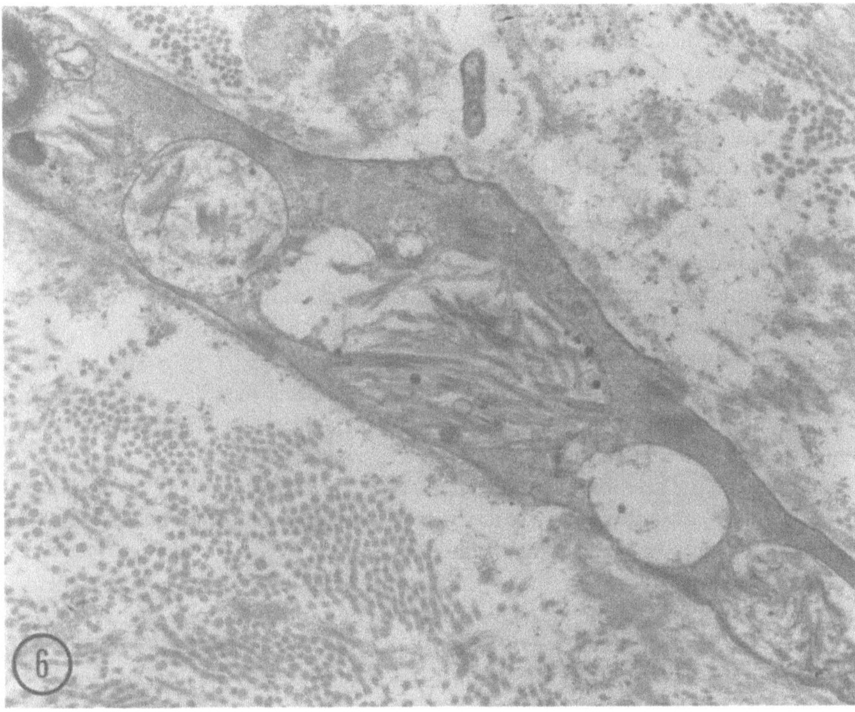
6

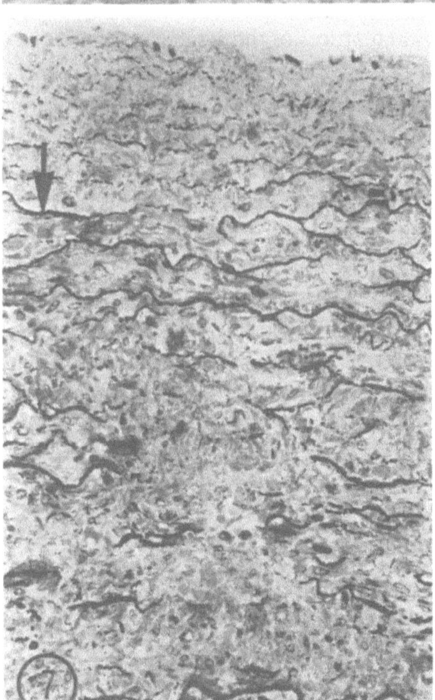
7

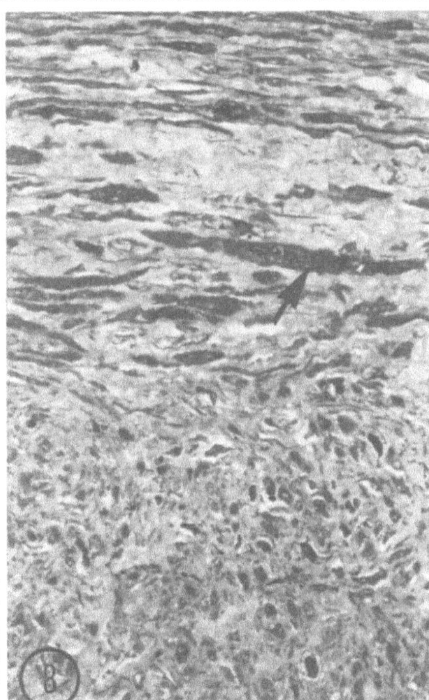
8

With advancing age the number of inclusions in individual cells, as well as the number of the SMCs affected, increases in both the intima and the media. The SMCs may be completely filled with these dense inclusions, thus resembling the cells of "low" intima and the media of coronary arteries with lesions characteristic for this disease (Fig. 7.8); these changes are identifiable even on light microscopic examination. Ultrastructurally (Figs. 7.10, 7.11), the inclusions in the aortic SMCs are in most instances still recognizable as consisting of membranous arrays (some have the appearance of "zebra bodies"), but in others are now electron-dense structureless bodies of complex variegated nature and probably represent degenerative end stages of the membranous arrays (Fig. 7.10). Distinct large vacuoles filled with finely filamentous or floccular substance were present in adventitial fibroblasts and/or macrophages – ie, in cells and location similar to those observed in the coronary arteries (see Haust,[55] Fig. 47, p 265). The content of these vacuoles resembles that present in hepatocytic vacuoles in this disorder[115,117,118] and is considered to represent the stored glycosaminoglycans, whereas the membranous inclusions of the aortic SMCs may be the GM_2, GM_3, and GD_3 or their respective derivatives – ie, materials found usually in the nervous system in the Hurler syndrome.

Ultrastructural studies of the alterations at various segments of the aorta, as well as the status of the extracellular mural components, are in progress.

Ehlers-Danlos syndrome (EDS) type IV is one of at least 13 forms of diseases grouped together because the formation of collagen fibrils is believed to be abnormal in all.[119-122] It has been suggested, however, that up to 50% of patients referred to genetic clinics with some features of the syndrome cannot be classified with any of the designated types.[123] Mutations in genes for type I or type III procollagens or defects of enzymes required for the processing of the procollagens (or their chains) are the underlying basis of tissue changes in EDS.[119,124-128] However, defects in the formation of collagen fibrils may result secondarily from aberration of copper metabolism – eg, in EDS type IX.[124] The designation "Ehlers-Danlos syndrome" may be considered to be a misnomer in view of the diverse diseases included in this group. Moreover, within a given type there may be a considerable genetic heterogeneity and clinical variability.[119,121,123-125,129]

Patients with EDS may show one, several, or all of the following features: thin and hyperextensible skin that bruises easily; ecchymoses; distension and tortuosity of superficial veins; and thin arterial walls (with or without dissection or

---

▶

FIGURE 7.9. Electron microscopy. Ultrastructure of aortic intima similar to that shown in Figure 7.7. Most smooth muscle cells have normal features. Membranous inclusions, empty vacuoles, and one vacuole filled with finely floccular material are present in one cell (left lower half of the photograph). Magnification ×14,300.

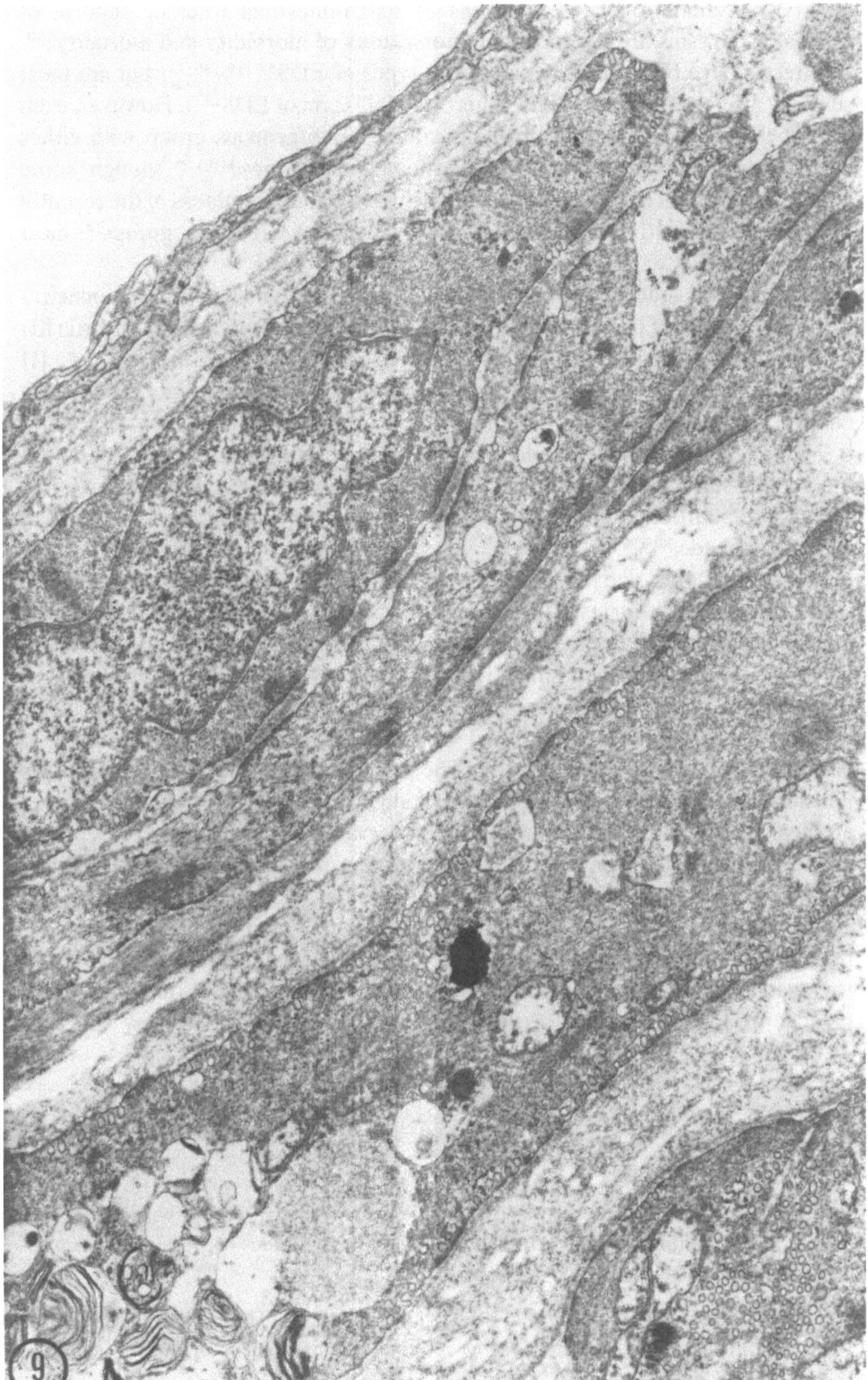
9

aneurysmal dilatations). Perforations of gastrointestinal tract or rupture of arterial aneurysms are the most common causes of morbidity and mortality.[130]

Arteries have been involved in several types of EDS[57,119,130-141] but are most severely affected in type IV EDS (thus "arterial" form of EDS[133]). However, even the type IV is clinically and biochemically a heterogeneous group with either autosomal-recessive or autosomal-dominant inheritance,[119,129] though some appear to represent de novo mutations. The validity and usefulness of the recently proposed classification of the type IV EDS into four (A to D) subgroups[142] must await further work.

Most patients studied showed a defect of type III procollagen, but biochemically not all were of the same nature. A decreased rate of synthesis of pro-αl (III) chains by cultured fibroblasts[129,143,144] or of secretion of type III procollagen[142,145,146] and abnormal amino acid composition of the pro-αl (III) chains[127,128] all have been reported.

With a few exceptions, detailed morphological studies in EDS type IV do not include the status of arteries other than those obviously altered. However, some reports are conflicting and provide only sparse or no illustrations in support of statements made.[57,130-141]

Most of the large-size muscular and elastic arteries, including the aorta, were studied in our laboratories. The aortic wall was relatively thinner than expected, but in its "normal" segments (not involved in aneurysmal dilatation) there were no changes on gross inspection. Microscopically, even in routinely prepared tissues, sections showed focal disorganization of lamellar pattern (Fig. 7.12) caused by "pools" of acellular foci of ground substance and associated fragmentation of elastic tissue elements (Fig. 7.13). The appearance of the mural SMCs was unusual with "depolarization" of their arrangement, bizarre shapes, and other atypical features. Ultrastructurally, the observations included the presence of abundant glycosaminoglycans (GAG) throughout the aortic wall (Figs. 7.14 to 7.15A), being particularly prominent in acellular foci (Fig. 7.15). This was astonishing in view of the fact that demonstration of GAG (or proteoglycans) at the electron microscopic level requires the use of special techniques.[147] SMCs in various stages of degeneration and necrosis, or their necrotic remnants, were present in or around the acellular foci (Fig. 7.15); at times, single "new" and well

---

►

FIGURE 7.10. Electron microscopy. Aortic tissue from a 15-year-old boy with Hurler syndrome. All the smooth muscle cells shown contain membranous or variegated electron-dense inclusions. Magnification ×10,000.

FIGURE 7.11. Electron microscopy. Tissue as in Figure 7.10. The smooth muscle cell is filled with membranous inclusions; some resemble "zebra bodies" (arrows). Magnification ×24,000.

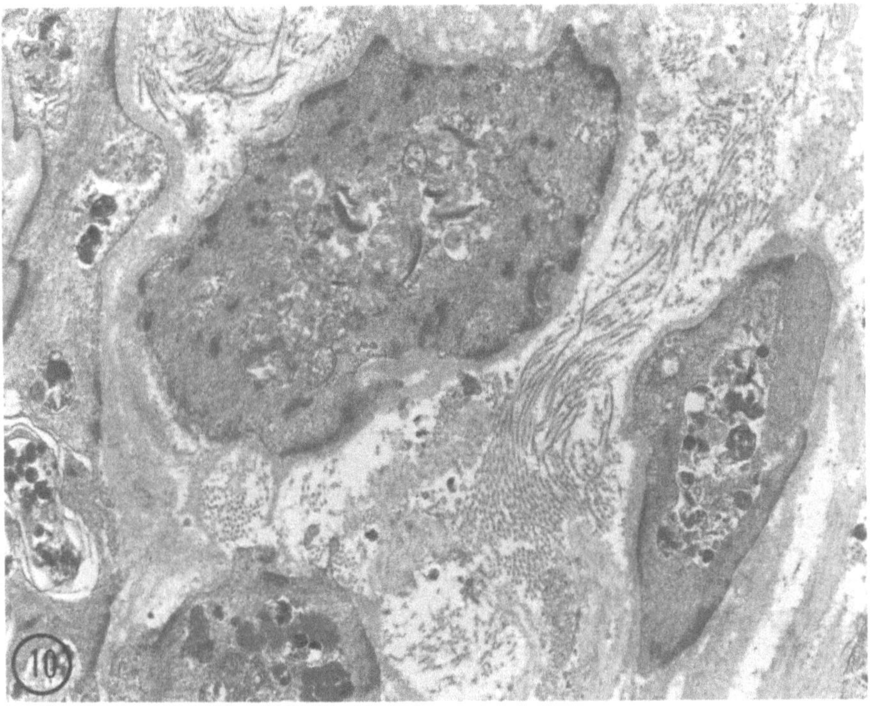
10

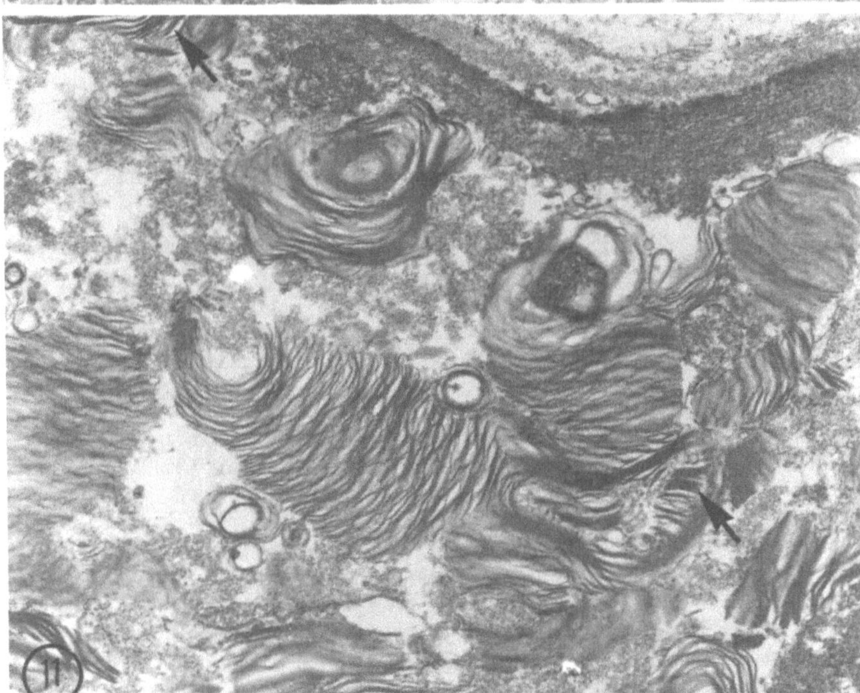
11

preserved cells occupied the interlamellar space, but they had only some features of SMCs (Fig. 7.14). Their nature is still under study. Bundles of collagen fibrils were absent in the acellular foci, and elsewhere in the wall they consisted of thin elements. This feature was striking in the aortic adventitial fibrous matrix, where a considerable variation in the diameter of collagen fibrils was apparent.

Since the collagen fibrils in the aorta (as well as in other arteries) are produced by the mural SMCs (rather than fibroblasts), it would appear that the arterial wall with its constituents could serve better in pursuing further studies of this as yet unresolved problem than will fibroblast-containing tissues.

Notes on Clinical Sequelae

Regardless of whether the arteries are affected primarily or secondarily in a given disease, their involvement may be a contributory cause to the ultimate morbidity or mortality. A few examples are: myocardial infarction occurring in such diverse diseases as in Fabry's disease or some forms of FHLP (because of mural changes in the coronary arteries) or in sickle cell trait (because of thrombosis); rupture of bowel (in certain types of Ehlers-Danlos syndrome with involvement of mesenteric circulation and ischemic necrosis of intestinal wall); uncorrected malformations (eg, the coarctation of aorta in Turner's syndrome); and ruptured aortic and other arterial aneurysms (eg, in tuberous sclerosis and in Marfan's syndrome and certain types of Ehlers-Danlos syndrome).

The affected arteries may also contribute to morbidity and eventual mortality in a more chronic rather than acute manner. Mental retardation and seizures in homocystinuria[148-150] do reflect the narrowing or occlusive vascular disease involving the central nervous system. Hypertension may be the outcome of such

---

►

FIGURE 7.12. Aorta in Ehlers-Danlos syndrome, type IV. Loss of stratification and polarity of smooth muscle cells. Small foci of pools of ground substance (arrows) are seen in intima and media. Hemalum, Phloxine, Saffron stains. Magnification ×150.

FIGURE 7.13. Tissue as in Figure 7.12. Foci of pools of ground substance, rarefaction of elastic lamellae, and paucity of cells are more apparent than in Figure 7.12. Weigert-Hart elastica - Nuclear Fast Red - Metanil Yellow stains. Magnification ×250.

FIGURE 7.14. Electron microscopy. Ultrastructure of an area of tissue as arrowed in Figure 7.12. There is a diffuse background of considerable amounts of glycosaminoglycans (tiny granules interconnected by filaments). They occupy the extracellular space between and beyond the elastic elements (E). The cell in center has a partial basement membrane (arrow) and the cytoplasmic filaments, suggesting a "relation" to smooth muscle cells. Magnification ×10,200.

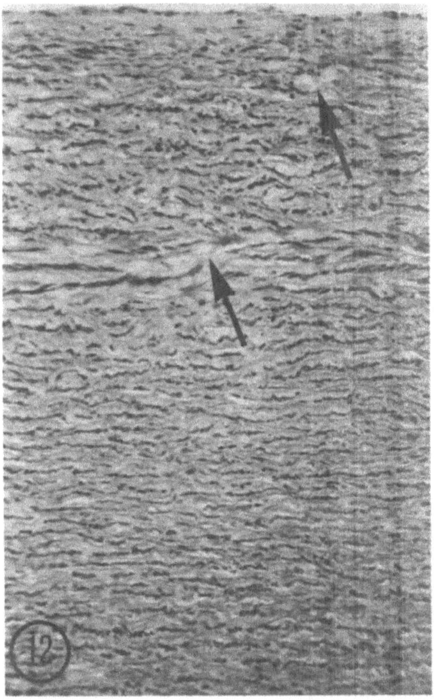
12

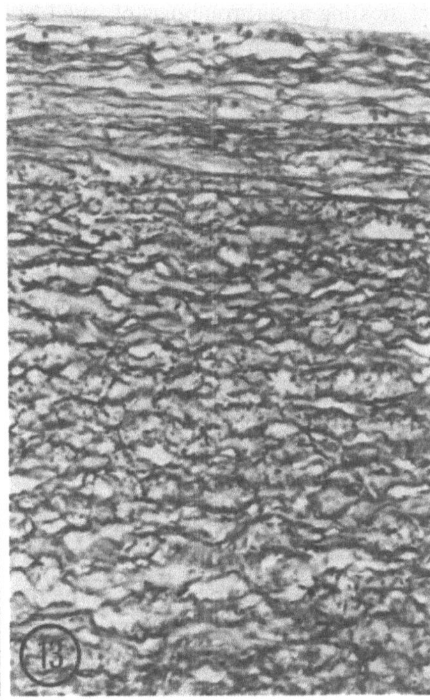
13

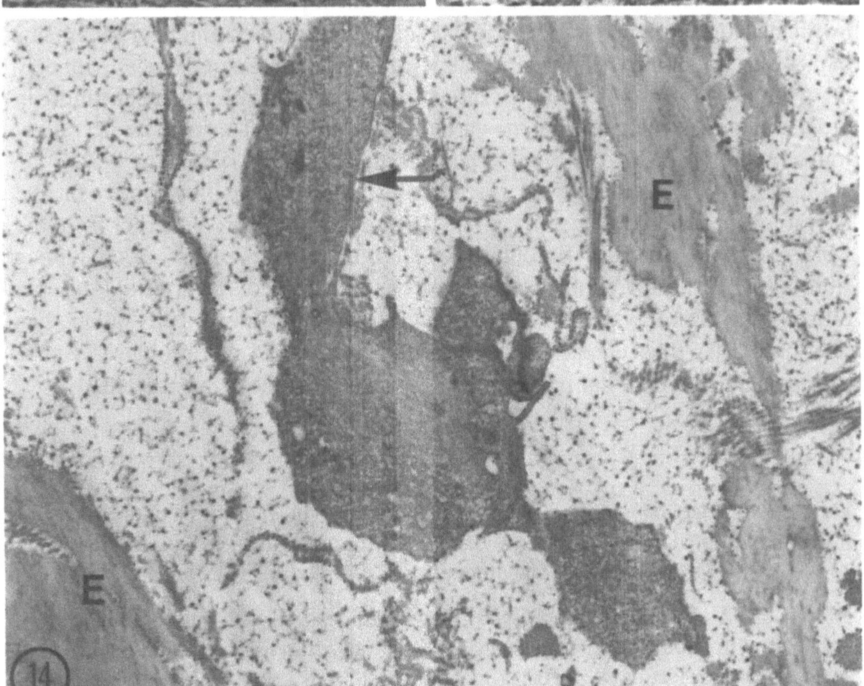
E
E
14

diverse disorders as sickle cell disease, secondary to repeated multiple episodes of sickling and thrombosis of small branches of pulmonary artery,[151,152] and in progeria in which the proliferative and calcific changes affect the walls of the pulmonary artery.[153-156] The thickening of the intima with narrowing of the coronary arteries plays a role in cardiac insufficiency in Hurler's syndrome[157] and in I-cell disease.[158-160] The deposition of oxalate crystals in arteriolar and capillary walls of extremities may cause narrowing (with acrocyanosis) or occlusion (with gangrene) in oxalosis.[32,33]

There are too many examples to be cited here, but one feature of interest should be added. In some genetic diseases, there is a "shift" from the arteries affected in homozygotes to other arteries in heterozygotes. For example, in sickle cell disease (SS hemoglobin), the multiple episodes of sickling and thrombosis affect primarily the small branches of pulmonary arteries[151,152] and the cerebral vasculature,[161] whereas in the sickle cell trait (SA hemoglobin) thrombosis involves the coronary arteries.[162,163]

Comments and Conclusions

It is apparent from the review of the literature that the existing data on the status of the arteries in genetic diseases are sketchy, incomplete, and often contradictory. Yet, much could be learned from systematic studies of the arterial wall. Such studies may prove important from the clinical point of view as exemplified by the recent experience with previously unsuspected development of aneurysms in tuberous sclerosis. Utilizing arterial tissues for ultrastructural assessment may draw attention to as yet unknown direction that further efforts might follow in order to identify the as yet unknown metabolic defects. This may be best illustrated by the studies in the Ehlers-Danlos syndrome, type IV. To the best of the author's knowledge much of the current information on the presumptive or real alterations in the procollagen III in this disease has been derived either from the work in tissue culture of fibroblasts or from extractions of tissues containing fibroblasts. Yet, the procollagens (of type I and type III) of the arterial (and specifically the aortic) wall are secreted by mural smooth muscle cells rather than by fibroblasts. It is uncertain whether data derived from fibroblasts can be extrapolated to functional properties of the arterial smooth muscle cells.

▶

FIGURE 7.15. Electron microscopy. Tissue as in Figure 7.14. In addition to the other features, the acellular space contains remnants of necrotic cellular cytoplasm (lower left corner of photograph; arrows). Magnification ×6,100.

FIGURE 7.15A. Electron microscopy. Higher magnification of the glycosaminoglycans (granules with interconnecting filaments) seen in the extracellular space in Figures 7.14 and 7.15. Magnification ×32,500.

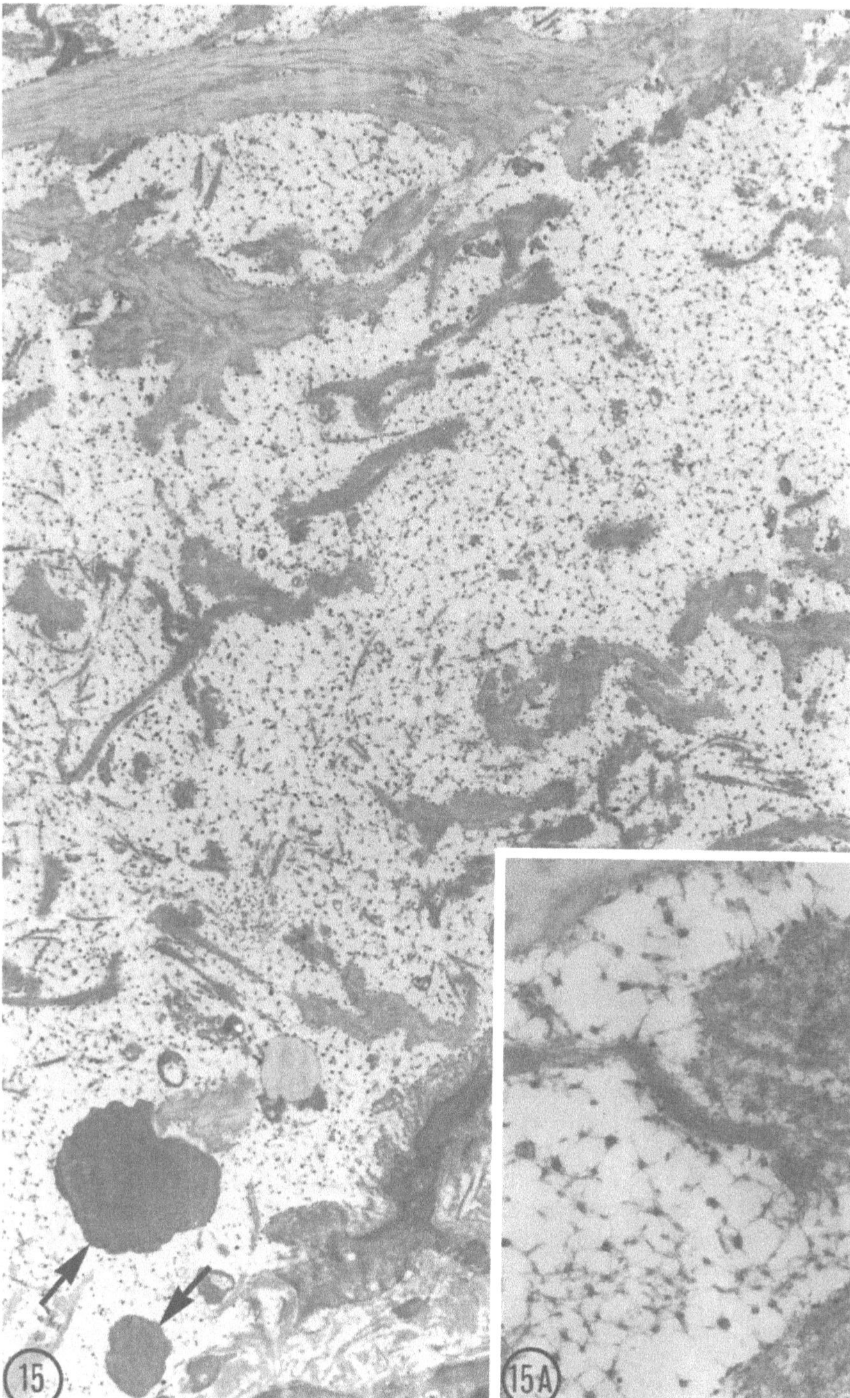
15
15A

The aortic wall in genetic disorders with known metabolic defect may provide some insight into diseases with incompletely understood pathogenesis—eg, atherosclerosis. Such studies could include tissue cultures or in situ hybridization of arterial cells with suitable manipulation relevant to atherosclerosis, and biochemical monitoring. Several excellent animal models of inborn errors of metabolism have been described[164-167] and these would provide additional opportunities for both in vivo and in vitro studies.

Acknowledgments. The author wishes to express her appreciation to Ms Irena Wojewodzka, Mr Roger Dewar, and Mrs Renate Feulgen for their expert technical assistance and library work, and to Miss Paula Fenner and Mrs Betty Gardiner for their efficient typing of this manuscript.

This work was supported by a grant in aid T.3-11 from the Heart and Stroke Foundation of Ontario, in Toronto, Canada.

References

1. Haust MD: Atherosclerosis in childhood. In Rosenberg HS, Bolande RP (eds): *Perspectives in Pediatric Pathology.* Chicago: Year Book, 1978, Vol 4, pp 155–216.
2. Char F: Tables of heritable cardiovascular conditions and associated syndromes. BDOAS 8:313–322, 1972.
3. Taylor WJ: Genetics and the cardiovascular system. In Hurst JW (ed): *The Heart, Arteries and Veins*, 4th Ed. New York: McGraw-Hill, 1978, p 753.
4. Rowe RD, Uchida IA, Char F: Heart disease associated with chromosomal abnormalities. In Keith JD, Rowe RD, Vlad P (eds): *Heart Disease in Infancy and Childhood*, 3d Ed. New York: Macmillan, 1978, pp 897–925.
5. Noonan JA: Association of congenital heart disease with syndromes or other defects. *Pediatr Clin North Am* 25:797–816, 1978.
6. Perloff JK: *The Clinical Recognition of Congenital Heart Disease*, 2d Ed. Philadelphia: Saunders, 1978.
7. Wald EB (Ed): *Heart Disease: A Textbook of Cardiovascular Medicine.* Philadelphia: Saunders, 1978.
8. Roberts WC (Ed): *Congenital Heart Disease in Adults.* Philadelphia: FA Davis, 1979.
9. Shows TB, McAlphine PJ: The 1979 catalog of human genes and chromosome assignments. *Cytogenet Cell Genet* 25:117–127, 1979.
10. Ferrans VJ, Boyce SW: Metabolic and familial diseases. In Silver MD (ed): *Cardiovascular Pathology.* New York: Churchill Livingstone, 1983, Vol 2, pp 945–1004.
11. Gerald PS: Sex chromosome disorders. *N Engl J Med* 294:706–708, 1976.
12. De Grouchy J, Turkleau C: *Clinical Atlas of Human Chromosomes.* New York: John Wiley, 1977.
13. Carr DH, Gideon M: Population cytogenetics of human abortuses. In Hook EB, Porter IH (eds): *Population Cytogenetics. Studies in Humans.* New York: Academic Press, 1977.
14. An international system for human cytogenetic nomenclature (1978). *BDOAS* XIV(8), 1978.

15. Grumbach MM, Conte FA: Disorders of sexual differentiation. In Wilson ID, Foster DW (eds): *Williams Textbook of Endocrinology*, 7th Ed. Philadelphia: Saunders, 1985, pp 312–401.
16. Breg WR: Down syndrome. A review of recent progress in research. *Pathobiol Annu* 7:257-303, 1977.
17. Fleisher GR, Buck BE, Cornfeld D: Primary intimal fibroplasia in a child with Down's syndrome. *Am J Dis Child* 132:700–703, 1978.
18. Martin GM, Hoehn H: Genetics and human disease. *Hum Pathol* 5:387-405, 1974.
19. Thompson JS, Thompson MW: *Genetics in Medicine*. Philadelphia: Saunders, 1980.
20. McKusick VA: The anatomy of the human genome. *Am J Med* 69:267-276, 1980.
21. Kronenberg HM: Looking at genes. *N Engl J Med* 307:50–52, 1982.
22. Storstein O, Rokseth R, Sörland S: Congenital heart disease in a clinical material. An analysis of 1,000 consecutive cases. *Acta Med Scand* 176:195–200, 1964.
23. Higgins ITT: The epidemiology of congenital heart disease. *J Chron Dis* 18: 699–721, 1965.
24. Nora JJ, Nora AH: The evolution of specific genetic and environmental counselling in congenital heart diseases. *Circulation* 57:205–213, 1978.
25. Friedman WF: Congenital heart disease in infancy and childhood. In Braunwald E (ed): *Heart Disease. A Textbook of Cardiovascular Medicine*. Philadelphia: Saunders, 1980, pp 967–1056.
26. Elliott LP, Newfeld HN, Anderson RC, Adams P, Edwards JE: Complete transposition of the great vessels. I. An anatomic study of sixty cases. *Circulation* 27:1105–1117, 1963.
27. Lev M, Alcalde VM, Baffes TG: Pathologic anatomy of complete transposition of the arterial trunks. *Pediatrics* 28:293–306, 1961.
28. Archer HE, Dormer AE, Scowen EF, Watts RWE: Primary hyperoxaluria. *Lancet* 273:320–322, 1957.
29. Stauffer M: Oxalosis. Report of a case, with a review of the literature and discussion of the pathogenesis. *N Engl J Med* 263:386–390, 1960.
30. Chisholm GD, Heard BE: Oxalosis. *Br J Surg* 50:78–92, 1962.
31. Hockaday TDR, Clayton JE, Frederick EW, Smith LH Jr: Primary hyperoxaluria. *Medicine* 43:315–345, 1964.
32. Blackburn WE, McRoberts JW, Bhathena D, Vazquez M, Luke RG: Severe vascular complications in oxalosis after bilateral nephrectomy. *Ann Intern Med* 82:44–46, 1975.
33. Williams HE, Smith LH Jr: Primary hyperoxaluria. In Stanbury JB, Wyngaarden JB, Fredrickson DS, Goldstein JL, Brown MS (eds): *The Metabolic Basis of Inherited Disease*, 5th Ed. New York: McGraw-Hill, 1983, pp 204–228.
34. Chaplin AJ: Histopathological occurrence and characterisation of calcium oxalate: A review. *J Clin Pathol* 30:800–811, 1977.
35. Beil E, Seibel K, Riecker G: Herzerkrankung bei primärer Oxalose. *Klin Wochenschr* 47:513–518, 1969.
36. Coltart DJ, Hudson REB: Primary oxalosis of the heart: A cause of heart block. *Br Heart J* 33:315–319, 1971.
37. Fayemi AO, Ali M, Braun EV: Oxalosis in hemodialysis patients. A pathologic study of 80 cases. *Arch Pathol Lab Med* 103:58–62, 1979.
38. Tonkin AM, Mond HG, Mathew TH, Solman JG: Primary oxalosis with myocardial involvement and heart block. *Med J Aust* 1:873–874, 1976.
39. West RR, Salyer WR, Hutchins GM: Adult-onset primary oxalosis with complete heart block. *Johns Hopkins Med J* 133:195–200, 1973.

40. Milch RA: Studies of alcaptonuria: Inheritance of 47 cases in eight highly interrelated Dominican kindreds. *Am J Hum Genet* 12:76–85, 1960.
41. Reginato A, Riera M, Martinez V, Ruiz F: Alkaptonuria, ochronotic arthropathy and aortic stenosis. *Rev Med Chile* 100:529–533, 1972.
42. Srsén S, Cisárik F, Pásztor L, Harmećko L: Alkaptonuria in the Trenćin district of Czechoslovakia. *Am J Med Genet* 2:159–166, 1978.
43. Moran TJ, Yunis EJ: Studies on ochronosis. 2. Effects of injection of homogentisic acid and ochronotic pigment in experimental animals. *Am J Pathol* 40:359–369, 1962.
44. Cooper JA, Moran TJ: Studies on ochronosis. I. Report of case with death from ochronotic nephrosis. *Arch Pathol* 64:46–53, 1957.
45. Beddard AP: Ochronosis associated with carboluria. *Q J Med* 3:329–336, 1910.
46. O'Brien WM, LaDu BN, Bunim JJ: Biochemical, pathologic and clinical aspects of alcaptonuria, ochronosis and ochronotic arthropathy: Review of world literature (1584–1962). *Am J Med* 34:813–838, 1963.
47. Bondurant RE, Henry JB: Pathogenesis of ochronosis in experimental alkaptonuria of the white rat. *Lab Invest* 14:62–69, 1965.
48. Attwood HD, Clifton S, Mitchell RE: A histological, histochemical and ultrastructural study of dermal ochronosis. *Pathology* 3:115–121, 1971.
49. Galdston M, Steele JM, Dobriner K: Alcaptonuria and ochronosis. With a report of three patients and metabolic studies in two. *Am J Med* 13:432–452, 1952.
50. Levine HD, Parisi AF, Holdsworth DE, Cohn LH: Aortic valve replacement for ochronosis of the aortic valve. *Chest* 74:466–467, 1978.
51. Lichtenstein L, Kaplan L: Hereditary ochronosis. Pathologic changes observed in two necropsied cases. *Am J Pathol* 30:99–125, 1954.
52. Buja LM, Khoi NB, Roberts WC: Clinically significant cardiac amyloidosis. Clinicopathologic findings in 15 patients. *Am J Cardiol* 26:394–405, 1970.
53. Mahloudji M, Teasdall RD, Adamkiewicz JJ, Hartmann WH, Lambird PA, McKusick VA: The genetic amyloidoses. With particular reference to hereditary neuropathic amyloidosis, type II (Indiana or Rukavina type). *Medicine* 48:1–37, 1969.
54. Hovig T, Gjone E: Familial lecithin: Cholesterol acyltransferase deficiency. *Scand J Clin Lab Invest* 33(Suppl 134–139):135–146, 1974.
55. Haust MD: Arterial involvement in genetic diseases. *Am J Cardiovasc Pathol* 1:231–285, 1987.
56. Beighton P: *The Ehlers-Danlos Syndrome*. London: William Heinemann, 1970.
57. Hunter GC, Malone JM, Moore WS, Misiorowski RL, Chvapil M: Vascular manifestations in patients with Ehlers-Danlos syndrome. *Arch Surg* 117:495–498, 1982.
58. Goodman RM, Smith EW, Paton D, et al: Pseudoxanthoma elasticum: A clinical and histopathological study. *Medicine* 42:297–334, 1963.
59. Swanton RH, Brooksby IAB, Davies MJ, Coltart DJ, Jenkins BS, Webb-Peploe MM: Systolic and diastolic ventricular function in cardiac amyloidosis. Studies in six cases diagnosed with endomyocardial biopsy. *Am J Cardiol* 39:658–664, 1977.
60. Factor SM, Biempica L, Goldfischer S: Coronary intimal sclerosis in Morquio's syndrome. Virchows Arch [Pathol Anat] 379:1–10, 1978.
61. Schenk EA, Haggerty J: Morquio's disease. A radiologic and morphologic study. *Pediatrics* 34:839–850, 1964.
62. James TN, Fisch C: Observations on the cardiovascular involvement in Friedreich's ataxia. *Am Heart J* 66:164–175, 1963.

63. James TN: Observations on the cardiovascular involvement, including the cardiac conduction system, in progressive muscular dystrophy. *Am Heart J* 63:48–56, 1962.
64. Perloff JK, DeLeon AC Jr, O'Doherty D: The cardiomyopathy of progressive muscular dystrophy. *Circulation* 33:625–648, 1966.
65. Danks DM, Campbell PE, Stevens BJ, Mayne V, Cartwright E: Menkes's kinky hair syndrome. An inherited defect in copper absorption with widespread effects. *Pediatrics* 50:188–201, 1972.
66. Martin JJ, Flament-Durnad J, Farriaux JP, Buyssens N, Ketelbant-Balasse P, Jansen C: Menkes kinky-hair disease. A report on its pathology. *Acta Neuropathol (Berl)* 42:25–32, 1978.
67. Oakes BW, Banks DM, Campbell PE: Human copper deficiency: Ultrastructural studies of the aorta and skin in a child with Menkes' syndrome. *Exp Mol Pathol* 25:82–98, 1976.
68. Wheeler EM, Roberts PF: Menkes's steely hair syndrome. *Arch Dis Child* 51: 269–274, 1976.
69. Desnick RJ, Sweeley CC: Fabry's disease: α-Galactosidase A deficiency. In Stanbury JB, Wyngaarden JB, Fredrickson DS, Goldstein JL, Brown MS (eds): *The Metabolic Basis of Inherited Disease*, 5th Ed. New York: McGraw-Hill, 1983, pp 906–944.
70. Parkinson JE, Sunshine A: Angiokeratoma corporis diffusum universale (Fabry) presenting as suspected myocardial infarction and pulmonary infarcts. *Am J Med* 31:951–958, 1961.
71. Becker AE, Schoorl R, Balk AG, Van der Heide RM: Cardiac manifestations of Fabry's disease. Report of a case with mitral insufficiency and electrocardiographic evidence of myocardial infarction. *Am J Cardiol* 36:829–835, 1975.
72. Desnick RJ, Blieden LC, Sharp HL, Hofschire PJ, Moller JH: Cardiac valvular anomalies in Fabry disease. Clinical, morphologic, and biochemical studies. *Circulation* 54:818–825, 1976.
73. Duncan C, McLeod GM: Angiokeratoma corporis diffusum universale (Fabry's disease): A case with gross myocardial involvement. *Aust Ann Med* 19:58–61, 1970.
74. Nikkilä EA: Familial lipoprotein lipase deficiency and related disorders of chylomicron metabolism. In Stanbury JB, Wyngaarden JB, Fredrickson DS, Goldstein JL, Brown MS (eds): *The Metabolic Basis of Inherited Diseases*, 5th Ed. New York: McGraw-Hill, 1983, pp 622–642.
75. Brown MS, Goldstein JL, Fredrickson DS: Familial type 3 hyperlipoproteinemia (dysbetalipoproteinemia). In Stanbury JB, Wyngaarden JB, Fredrickson DS, Goldstein JL, Brown MS (eds): *The Metabolic Basis of Inherited Diseases*, 5th Ed. New York: McGraw-Hill, 1983, pp 655–671.
76. Goldstein JL, Kita T, Brown MS: Defective lipoprotein receptors and atherosclerosis. Lessons from an animal counterpart of familial hypercholesterolemia. *N Engl J Med* 309:288–296, 1983.
77. Goldstein JL, Brown MS: Familial hypercholesterolemia. In Stanbury JB, Wyngaarden JB, Fredrickson DS, Goldstein JL, Brown MS (eds): *The Metabolic Basis of Inherited Diseases*, 5th Ed. New York: McGraw-Hill, 1983, pp 672–712.
78. Lippel K, Tyroler H, Eder H, Gotto A Jr, Vahouny G: Relationship of hypertriglyceridemia to atherosclerosis. *Arteriosclerosis* 1:406–417, 1981.
79. Grundy SM: Pathogenesis of hypertriglyceridemia in man. In Carlson LA, Olsson AG (eds): *Treatment of Hyperlipoproteinemia*. New York: Raven Press, 1984, pp 21–34.

80. Schaefer EJ, Levy RI: Pathogenesis and management of lipoprotein disorders. *N Engl J Med* 312:1300–1310, 1985.
81. Goldstein JL, Brown MS: Familial hypercholesterolemia: pathogenesis of a receptor disease. *Johns Hopkins Med J* 143:8–16, 1978.
82. Morganroth J, Levy RI, Fredrickson DS: The biochemical, clinical and genetic features of type III hyperlipoproteinemia. *Ann Intern Med* 82:158–174, 1975.
83. Roberts WC, Levy RI, Fredrickson DS: Hyperlipoproteinemia. A review of the five types with first report of necropsy findings in type 3. *Arch Pathol Lab Med* 90:45–56, 1970.
84. Haust MD, Gilbert EF, Levy J, Hahn MF: Hypoplastic aorta—a failure of remodelling. *Pediatr Pathol* 6:101–108, 1986.
85. Haust MD: Genetic diseases and atherosclerotic lesions. In Crepaldi G, Gotto AM, Manzato E, Baggio G (eds): *Atherosclerosis VIII*. Amsterdam: Excerpta Medica, International Congress Series 817, 1989, pp 3–10.
86. Gomez MR: *Tuberous Sclerosis*. New York: Raven Press, 1979.
87. Comings DE: Review of Gomez's "Tuberous Sclerosis." *Am J Hum Genet* 32:285–286, 1980.
88. Wilson J, Carter C: Genetics of tuberose sclerosis. (Letter.) *Lancet* 1:340, 1978.
89. Sybert VP, Hall JG: Inheritance of tuberous sclerosis. (Letter.) *Lancet* 1:783, 1979.
90. Bender BL, Yunis EJ: The pathology of tuberous sclerosis. *Pathol Annu* 1:339–382, 1982.
91. Anderson DE, Tannen RL: Tuberous sclerosis and chronic renal failure. Potential confusion with polycystic kidney disease. *Am J Med* 47:163–168, 1969.
92. McWilliam RC, Stephenson JBP: Depigmented hair: The earliest sign of tuberous sclerosis. *Arch Dis Child* 53:961–963, 1978.
93. Freycon F, Mollard PC, Hermier M, et al: Anevrysme de l'aorte abdominale au cours d'une sclerose tubereuse de Bourneville. *Pediatrie* 26:421–427, 1971.
94. Larbre F, Loire R, Guibaud P, Lauras B, Weill B: Observation clinique et anatomique d'un anevrysme de l'aorte au cours d'une sclerose tubereuse de Bourneville. *Arch Fr Pediatr* 28:975–984, 1971.
95. Dutton RV, Singleton EB: Tuberous sclerosis: A case report with aortic aneurysm and unusual rib changes. *Pediatr Radiol* 3:184–186, 1975.
96. Hagood CO, Garvin DD, Lachina FM, Polsky WS, Ball TP, Bobroff LM: Abdominal aortic aneurysm and renal hamartoma in an infant with tuberous sclerosis. *Surgery* 79:713–715, 1976.
97. Imaizumi M, Nukada T, Yoneda S, Takano T, Hasegawa K, Abe H: Tuberous sclerosis with moyamoya disease: Case report. *Med J Osaka Univ*, 28:345–353, 1978.
98. Hurst JW (ed): *The Heart, Arteries and Veins*, 4th Ed. New York: McGraw-Hill, 1978.
99. Schwartz PL, Beards JA, Maris PJG: Tuberous sclerosis associated with a retinal angioma. *Am J Opthalmol* 90:485–488, 1980.
100. Rolfes DB, Towbin R, Bove KE: Vascular dysplasia in a child with tuberous sclerosis. *Pediatr Pathol* 3:359–373, 1985.
101. Stanley JC, Gewertz BL, Bove EL, Sottiurai V, Fry WJ: Arterial fibrodysplasia: Histopathologic character and current etiologic concepts. *Arch Surg* 110:561–565, 1975.
102. Sottiurai VS, Fry WJ, Stanley J: Ultrastructure of medial smooth muscle and myofibroblasts in human arterial dysplasia. *Arch Surg* 113:1280–1288, 1978.

103. O'Brien JS: The gangliosidoses. In: Stanbury JB, Wyngaarden JB, Fredrickson DS, Goldstein JL, Brown MS (eds): *The Metabolic Basis of Inherited Disease*, 5th Ed. New York: McGraw-Hill, 1983, pp 945–969.
104. Landing BH, Silverman FN, Craig JM, Jacoby MD, Lahey ME, Chadwick DL: Familial neurovisceral lipidosis. *Am J Dis Child* 108:503–522, 1964.
105. Suzuki K, Suzuki K, Chen GC: Morphological, histochemical and biochemical studies on a case of systemic late infantile lipidosis (generalized gangliosidosis). *J Neuropathol Exp Neurol* 27:15–38, 1968.
106. Yamano T, Shimada M, Okada S, et al: Ultrastructural study on nervous system of fetus with GM_1-gangliosidosis type I. *Acta Neuropathol (Berl)* 61:15–20, 1983.
107. Abu-Dalu KI, Tamary H, Livni N, Rivkind AI, Yatziv S: GM_1 gangliosidosis presenting as neonatal ascites. *J Pediatr* 100:940–943, 1982.
108. Benson PF, Babarik A, Brown SP, Mann TP: GM_1-generalized gangliosidosis variant with cardiomegaly. *Postgrad Med J* 52:159–165, 1976.
109. Kohlschütter A, Sieg K, Schulte FJ, Hayek HW, Goebel HH: Infantile cardiomyopathy and neuromyopathy with β-galactosidase deficiency. *Eur J Pediatr* 139:75–81, 1982.
110. Nakano T, Ikeda S, Kondo K, Yanagisawa N, Tsuji S: Adult GM_1-gangliosidosis: Clinical patterns and rectal biopsy. *Neurology* 35:875–880, 1985.
111. Yamano T, Shimada M, Okada S, Yutaka T, Kato T, Yabuuchi H: Ultrastructural study of biopsy specimens of rectal mucosa. Its use in neuronal storage diseases. *Arch Pathol Lab Med* 106:673–677, 1982.
112. Takahashi K, Naito M: Lipid storage disease. II. Ultrastructural pathology of lipid storage cells in sphingolipidoses. *Acta Pathol Jpn* 35:385–408, 1985.
113. Spycher MA: Electron microscopy: A method for the diagnosis of inherited metabolic storage diseases. Electron microscopy in diagnosis. *Pathol Res Pract* 167: 118–135, 1980.
114. Elleder M: Ito cells in lysosomal storage disorders. An ultrastructural study. *Virch Arch [Cell Pathol]* 46:13–19, 1984.
115. Haust MD: The genetic mucopolysaccharidoses (GMS). *Int Rev Exp Pathol* 12:251–314, 1973.
116. McKusick VA, Neufeld EF: The mucopolysaccharide storage diseases. In Stanbury JB, Wyngaarden JB, Fredrickson DS, Goldstein JL, Brown MS (eds): *The Metabolic Basis of Inherited Diseases*, 5th Ed. New York: McGraw-Hill, 1983, pp 751–777.
117. Orizaga M, Haust MD, Bryans AM, Frank H: Electron microscopic study of liver in Hurler's syndrome. *Fed Proc* 22:484, 1963.
118. Haust MD, Orizaga M, Bryans AM, Frank HF: The fine structure of liver in children with Hurler's syndrome. *Exp Mol Pathol* 10:141–161, 1969.
119. McKusick VA: *Mendelian Inheritance in Man. Catalog of Autosomal Dominant, Autosomal Recessive, and X-Linked Phenotypes*, 6th Ed. Baltimore: Johns Hopkins University Press, 1983, pp 151–153, 316–317, 695–697, 958, 1004, 1009.
120. Cupo LN, Pyeritz RE, Olson JL, McPhee SJ, Hutchins GM, McKusick VA: Ehlers-Danlos syndrome with abnormal collagen fibrils, sinus of Valsalva aneurysms, myocardial infarction, panacinar emphysema and cerebral heterotopias. *Am J Med* 71:1051–1058, 1981.
121. Sulh HMB, Steinmann B, Rao VH, Dudin G, Zeid JA, Slim M, DerKaloustian VM: Ehlers-Danlos syndrome type IV D: An autosomal recessive disorder. *Clin Genet* 25:278–287, 1984.

122. Arneson MA, Hammerschmidt DE, Furcht LT, King RA: A new form of Ehlers-Danlos syndrome: Fibronectin corrects defective platelet function. *JAMA* 244: 144–147, 1980.
123. Hollister DW: Heritable disorders of connective tissue: Ehlers-Danlos syndrome. *Pediatr Clin North Am* 25:575–591, 1978.
124. Prockop DJ, Kivirikko KI: Heritable diseases of collagen. *N Engl J Med* 311: 376–386, 1984.
125. Hollister DW, Byers PH, Holbrook KA: Genetic disorders of collagen metabolism. *Adv Hum Genet* 12:1–87, 1982.
126. Minor RR: Collagen metabolism. *Am J Pathol* 98:225–280, 1980.
127. Pyeritz RE, Stolle CA, Parfrey NA, Myers JC: Ehlers-Danlos syndrome IV due to a novel defect in type III procollagen. *Am J Med Genet* 19:607–622, 1984.
128. Stolle CA, Pyeritz RE, Myers JC, Prockop DJ: Synthesis of an altered type III procollagen in a patient with type IV Ehlers-Danlos syndrome. *J Biol Chem* 260:1937–1944, 1985.
129. Pope FM, Nicholls AC, Jones PM, Wells RS, Lawrence D: EDS IV (acrogeria): New autosomal dominant and recessive types. *J R Soc Med* 73:180–186, 1980.
130. Beighton P: Lethal complications of Ehlers-Danlos syndrome. *Br Med J* 3:656–659, 1968.
131. Schoolman A, Kepes JJ: Bilateral spontaneous carotid-cavernous fistulae in Ehlers-Danlos syndrome. Case report. *J Neurosurg* 26:82–86, 1967.
132. Umlas J: Spontaneous rupture of the subclavian artery in the Ehlers-Danlos syndrome. *Hum Pathol* 3:121–126, 1972.
133. Barabas AP: Vascular complications in the Ehlers-Danlos syndromes. With special reference to the "arterial type" or Sack's syndrome. *J Cardiovasc Surg (Torino)* 13:160–167, 1972.
134. Dalton ML, Bricker DL, Nannini L: Spontaneous rupture of the subclavian artery and innominate vein. *Arch Surg* 109:552–554, 1974.
135. Krane SM, Trelstad RL: Case records of the Massachusetts General Hospital, case 3-1979. *N Engl J Med* 300:129–135, 1979.
136. Rudd NL, Nimrod C, Holbrook KA, Byers PH: Pregnancy complications in type IV Ehlers-Danlos syndrome. *Lancet* 1:50–53, 1983.
137. Sheiner NM, Miller N, Lachance C: Arterial complications of Ehlers-Danlos syndrome. *J Cardiovasc Surg* 26:291–296, 1985.
138. Imahori S, Bannerman RM, Graf CJ, Brennan JC: Ehlers-Danlos syndrome with multiple arterial lesions. *Am J Med* 47:967–977, 1969.
139. Burnett HF, Bledsoe JH, Char F, Williams GD: Abdominal aortic aneurysmectomy in a 17-year-old patient with Ehlers-Danlos syndrome: Case report and review of the literature. Surgery 74:617–620, 1973.
140. Williams JL: Multiple aneurysms in a child. *Proc R Soc Med* 68:523–525, 1975.
141. Short DW: Multiple congenital aneurysms in childhood: Report of a case. *Br J Surg* 65:509–512, 1978.
142. Byers PH, Holbrook KA, McGillivray B, MacLeod PM, Lowry RB: Clinical and ultrastructural heterogeneity of type IV Ehlers-Danlos syndrome. *Hum Genet* 47: 141–150, 1979.
143. Pope FM, Martin GR, Lichtenstein JR, et al: Patients with Ehlers-Danlos syndrome type IV lack type III collagen. *Proc Natl Acad Sci USA* 72:1314–1316, 1975.
144. Byers PH, Barsh GS, Holbrook KA: Molecular mechanisms of connective tissue abnormalities in the Ehlers-Danlos syndrome. *Coll Relat Res* 1:475–489, 1981.

145. Clark JG, Kuhn C III, Uitto J: Lung collagen in type IV Ehlers-Danlos syndrome: Ultrastructural and biochemical studies. *Am Rev Respir Dis* 122:971- 978, 1980.
146. Byers PH, Holbrook KA, Barsh GS, Smith LT, Bornstein P: Altered secretion of type III procollagen in a form of type IV Ehlers-Danlos syndrome. Biochemical studies in cultured fibroblasts. *Lab Invest* 44:336-341, 1981.
147. Huang W, Haust MD: Proteoglycans in human atherosclerotic lesions – a pilot quantitative study by ruthenium red. *Histopathology* 8:835-845, 1984.
148. Grieco AJ: Homocystinuria: Pathogenetic mechanisms. *Am J Med Sci* 273:120-132, 1977.
149. Carson NAJ, Dent CE, Field CMB, Gaull GE: Homocystinuria. Clinical and pathological review of ten cases. J Pediatr 66:565-583, 1965.
150. Gibson JB, Carson NAJ, Neill DW: Pathological findings in homocystinuria. *J Clin Pathol* 17:427-437, 1964.
151. Lindsay J Jr, Meshel JC, Patterson RH: The cardiovascular manifestations of sickle cell disease. *Arch Intern Med* 133:643-651, 1974.
152. Rubler S, Fleischer RA: Sickle cell states and cardiomyopathy. Sudden death due to pulmonary thrombosis and infarction. *Am J Cardiol* 19:867-873, 1967.
153. Atkins L: Progeria. Report of a case with postmortem findings. *N Engl J Med* 250:1065-1069, 1954.
154. Gabr M, Hashem N, Hashem M, Fahmi A, Safouh M: Progeria, a pathologic study. *J Pediatr* 57:70-77, 1960.
155. Makous N, Friedman S, Yakovac W, Maris EP: Cardiovascular manifestations in progeria. Report of clinical and pathologic findings in a patient with severe arteriosclerotic heart disease and aortic stenosis. *Am Heart J* 64:334-346, 1962.
156. Reichel W, Garcia-Bunuel R: Pathologic findings in progeria: Myocardial fibrosis and lipofuscin pigment. *Am J Clin Pathol* 53:243-253, 1970.
157. Perkins DG, Haust MD: Ultrastructure of myocardium in the Hurler Syndrome: Possible relation to cardiac function. *Virchows Arch A* 394:195-205, 1982.
158. Blank E, Linder D: I-cell disease (mucolipidosis II): A lysosomopathy. *Pediatrics* 54:797-805, 1974.
159. Glaser JH, McAlister WH, Sly WS: Genetic heterogeneity in multiple lysosomal hydrolase deficiency. *J Pediatr* 85:192-198, 1974.
160. Nagashima K, Sakakibara K, Endo H, Konishi Y, Nakamura N, Suzuki Y, Abe T: I-cell disease (mucolipidosis II). Pathological and biochemical studies of an autopsy case. *Acta Pathol Jpn* 27:251-264, 1977.
161. Wood DH: Cerebrovascular complications of sickle cell anemia. *Stroke* 9:73-75, 1978.
162. Botreau-Rousell P, Drobinski G, Lévy R, Vachon JM, Nivet M, Grosgogeat Y: Infarctus du myocarde et drépanocytose hétérozygote. A propos de 2 cas. *Arch Mal Coeur* 70:141-147, 1977.
163. Fleischer RA, Rubler S: Primary cardiomyopathy in nonanemic patients. Association with sickle cell trait. *Am J Cardiol* 22:532-537, 1968.
164. Walkley SU, Wurzelmann S, Purpura DP: Ultrastructure of neurites and meganeurites of cortical pyramidal neurons in feline gangliosidosis as revealed by the combined Golgi-EM technique. *Brain Res* 211:393-398, 1981.
165. Rodrigues M, O'Brien JS, Garrett RS, Powell HC: Canine GM_1 gangliosidosis. An ultrastructural and biochemical study. *J Neuropathol Exp Neurol* 41:618-629, 1982.

166. Shull RM, Helman RG, Spellacy E, Constantopoulos G, Munger RJ, Neufeld EF: Morphologic and biochemical studies of canine mucopolysaccharidosis I. *Am J Pathol* 114:487–495, 1984.
167. Damle SP, Minor RR, Gregory JD: Proteoglycans in dog skin in a genetic dominant trait that shows defects in collagen fibrillogenesis. In Davidson EA, Williams JC, Di Ferrante NM (eds): *Glycoconjugates. Proceedings of the VIIIth International Symposium*. New York: Praeger, 1985, Vol 1, p 301.

8
Immunoregulatory CD4⁺ T Cell Subpopulations: Enumeration, Activation, and Functional Analyses in Normals and Autoimmune Disease

DOUGLAS J. BARRETT, DESMOND A. SCHATZ,
JOHN W. SLEASMAN

Introduction

Our understanding of the regulation of the normal immune response by T cells has been advanced enormously by the recognition of two distinct subsets of mature T cells. Inducer T cells that express the CD4 cell surface glycoprotein recognize antigen when it is presented by accessory cells in the context of class II self-histocompatibility determinants—eg, HLA-DR, -DQ, -DP.[1] Suppressor/cytotoxic T cells that bear the CD8 surface molecule recognize antigen along with MHC class I determinants—eg, HLA-A and -B.[1] It is now clear that $CD4^+$ T cells play a pivotal role in the induction and regulation of a variety of immunological events. These include antigen-specific or polyclonal B cell activation, proliferation and differentiation of B cells into immunoglobulin producing cells, delayed type hypersensitivity, induction of $CD8^+$ suppressor or cytotoxic T cells, and killing of appropriate target cells.

Recent studies indicate that the multiple functions performed by inducer T cells are due to distinct subpopulations of the $CD4^+$ subset. $CD4^+$ T cells can be divided into two subpopulations according to the expression of different isoforms of the common leukocyte antigen, T200 or CD45.[2-8] These phenotypically distinct subpopulations also appear to be functionally distinct. $CD4^+$ T cells that express the high-molecular-weight isoform of the leukocyte common antigen ($CD4^+CD45R^+$) function as suppressor-inducer T cells in that they are required to induce $CD8^+$ T cells to express suppressor cell function.[2] In contrast, $CD4^+$ T cells that do not express the high-molecular-weight isoform of the common leukocyte antigen ($CD4^+CD45R^-$ T cells) proliferate in response to soluble recall antigen and provide help for B cell immunoglobulin synthesis; ie, they function as memory or helper-inducer T cells.[3-5] Most of the $CD4^+CD45R^-$ T cells also express the CDw29 marker ($CD4^+CD45R^-CDw29^+$).

From the Division of Immunology and Transplantation, Department of Pediatrics, University of Florida College of Medicine, Gainesville, Florida.
Presented by Dr Barrett in honor of Lewis A. Barness, MD, November 12, 1988.

The studies described in this paper were performed to determine whether these $CD4^+$ T cell subpopulations could be selectively activated and expanded by in vitro stimulation. In addition, we attempted to determine if there were abnormalities in the number or function of the $CD4^+CD45R^+$ or $CD4^+CD45R^-$ subpopulations in autoimmune disease using type I insulin-dependent diabetes mellitus (IDDM) as a model.

Materials and Methods

Study Subjects

Healthy adult volunteers were recruited for studies of normal inducer T lymphocytes, according to protocols approved by the Institutional Review Board of the University of Florida College of Medicine. To study the role of inducer T cells in the pathogenesis of autoimmune diabetes, 25 nondiabetic subjects at high risk for the development of IDDM were selected for study on the basis of consistently positive serum tests for islet cell antibodies (ICA).[9-11] These individuals had no clinical or laboratory evidence of diabetes. There were 15 females and 10 males with a mean age of 15.6 years (age range 6 to 41 years). ICA were determined according to previously described methods.[12]

Monoclonal Antibodies

Murine monoclonal antibodies used for lymphocyte separation and for enumeration studies included anti-CD3 (anti-T3; Coulter or OKT3; Ortho), anti-CD4 (Leu 3; Becton Dickinson), anti-CD8 (OKT8; Ortho), anti-CD20 (anti-B1; Coulter), anti-CDw29 (anti-4B4; Coulter), and anti-CD45R (anti-2H4; Coulter). A mitogenic anti-CD3 antibody, RW28C8, was graciously provided by Dr Stuart Schlossman, Dana Farber Cancer Institute, Boston. All antibodies were used at concentrations determined to be optimal in preliminary experiments.

Lymphocyte Isolation

Peripheral blood mononuclear cells (PBMC) were isolated from heparinized whole blood by Ficoll-Hypaque (Pharmacia, Piscataway, NJ) density gradient centrifugation. After three washes in Hanks Balanced Salt Solution (Mediatech, Washington, DC), the cells were depleted of macrophages by adherence to plastic at 37°C. Ten million unfractionated PBMC were removed for cytofluorographic analysis of the $CD4^+$ T cell subpopulations. The remaining PBMCs were separated into T cell–enriched and T cell–depleted populations by rosetting with 1% AET-treated sheep erythrocytes.[13] The T cell population was further purified by treatment with anti-B1 monoclonal antibody and noncytotoxic rabbit complement (Pel Freeze Biologicals, Rogers, AR) to deplete residual B cells.[14] The non-

T cell fraction was further enriched for B cells by lysing the remaining T cells using a lytic anti-CD3 monoclonal antibody (OKT3) and complement.

$CD4^+$ T lymphocytes were isolated from the T cell fraction by lysing the reciprocal $CD8^+$ subset using lytic anti-CD8 monoclonal antibody and complement.

For some experiments, the $CD4^+$ purified T cells were further separated into $CD4^+CD45R^-$ and $CD4^+CD45R^+$ cells by "panning."[15] Following a 45-minute incubation with anti-CD45R monoclonal antibody (anti-2H4) at 4°C, the CD4+ T cells were placed on a plastic tissue culture plate (Fisher Scientific, Pittsburgh, PA) precoated with goat anti-mouse Ig antibodies (Tago, Burlingame, CA). The antibody-coated cells were panned for 70 min at 4°C. The nonadherent cells ($CD4^+CD45R^-$) were then removed by decanting. The plates were washed five times with phosphate-buffered saline containing 2% newborn calf serum to remove semiadherent cells. Adherent $CD4^+CD45R^+$ cells were then collected by scraping the plate. Both subpopulations of $CD4^+$ cells were washed and resuspended in enriched tissue-cultured media.

Immunofluorescent Labeling and Cytofluorographic Analysis

Two-color cytofluorographic analyses were performed on unfractionated PBMC for enumeration of $CD4^+$ T cell subpopulations.[15] Briefly, a 100-μl suspension of PBMC at 1×10^6 cells/ml was added to a test tube on ice. The cells were labeled with 20 μl of anti-CD4 monoclonal antibody coupled to phycoerythrin (Leu 3-PE; Becton Dickinson), mixed, and incubated at 4°C for 30 min in the dark. The cells were then washed three times, and 10 μl of fluorescein isothiocyanate (FITC)-conjugated anti-2H4 or FITC-conjugated anti-4B4 (Coulter) was added to identify the $CD4^+CD45R^+$ cells or the reciprocal $CD4^+CD45R^-CDw29^+$ lymphocyte population, respectively. Cells were incubated for an additional 30 min in the dark and washed as above. FITC- or PE-conjugated mouse immunoglobulins that were unreactive with human PBMC served as negative controls. Samples were analyzed using a FACStar flow cytometer (Becton Dickinson Immunocytometry Systems, Mountain View, CA) equipped with an argon ion laser (Spectra Physics, Mountain View, CA). Excitation of FITC and PE was at 488 nm light (250 mW). Fluorescence emitted from FITC and PE was distinguished using 530 and 575 band pass filters. Markers were set so that less than 5% of the cells stained with control antibodies were to the right of the channel marker. Light scatter and fluorescence data were stored in the list mode of a Consort 30 computer system (Becton Dickinson Immunocytometry Systems). Data obtained on 1×10^5 cells for each sample were presented as a two-dimensional contour map.

Mitogen-Induced Lymphocyte Activation

Purified populations of $CD4^+$ T cells, with 5% autologous monocytes, were placed at 1×10^6 cells/ml in enriched culture media consisting of RPMI 1640 (Mediatech) with 200 mM L-glutamine (Gibco), 200 units penicillin/ml (Gibco), 200 μg streptomycin/ml (Gibco), and 10% fetal bovine serum (Hyclone; Logan, UT). The cells were incubated at 37°C and 5% CO_2 in 100% humidity with phytohemagglutinin (PHA, 10 μg/ml; Gibco), pokeweed mitogen (PWM; 10 μg/ml; Sigma), concanavalin A (Con A, 10 μg/ml; Calbiochem), RW28C8 mitogenic anti-CD3 antibodies (1:200 final dilution), or medium alone. After 48 h, the cells were pulsed with 1.0 μCi of tritiated thymidine and harvested onto glass fiber filter spots 18 h later with a PHD cell harvester (Cambridge Technologies, Cambridge, MA). Tritium incorporation was measured in a Beckman LS250 scintillation counter.

Con A Stimulation of Suppressor-Inducer T Cells

Purified $CD4^+$ cells were suspended in enriched RPMI medium at 1×10^6 cells/ml plus 5% macrophages. Two-milliliter aliquots of cell suspension were placed in 12 × 72 plastic culture tubes containing either 10 μg/ml of Con A, 10 μg/ml of PHA, or no mitogen. After a 48-h incubation at 37°C, with 5% CO_2, and 100% humidity, the cells were harvested and treated with 0.1 M α-methyl-D-mannoside for 30 min. The viable cells were resuspended in enriched RPMI media at 1×10^6 cells/ml. Autologous T cells, B cells, or purified $CD4^+$ cells were prepared as described above and suspended in enriched RPMI media at 1 × 10 cells/ml. Combinations of fresh T cells, purified $CD4^+$ T cells, or mitogen-activated $CD4^+$ cells were cultured with normal B cells and PWM, as described below, to assay T cell help for B cell differentiation.

B Cell Differentiation Assay

Helper-inducer $CD4^+$ function was determined by assessing T cell help for B cell immunoglobulin secretion in a PWM driven coculture system.[16] Previous studies have shown that helper-inducer function in this assay is expressed predominantly by the $CD4^+CD45R^-$ ($CD4^+CDw29^+$) lymphocyte population.[3,5,7,8] Unfractionated T cells, $CD4^+$ T cells, or purified subpopulations of $CD4^+$ cells (1×10^6/ml) were cocultured with an equal number of B cells plus 5% monocytes and 10 μg/ml of PWM in enriched RPMI medium. The cells were placed in round-bottom microtiter plates (Costar, Cambridge, MA) in 200 μl final volume. Cultures were maintained in 100% humidified atmosphere with 5% CO_2. On day 7 of culture, the acellular supernatant was collected, and the concentration of IgG in the supernatant was quantified by an enzyme-linked immunosorbent assay as previously described.[17] Helper-inducer function was assessed by the ability of T cells or T cell subpopulations to provide help for B cell immunoglobulin production over and above that found in cultures of B cells alone.

Autologous Mixed Lymphocyte Reaction (AMLR)

Suppressor-inducer function was determined in the AMLR as previously described.[18] The $CD4^+CD45R^+$ suppressor-inducer T lymphocyte subpopulation has been shown to selectively proliferate in this assay system.[18] Briefly, responder

TABLE 8.1. Proliferation of CD4+ T cell subpopulations in response to mitogens.

Mitogen	Unfractionated CD4+	CD4+ subpopulations: CD45R-CDw29+	CD4+ subpopulations: CD45R+
None	2,072 ± 1,657	2,315 ± 1,117	3,900 ± 3,402
Anti-CD3	51,108 ± 15,247	57,742 ± 12,023	40,681 ± 13,207
PHA	59,598 ± 476	96,010 ± 1,360	106,000 ± 1,552
Con A	25,671 ± 2,557	22,400 ± 4,322	35,164 ± 7,317
PWM	53,282 ± 8,069	40,361 ± 3,876	37,821 ± 5,963

T cells were suspended in enriched media (1 × 10^6 cells/ml) and were mixed with an equal number of irradiated (3,000 rads) autologous B cells containing 5% monocytes. Control wells containing only responder T cells or stimulator B cells were set up in parallel. After 6 days the cultures were pulsed with tritiated thymidine, and the radioactivity incorporated into DNA was measured as described earlier. The results were expressed as a stimulation index of triplicate cultures.[19]

Statistical Analyses

Analysis of the data was performed using a computer-assisted statistical package (ED-SCI Development, Modesto, CA). Parametric data were expressed as means ± standard error. Student's t-test was used for comparison of means. In the assessment of helper-inducer function where the data did not conform to a normal Gaussian distribution, statistical differences were determined using the nonparametric Wilcoxon Rank Sum Test.

Results

Mitogenic Activation of CD4 Subpopulations

Following panning with monoclonal antibody to CD45R, more than 90% of the adherent cells expressed the CD45R determinant by reanalysis with anti-2H4 antibody. In the reciprocal nonadherent subpopulation of CD4+ cells, over 90% were enriched for CD4+CD45R- cells that expressed the CDw29 determinant identified by anti-4B4. Both the CD45R+ and the CD45R-CDw29+ subpopulations, as well as unfractionated CD4+ lymphocytes, were then activated by a variety of mitogens. As shown in Table 8.1, both the CD4+CD45R+ and the CD4+CD45R-CDw29+ subpopulations proliferated following stimulation with mitogenic anti-CD3 antibody, PHA, Con A, and PWM.

Since T cell activation by the Con A is known to induce suppressor cell activity,[20,21] we sought to determine whether the suppression induced by Con A was due to expansion of the CD4+CD45R+ suppression-inducer lymphocyte subpopulation. Enumeration of the CD4+CD45R+ suppressor-inducer and the reciprocal CD4+CDw29+ helper-inducer T lymphocyte subpopulations before

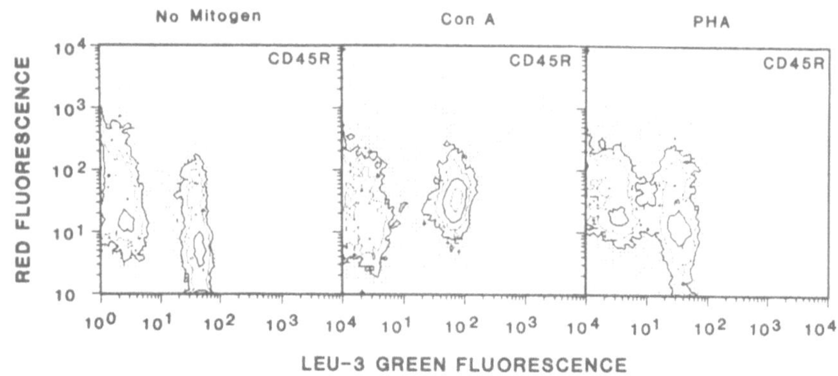

FIGURE 8.1. Two-color immunofluorescence was used to enumerate the percentage of CD4⁺ inducer T lymphocytes expressing the CD45R determinant both before and 48 h after mitogen stimulation. Lymphocytes were cultured with either no mitogen, Con A, PHA, or mitomycin C and Con A.

and after mitogen stimulation of PBMC is shown in Figure 8.1 and Table 8.2. Two-color immunofluorescence contour plots before and following Con A and PHA activation demonstrate a specific increase in the number of $CD4^+CD45R^+$ lymphocytes following Con A activation, as shown in Figure 8.1. This was not seen following PHA stimulation.

Summarized analyses of seven such experiments are shown in Table 8.2. Prior to mitogen stimulation, 36% to 40% of the $CD4^+$ inducer T lymphocytes expressed either the $CD4^+CD45R^-$ suppressor-inducer phenotype or the $CD4^+CD45R^-CDw29^+$ helper-inducer phenotype. Incubating the cells for 48 h in mitogen-free enriched media alone produced no significant change in either subpopulation of $CD4^+$ cells. However, after a 48-h incubation with Con A, there was a significant increase in $CD45R^+$ but no change in the reciprocal $CD45R^-$ ($CDw29^+$) expression. The change was specific for Con A activation since incubation of cells with PHA resulted in a nonspecific increase in both $CD45R^+$ and $CDw29^+$ expression.

The Con A–induced increase in the percentage of $CD4^+CD45R^+$-bearing lymphocytes could be explained either by proliferation of the $CD45R^+$ suppressor-

TABLE 8.2. Expression of CD45R and CDw29 on $CD4^+$ T lymphocytes before and after mitogenic stimulation.

	Prior to mitogen	After 48 h: No mitogen	Con A	PHA	Con A/ mitomycin
$CD45R^+$	36 ± 13%	39 ± 11%	85 ± 7%	76 ± 17%	24 ± 11%
$CD45R^-CDw29^+$	40 ± 11%	46 ± 13%	49 ± 22%	74 ± 11%	36 ± 12%

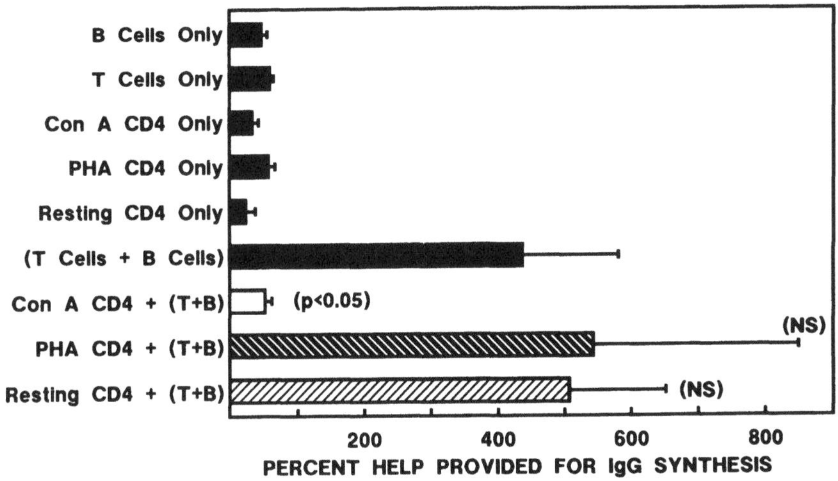

FIGURE 8.2. Pokeweed mitogen–induced immunoglobulin synthesis by B cells in coculture with autologous T cells. Unfractionated T cells, resting CD4+ T cells, and mitogen-activated CD4+ T cells were cultured alone or cocultured with autologous B cells in the presence of PWM. At the end of 7 days of culture, the concentration of IgG in the culture supernatant was measured by ELISA. T cell help for B cell immunoglobulin synthesis was calculated as:

$$\text{Percent help} = \frac{\begin{array}{c}\text{IgG (ng/ml) produced by}\\ \text{Coculture of T cells plus B cells}\end{array}}{\begin{array}{c}\text{IgG (ng/ml) from T cells alone}\\ + \text{IgG (ng/ml) from B cells alone}\end{array}} \times 100$$

The results shown represent the mean (± SEM) for three separate experiments.

inducer subset or a selective loss of CDw29+ helper-inducer cells. To determine if CD4+CD45R+ proliferation was occurring, lymphocytes were incubated with Con A in the presence of mitomycin C to inhibit cellular proliferation. As shown in Table 8.2, there was an actual decrease in the percentage of CD4+CD45R+-bearing cells but no change in the percentage of cells expressing the CDw29+ cell surface marker when cells were incubated with Con A plus mitomycin C, confirming selective proliferation of CD4+CD45R+ cells after Con A activation.

Functional Activity of Con A–Activated CD4+ T Cells

The functional helper cell activity of CD4+CD45R+ and CD4+CD45R−CDw29+ T cells was measured using a PWM-induced T plus B cell coculture. As shown in Figure 8.2, the addition of Con A–activated CD4+ cells to a coculture of autologous T cells plus B cells led to suppression of B cell immunoglobulin synthesis.

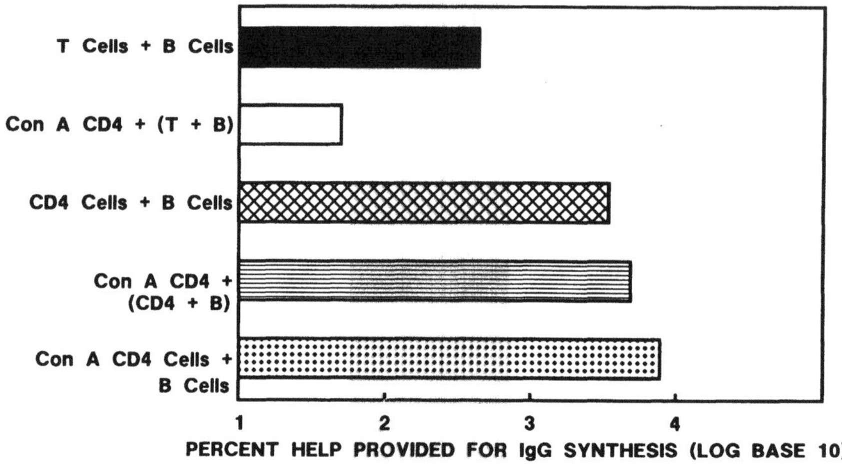

FIGURE 8.3. Pokeweed mitogen-induced immunoglobulin synthesis by B cells in coculture with autologous CD4 cells. The percent help that T cells provided for B cell IgG synthesis was calculated as described in Methods and in the legend to Figure 8.2.

This was not seen when PHA-stimulated CD4⁺ cells were added to the same T–B cell coculture, nor was it seen when resting CD4⁺ cells were added.

To determine whether Con A–activated CD4⁺ lymphocytes required the presence of CD8⁺ suppressor-effector T cells for suppression of B cell IgG production, or alternatively, whether the Con A–activated CD4⁺ cells were suppressive alone, Con A–activated CD4⁺ lymphocytes were added to a coculture of B cells with pure CD4⁺ T cells (depleted of CD8⁺ T cells). As seen in Figure 8.3, the addition of Con A–activated CD4⁺ lymphocytes to the coculture of purified CD4⁺ T cells plus B cells produced no suppression of IgG synthesis but, rather, increased B cell immunoglobulin synthesis. Thus, in order for the Con A–activated CD4⁺ cells to effect suppression, CD8⁺ suppressor-effector cells are required in the culture.

Helper-Inducer and Suppressor-Inducer CD4⁺ T Cell Subpopulations in Autoimmunity

Abnormalities in immunoregulatory T cell function have been hypothesized to play a role in the pathogenesis of autoimmune disease. Defects in the CD4⁺CD45R⁺ suppressor-inducer and CD4⁺CDw29⁺ helper-inducer subpopulations of T cells have recently been reported in several autoimmune disorders including Graves disease,[22] systemic lupus erythematosus,[23] rheumatoid arthritis,[24] and multiple sclerosis.[25] Similarly, abnormalities in Con A–activated suppressor cell function have previously been reported in autoimmune type I diabetes.[26] Most of these studies attempting to define the role of T cell regulation in

TABLE 8.3. Enumeration of CD4+ subpopulations in autoimmune ICA+ subjects.

	CD4+CD45R+	CD4+CDw29+
ICA+ subjects	20 ± 3%	30 ± 2%*
Normals	23 ± 4%	39 ± 3%

*$p < .05$ compared to normals.

autoimmune diseases have been confounded by the possible effects of overt inflammatory disease and/or metabolic abnormalities on the immune system.[26] Since nondiabetic persons whose sera contain ICA have been shown to be at high risk for the subsequent development of IDDM,[9-11] we chose to study the immunoregulatory T cell number and function in such individuals with serologic autoimmunity before they developed clinically apparent diabetes.

Enumeration of helper-inducer and suppressor-inducer CD4+ T cell subpopulations in 25 ICA+ individuals and matched controls are shown in Table 8.3. The helper-inducer CD4+CDw29+ subpopulation in individuals who are ICA+ were decreased (mean 30 ± 2%) compared to those of controls (mean 29 ± 3%; $p <$ .05). In contrast, enumeration of the CD4+CD45R+ suppressor-inducer subpopulation was similar between ICA+ subjects and controls.

Helper-inducer T cell function in ICA+ subjects was assessed in PWM-stimulated T plus B cell cocultures. Comparison of helper-inducer function of T cells from ICA+ subjects with those of controls is shown in Figure 8.4. T cells from six ICA+ subjects and matched controls were cocultured with allogeneic B cells from a single, normal individual. T cells from the ICA+ subjects provided less helper function than did the T cells from ICA− controls ($p < .0025$). To ensure that the ICA+ subjects did not have excessive T cell–mediated suppressor activity which would produce similar results in the coculture experiments, T cells from the ICA+ subjects were cocultured with B cells from the control together with T cells from the same control to provide normal T cell help. Neither normal individuals' T cells nor the ICA+ subjects' T cells tested in this coculture system demonstrated allogeneic suppression (% IgG expected in ICA subjects was 1,789 ± 443 vs controls 1,664 ± 1,010).

Further evidence for a specific fundamental defect in the CD4+ helper-inducer T cell subpopulation from ICA+ subjects was provided by culturing fractionated pure CD4+ T cells from both ICA+ subjects and in controls with normal allogeneic B cells. In three such experiments, the same defect in helper-inducer T cell function in ICA+ subjects was found when purified CD4+ T cells were used in place of the unfractionated T cells in the assay (ICA+ subjects 1,075 ± 842 vs controls 8,156 ± 2,431).

The function of the CD4+CD45R+ suppressor-inducer T lymphocyte subpopulation was assessed by T cell proliferation in the AMLR. No difference in T cell proliferation between ICA+ subjects and controls was noted (data not shown).

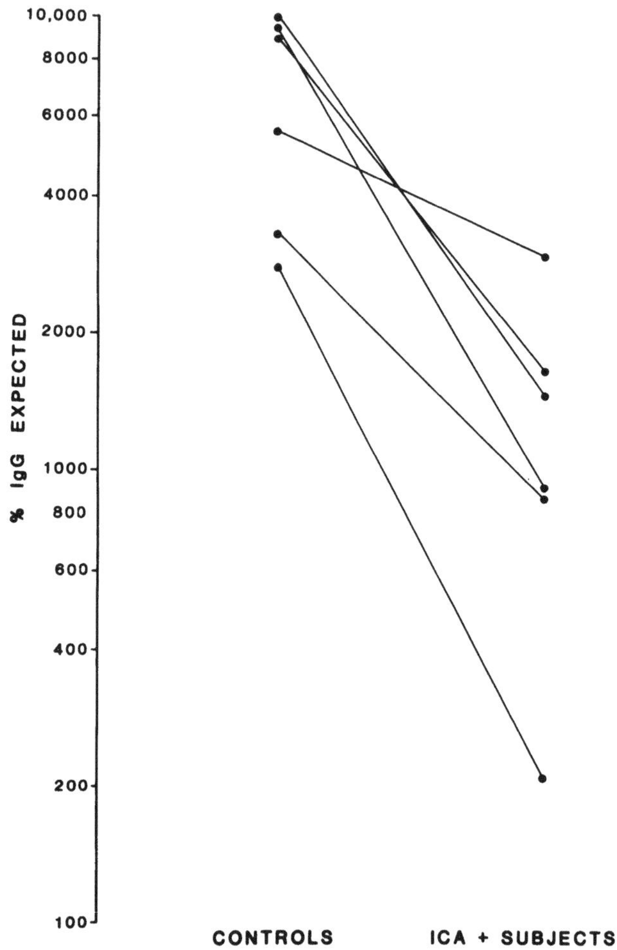

FIGURE 8.4. Helper-inducer T cell function using allogeneic B cells. T cells from ICA$^+$ subjects and from ICA$^-$ controls were cocultured with allogeneic B cells isolated from a single, healthy, third-party control in the presence of PWM. After 7 days, IgG secretion into the coculture was quantified and expressed as a percentage of the IgG expected, based on that produced by individual cultures of T cells alone and B cells alone. Values above 100% represent a helper T cell effect. ICA$^+$ subjects had diminished helper-inducer T cell function compared to the controls ($p < .0025$).

Discussion

Monoclonal antibodies to CD4$^+$ inducer T lymphocyte subpopulations are useful in identifying phenotypically distinct subpopulations that have different functional roles in B cell activation and differentiation. Further, these antibodies can be used to isolate and purify CD4$^+$ T cell subpopulations based on the expression of the CD45R molecule.[2-8] Our results confirm that both the $CD4^+CD45R^+$ and the $CD4^+CD45R^-$ inducer T cell subpopulations are capable of providing the signals necessary for T cell–dependent B cell proliferation.[4,5,15] In contrast, only the $CD45R^-$ subpopulation of $CD4^+$ cells can induce T cell–dependent B cell differentiation to immunoglobulin secretion.[3,5,6-8,15] We have further demonstrated that Con A selectively activates the $CD45R^+$ subpopulation and increases the ability of those cells to induce $CD8^+$ suppressor cell function. Thus, these phenotypically distinct subpopulations of $CD4^+$ T cells can be differentially activated in vitro by mitogens to express distinct immunoregulatory activities.

The second part of our study was designed to determine if abnormalities in these $CD4^+$ T lymphocyte subpopulations are present in subjects with autoimmune diabetes. Individuals with impending IDDM were chosen for study for several reasons. First, ICA are expressed in the sera of these individuals long before the onset of overt diabetes.[9-11] Second, while these individuals express autoimmune phenomena (ie, autoantibodies), they do not have inflammatory or metabolic derangement which might complicate interpretation of results. Third, abnormalities in $CD4^+$ lymphocyte function are known to occur in the NOD mouse model of human IDDM.[27-28]

Our results demonstrated that both the number and the function of the helper-inducer $CD4^+CD45R^-CDw29^+$ T cell subpopulation were diminished in individuals with prediabetes. We found no abnormality in the number of function of the reciprocal suppressor-inducer $CD4^+CD45R^+$ subpopulation.

Controversy exists as to whether these $CD4^+$ lymphocyte subpopulations are separate and distinct T cell lineages or, rather, represent different stages of maturation along a common pathway of T cell differentiation. $CD4^+CD45R^-CDw29^+$ T cells have the property of memory cells in that they proliferate vigorously when exposed to recall antigens.[3,5,6] In contrast, $CD4^+CD45R^+$ T cells do not respond to soluble antigens,[2,5,6] but they can be induced to express the $CD45R^-CDw29^+$ phenotype upon activation with certain mitogens.[5,6] It has thus been proposed that the $CD4^+CD45R^+$ and $CD4^+CD45R^-CDw29^+$ subpopulations can be more generally designated as naïve T cells (encompassing cells with suppressor-inducer activity) and memory T cells (encompassing cells with helper-inducer activity), respectively.[5,6]

If this hypothesis is correct, the selective abnormality in $CD45R^-CDw29^+$ cells that we observed among autoimmune prediabetic ICA^+ subjects in this study may reflect a maturational defect in antigen-specific T cell activation from the naïve to the memory state. This could result in a failure to eradicate a potentially offending diabetogenic agent, such as a virus or toxin.[29] Alternatively, abnormal $CD45R^-CDw29^+$ T cell function might lead to a disturbance in B cell immunoregulation and a deranged autoimmune process resulting from a failure to induce normal immunoregulatory networks such as idiotypic antiidiotypic circuits capable of inhibiting autoreactive B cell clones. Additional study of these possible mechanisms may give insight into the autoimmune pathogenic events leading to IDDM and, furthermore, could provide important additional markers for disease susceptibility.

In summary, we have used a panel of monoclonal antibodies to identify and purify distinct phenotypic and functional subpopulations of $CD4^+$ T lymphocytes. The subpopulations can be selectively activated to express some of the differential functions of inducer T cells that are important for normal immunoregulation. Finally, we have demonstrated that individuals with autoimmune prediabetes have a disturbance in the number and function of $CD4^+CD45R^-CDw29^+$ helper-inducer $CD4^+$ T lymphocytes. These abnormalities may be important in the initial pathogenic events leading to IDDM.

References

1. Schwartz RH: T lymphocyte recognition of antigen in association with gene products of the major histocompatibility complex. *Ann Rev Immunol* 3:237, 1985.
2. Morimoto C, Letvin NL, Distaso JA, Aldrich WC, Schlossman SF: The isolation and characterization of the human suppressor inducer T cell subset. *J Immunol* 134:1508–1515, 1985.
3. Morimoto C, Letvin NL, Boyd AW, et al: The isolation and characterization of the human inducer T cell subset. *J Immunol* 134:3762–3769, 1985.
4. Tedder TF, Cooper MD, Clement LT: Human lymphocyte differentiation antigens HB-10 and HB-11. II. Differential production of B cell growth and differentiation factors by distinct helper T cell subpopulations. *J Immunol* 134(5):2989–2994, 1985.
5. Clement LT, Yamashita N, Martin AM: The functionally distinct subpopulations of human $CD4^+$ helper/inducer T lymphocytes defined by anti-CD45R antibodies derive sequentially from a differentiation pathway that is regulated by activation-dependent post-thymic differentiation. *J Immunol* 141(5):1464–1470, 1985.
6. Sanders ME, Malegapuru WM, Shaw S: Human naïve and memory T cells: Reinterpretation of helper-inducer and suppressor-inducer subsets. *Immunol Today* 9:195–199, 1988.
7. Bottomly K: A functional dichotomy in $CD4^+$ T lymphocytes. *Immunol Today* 9: 268–274, 1988.
8. Powrie F, Mason D: Phenotypic and functional heterogeneity. *Immunol Today* 9: 274–277, 1988.
9. Riley WJ, Krischer J, Clarke DW, et al: Islet cell antibodies (ICA): Relative risk (RR) of developing insulin dependent diabetes (IDD) is 166. *Diabetes* 36:278A, 1987.
10. Tarn AC, Dean BM, Schwarz G, et al: Predicting insulin-dependent diabetes. *Lancet* 845–850, 1988.
11. Neufeld M, Maclaren NK, Riley WJ, et al: Islet cell antibodies in U.S. Caucasians and blacks with insulin dependent diabetes mellitus. *Diabetes* 29:589–592, 1980.
12. Van Rood, Van Leeuman A, Phoem J: A method to test simultaneously two cell populations by two-color fluorescence. *Nature* 262:795–797, 1976.
13. Saxon A, Feldhouse J, Robins A: Single step separation of human T cells using AET treated SRBC rosettes. *J Immunol Methods* 12:285–288, 1976.
14. Reinherz EL, Morimoto C, Fitzgerald KC, Husseyre J, Daley JA, Schlossman SF: Heterogeneity of human $T4^+$ inducer T cells as defined by monoclonal antibody that delineates two functionally distinct subpopulations. *J Immunol* 128:463–468, 1982.
15. Sleasman JW, Morimoto C, Schlossman SF, Tedder TF: The role of functionally distinct helper T lymphocyte subpopulations in the induction of human B cell differentiation. *J Immunol* (in press).

16. Saxon A: Assessment of T-cell help and suppression of B-cell function. In Rose NR, Friedman H (eds): *Manual of Clinical Immunology.* Washington, DC: American Society for Microbiology, 1980, pp 151–156.
17. Barrett DJ, Edwards JR, Pietrantuono BA, Ayoub EM: Inhibition of human leukocyte activation by wheat germ agglutinin: A model of saccharide specific suppressor factors. *Cell Immunol* 81:287–297, 1983.
18. Damle NK, Gupta S: Autologous mixed lymphocyte reaction in man. V. Functionally and phenotypically distinct human T cell subpopulations respond to non T and activated T cells in AMLR. *Scand J Immunol* 16:59–68, 1982.
19. Maluish AE, Strong DM: Lymphocyte proliferation. In Rose NK, Friedman H, Fahey JL (eds): *Manual of Clinical Laboratory Immunology,* 3d Ed. Washington, DC: American Society for Microbiology, 1986, pp 274–287.
20. Dutton RW: Inhibitory and stimulatory effects of concanavalin A on the response of mouse spleen cell suspension to antigen. I. Characterization of the inhibitory cell activity. *J Exp Med* 136:1445, 1972.
21. Shou L, Schwartz SA, Good RA: Suppressor cell activity after concanavalin A treatment of lymphocytes from normal donors. *J Exp Med* 143:1100–1110, 1976.
22. Ishikawa N, Eguchi K, Otsubo T, et al: Reduction in the suppressor-inducer T cell subset and increase in the helper T cell subset in thyroid tissue from patients with Graves disease. *J Clin Endocrinol Metab* 65:17–23, 1987.
23. Morimoto C, Steinberg AD, Letvin NL, et al: A defect of immunoregulatory T cell subsets in systemic lupus erythematosus patients demonstrated with anti-2H4 antibody. *J Clin Invest* 79:762–768, 1987.
24. Emery P, Gentry KC, Mackay IR, Muirden KD, Rowley M: Deficiency of the suppressor-inducer subset of T lymphocytes in rheumatoid arthritis. *Arthritis Rheum* 30:849–856, 1987.
25. Morimoto C, Hafler DA, Weiner HL, et al: Selective loss of the suppressor-inducer T cell subset in progressive multiple sclerosis. *N Engl J Med* 316:67–72, 1987.
26. Crosti F, Secchi A, Ferrero E, et al: Impairment of lymphocyte-suppressive system in recent onset insulin-dependent diabetes mellitus. Correlation with metabolic control. *Diabetes* 35:1055–1057, 1986.
27. Charlton B, Mandel TE: Progression from insulitis to B-cell destruction in NOD mouse requires L3T4⁺ T lymphocytes. *Diabetes* 37:1108–1112, 1988.
28. Shizuru JA, Taylor-Edwards C, Banks B, Gregory AK, Fathman CA: Immunotherapy of the nonobese diabetic mouse: Treatment with antibody to T-helper lymphocytes. *Science* 241:659–661, 1988.
29. Pak CY, Eun H-M, McArthur RG, Yoon JW: Association of cytomegalovirus infection with autoimmune type I diabetes. *Lancet* 2:1–4, 1988.

9
A Perspective on Pediatric AIDS

C. Everett Koop

From the early days of the epidemic of acquired immune deficiency syndrome (AIDS) until now, there have been 1,013 cases of AIDS among children under the age of 13. This represents less than 2% of the total. In a society fascinated by numbers, 2% is not very much, but each child with AIDS presents our society with a special medical and social challenge, one, I hasten to add, that we are still generally unprepared to meet.

Of the total number of children thus far reported as having AIDS (1,013), 60% have died. This rate is, however, subject to change, and not for the better. If the mortality among children with AIDS parallels that of infected adults, then it will rise to more than 90%, the mortality rate for adults diagnosed as early as 1981 and 1982.

We estimate that, by 1991, the cumulative total of children with AIDS symptomatology will rise to 3,000. However, the number of HIV-positive children may be as high as 10,000 by then.

Of the current total, the largest number by far, 779, are children whose mothers *have, have had*, or are *at risk for having* AIDS. These children acquired the virus either in utero or during labor and delivery. Although an infected mother will not *always* transmit the virus to her child, the odds are as high as 1 in 2.

There are still a great many unknowns in this area. For example, we do not really know the role of the placenta as a vector or as an inhibitor. We are not clear as to the numbers of cases in which transmission from mother to child was transplacental, as opposed to perinatal or even postnatal.

We are starting our research in pediatric AIDS with a data base that reflects the activity of the HIV in adults. We are finding out that, in AIDS as in so many other diseases, children are "little adults." There are medical differences in the way the disease is manifest in children; for example, lymphocytic interstitial pneumonia

---

Adapted from a talk given at Georgetown University, Washington, DC, June 1988.
From the Office of the Surgeon-General, United States Public Health Service, Rockville, Maryland.
Submitted in honor of Lewis A. Barness, MD, November, 1988.

(LIP) is characteristic of children with HIV, although it is rarely seen in adults. On the other hand, Kaposi's sarcoma is common among homosexual men with AIDS but is an infrequent manifestation among children.

Recurrent bacterial infections are more prominent among children than among adults with AIDS. Many children also exhibit a characteristic encephalopathy leading to developmental delays or even to loss of developmental milestones.

Although we recognize these and other differences, we have no explanation as yet for them. For these and other reasons, we are just at the "starting gate" when it comes to research for the diagnosis and treatment of children with AIDS.

So far, I have just touched upon some areas of biomedical interest. However, this is a very narrow frame of reference, because children with AIDS present a range of special problems not only to the biomedical community but also to the community at large. For example:

- They are totally dependent on others for help, unlike the adult.
- They tend to be from families that are themselves under stress of poverty or disease, or they are the children of single women who cannot provide home or family support.
- They are unfairly stigmatized. Hence, although they may be asymptomatic for many years, the stigma of seropositivity clouds their social development at every step of the way.

Last year, I convened a "Surgeon General's Workshop on Pediatric AIDS" in order to arrive at some baseline agreements among medical and social service professionals as to *where we were* in our understanding of the problem and *where we ought to be* in the years ahead. It was a very fruitful meeting and led to a number of useful developments. The most significant was the establishment of a special, departmentwide initiative on pediatric HIV disease by Dr Otis R. Bowen, the Secretary of Health and Human Services (HHS).

The director of the work group under this initiative is Dr Antonia Novello, who is also the Deputy Director of the National Institute of Child Health and Human Development. My role is as the Senior Scientific Advisor to the work group. Thus far, we have laid out a research agenda in the area of pediatric AIDS, within the context of the overall research effort in AIDS. We have not yet assigned priorities in pediatric AIDS research, but this may be possible in the first report to the Secretary.

The research agenda includes not only the expected items of cofactors, virology, and therapeutics, but also research that might help us to integrate more effectively the biomedical and biobehavioral research with a variety of research and demonstration efforts in family services, legal aid, human sexuality, ethics, and funding.

Appropriate funding is important because, as closely as we can calculate today, only about 4% of the overall HHS budget for AIDS is devoted to research peculiar to pediatric AIDS. Yet, the cost of diagnosis, treatment, and placement of infected infants and children is rising significantly.

Should that 4% figure be higher? I think everyone would agree that it should. However, the availability of more money will not, by itself, answer those questions of ethics, law, and medicine that now circumscribe pediatric research *in general*—not just relative to the epidemic of AIDS.

For example, we would not permit expeditious drug testing in children under the kind of "humane IND" that has been used for AZT in adult AIDS patients. Moreover, there are good ethical reasons for limiting clinical drug trials in infants and children. I do not know how to resolve this particular problem, but I know we will have to confront it the moment a researcher comes up with a drug that just might alleviate, or possibly reverse, an AIDS-related condition in children.

We also have to face the fact that nearly all the children born with AIDS thus far are in those major metropolitan areas with high concentrations of black and Hispanic minorities: New York City, Miami, Los Angeles, Washington, DC, and Newark, New Jersey, for example. These are the same areas in which medical and public health personnel have been fighting enormous odds in their day-to-day effort to deliver effective primary health care: well-baby care, hypertension screening, maternal and child nutrition, treatment for substance abuse, and so on.

The tasks associated with AIDS are a hundred times more complex than the others, not only for health professionals but also for the community residents themselves. Suspicion, denial, guilt, frustration, anger, the feelings that already cloud the public health picture in these inner-city environments are even more evident when the subject is AIDS.

These issues and questions are on our pediatric AIDS agenda. *None* of them is easy to approach. I wish I were in a position to recite a number of major advances, research breakthroughs, or other evidence of dramatic progress. We just are not there yet. However, the breakthroughs will come, as a result of new interest and attention by the pediatric profession, not only by its leadership but also by the young men and women just entering the field.

I have said that our best hope in the battle against AIDS is education, education, and more education, so that people will avoid those behaviors that lead to the transmission of the AIDS virus. I still believe that is the case.

In the meantime, the toll of AIDS among children continues to rise. Yesterday, there were a few hundred, today the number is over a thousand, and tomorrow there may possibly be 10,000 or 20,000 children infected with HIV. They will need our help. And we *must* be prepared to provide all the help we can.

10
Insulin-Containing Pancreatic Islet Cells in the Sudden Infant Death Syndrome

MARIE VALDES-DAPENA, CARMEN PATRICIA VALDES-DAPENA, MEHRDAD NADJI, PARVIN GANJEI, JUAN CUETO

Introduction

In 1976, in a letter to the editor of Lancet, Cox et al[1] reported a study of the pancreas in 25 so-called cot deaths, infants who had died of the sudden infant death syndrome (SIDS). Those authors claimed that 9 of the 25 (36%) had islet cell hyperplasia and nesidioblastosis. They attributed those nine deaths to hypoglycemia secondary to pancreatic lesions. They defined nesidioblastosis as multifocal budding of endocrine cells from ductal or ductular epithelium, or interposition of endocrine cells in the midst of ductal or ductular epithelium, together with diffuse proliferation of single endocrine cells or small cell nests in the midst of parenchyma and apart from clearly defined islets. The conviction of these investigators was apparently supported, at least in part, by an earlier report that many SIDS victims have abnormally low levels of glucose in the vitreous humor.[2]

That same year and two years later, Polak et al[3,4] published their findings in two infants who had died suddenly and unexpectedly. In one, they found the total endocrine cell population to be 10.8 ± 1.2% of all pancreatic tissue, and in the other, 5.46 ± 3.07%. In contrast, they determined the proportion of all islet cells in seven control infants to be 2.13 ± 0.29%. They concluded that the apparent fivefold increase in islet tissue in the SIDS babies constituted a pathologic lesion reflecting mortal hypoglycemia. They seem to have relied on the earlier report of Swift and Emery[2] regarding low levels of glucose in the vitreous humor of crib death victims.

Prior to those two reports, several groups of investigators had described the range of normal for infants in the first year of life as being between 1.3% and 3.0% of total pancreatic tissue (Table 10.1).[5-10] In 1977, Heitz, using immunohistochemistry and a television image conversion analyzer and calculator,

---

From the Department of Pathology, University of Miami School of Medicine, Miami, Florida, and the Underwood Hospital, Underwood, New Jersey.
Presented by Dr Marie Valdes-Dapena in honor of Lewis A. Barness, MD, November 11, 1988.

TABLE 10.1. Mean relative area of all endocrine cells in controls.

Author	Year	Ref	No. pts.	Age	Range	Mean
Gepts	1965	5	3	1 yr	1.3–3.1%	–
Van Assche	1970	6	41	7–10 mo	1.9–9.8%	–
Kloppel et al	1975	7	10	4–8 mo	1.3–3.0%	1.8%
Slovik et al	1975	8	10	1–8 mo	1.3–3.0%	2.0%
Kissane	1975	9	–	Neonates	–	2.0%

Source: Jaffe et al.[10]

ascertained the range of normal for all pancreatic endocrine cells in late fetal life to be 1.5% to 3.4% with a mean of 2.4.[11]

In 1978 Aynsley-Green et al[12] described an "averted sudden neonatal death" in an infant who was severely hypoglycemic, presumably because of hyperinsulinemia. The child's death was averted by total pancreatectomy; the reported pathologic diagnosis for the pancreas was nesidioblastosis together with a microadenoma. On the basis of that experience, those authors recommended that insulin-specific staining methods be used to examine the pancreata of all infants who die suddenly and unexpectedly.

In 1982, Jaffe et al[13] published the results of their detailed, comprehensive study of the normal histology of pancreatic islets in infants. In their study they included a discussion of the islets in SIDS infants. Using indirect antibody staining for glucagon, somatostatin, human pancreatic polypeptides, and insulin combined, they found *no* evidence of any relationship between islet cell hyperplasia or "nesidioblastosis" and SIDS. In their view, "nesidioblastosis" is part of the normal development of the human infant pancreas. However, in striking contrast to *all* of the earlier works mentioned above, these authors reported the normal range for the relative percent area of all endocrine cells in late fetal life and in liveborns less than 2 months of age to be 6.1% to 12.9% of total pancreatic parenchyma with a mean of 9.5. Not only did they find the relative amount of islet tissue in SIDS infants to be within that range of normal, but they also indicated that the islets in SIDS infants are normal in regard to morphology as well.

We undertook this study to examine specifically the fractional percent area of the pancreas occupied by *insulin-containing* islet cells, in a large number of SIDS patients and controls, in order to assess more critically the likelihood of excess insulin production in infants who die of crib death.

Materials

All of the tissues for this study, from both SIDS and control infants, were obtained from autopsies performed at the Office of the Medical Examiner for the State of Maryland, in Baltimore. The 97 autopsies were reviewed in their entirety, a second time, by one pediatric pathologist to ensure accuracy and consistency of diagnoses.

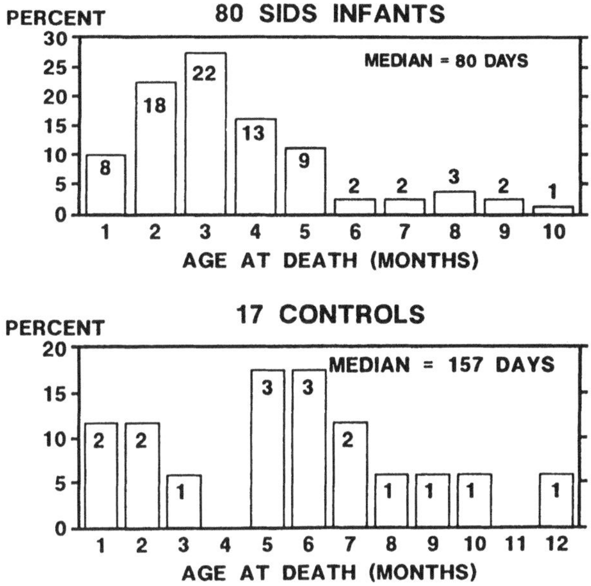

FIGURE 10.1. Distribution of SIDS and control infants by age.

In each case, the pancreas was gleaned intact, at the time of necropsy, and all or almost all of it was placed, in one piece, into a container of buffered formalin. After fixation it was divided into three portions—roughly the head, the body, and the tail. The three pieces were then embedded longitudinally in a single block of paraffin for histologic sectioning. Thus, each case was represented by one paraffin block in which were mounted three longitudinal (coronal) segments of that pancreas. Individual cases were identified by their autopsy numbers only, and thus all of the work on the sections was conducted as a blind study.

The subjects of the study were 80 infants who had died of SIDS and 17 who had succumbed to recognized diseases. The causes for the deaths of the latter group included an accident (1), acute respiratory illnesses (4), acute diseases of the central nervous system (5), other acute illnesses (2), chronic problems involving either the central nervous system or the heart (4), and one identified only as "non-SIDS" (1). None of the conditions included would have been expected to alter the number, the morphology, or the function of any of the islet cells.

The control infants were *not* age-matched for the SIDS; however, all SIDS and control infants were under 1 year of age. The mean age for the SIDS victims was 94.8 days + 60.9; the median was 80 days. The mean age for the controls was 156.1 days + 93.1; the median was 157 (Fig. 10.1).

Approximately two thirds of both groups were male (Table 10.2), and there were roughly equal numbers of black and white infants in each group (Table 10.3).

TABLE 10.2. Sex distribution of SIDS infants and controls.

Sex	80 SIDS infants	17 Controls
Male	53 (65%)	11 (65%)
Female	27 (34%)	5 (29%)
Unspecified	1 (1%)	1 (6%)

Methods

Eight microscopic slides were prepared from each block (and thus for each case); each bore three sections as described above–one of head, one of body, and one of tail. Each segment was readily recognized grossly because of its relative size and its shape.

The paraffin sections of formalin-fixed pancreatic tissue were then subjected to immunoperoxidase staining using antisera specific for insulin, human pancreatic polypeptide (HPP), gastrin, glucagon, and somatostatin (Fig. 10.2). Matching sections were also stained with hematoxylin and eosin, and two unstained sections from each block were saved; these were used later in restaining for insulin and HPP to achieve greater contrast for the Quantimet assays.

The peroxidase antiperoxidase procedure was performed in the standard fashion.[14] Briefly, following the blockage of endogenous peroxidase activity by a mixture of methanol and hydrogen peroxide, the sections were treated sequentially with bovine albumin, primary antibody, linking antibody, and peroxidase-antiperoxidase complex. Diaminobenzidine was used as chromogen in the presence of hydrogen peroxide. Antibody control slides consisted of replacement of the primary antibody with nonimmune rabbit serum of equal concentration. All incubations were for 30 min in a humidity chamber at room temperature (22 °C). All washes and dilutions were made with phosphate-buffered saline, pH 7.4. All immunologic reagents were from DAKO, Santa Barbara, CA.

The embryonic ventral and dorsal lobes of the pancreas give rise to two adult regions of the pancreas which are separable only histologically; one is rich in pancreatic polypeptides (PP) and the other, poor in PP.[15] It has been established that only the ventrally derived portion of the head of the pancreas contains islets that are PP rich. The remainder of the head, derived from the dorsal duct, the body, and the tail, contains only PP-poor islets. Because at the outset, there was no bias as to whether or not these two types of islets contained different complements of beta cells, assays were done on islets of both types. Scanning the

TABLE 10.3. Race distribution of SIDS infants and controls.

Race	80 SIDS infants	17 controls
Black	36 (45%)	11 (65%)
White	41 (51%)	5 (29%)
Other	3 (4%)	1 (6%)

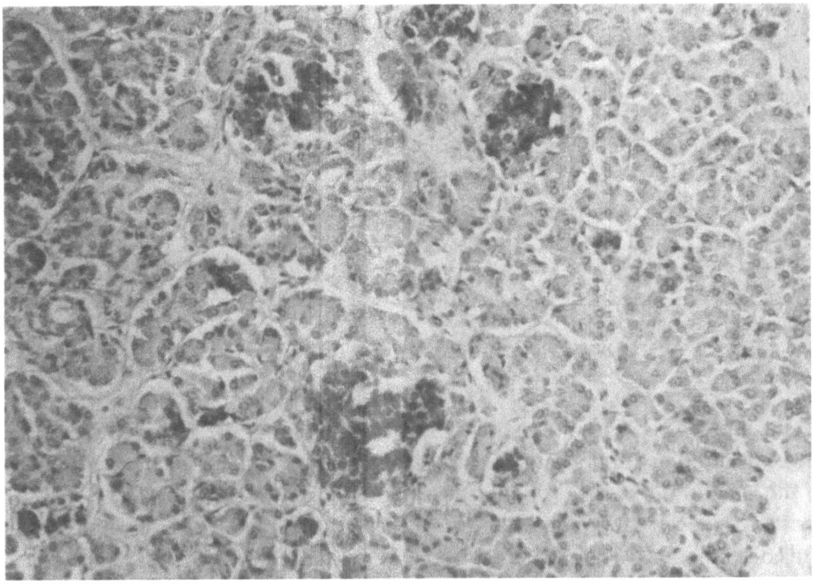

FIGURE 10.2. Photomicrograph of immunoperoxidase staining for insulin in acinar cells of the pancreas.

polypeptide-stained sections at low power, the examiner divided them into PP-rich and PP-poor regions. The identified regions were outlined with a mapping pen on that slide. Identical slides, stained to detect insulin, were superimposed on the pancreatic polypeptide "mapped" slides so that the PP-poor and PP-rich mapping could be transferred to them. Using the slides stained for insulin, the fractional surface area of each of the three pancreatic segments (head, body, and tail) occupied by immunostained cytoplasm (containing insulin) was measured using the Quantimet Automatic Image Analyzer (100 fields = 38.5 mm^2). In every case when feasible, up to three fields of each type—PP-poor and PP-rich—were assayed. Only in the head could both types be assessed; in the body and in the tail, only PP-poor islets were assayed. When two or three determinations of one type were made in one segment of the pancreas, they did not vary much from one to another.

Results

Statistical analysis of the data showed no significant difference in the fractional percent area of insulin-containing cells between SIDS and control infants in either the PP-poor or the PP-rich areas individually (Table 10.4) If the relative area occupied by beta cells reflects that occupied by the entire endocrine cell mass, then the tail of the pancreas in the infant, as in the adult, seems to contain the greatest numbers of islet cells (Table 10.4) as previously shown by Heitz et al.[11]

TABLE 10.4. Fractional percent area occupied by insulin-containing cells.

		SIDS cases	Control cases	p
Head	n[a]	65	17	
PP-poor	x[b]	1.87 + 0.58	1.98 + 0.58	.5
Body	n	36	7	
PP-poor	x	2.18 + 0.67	2.03 + 0.52	.6
Tail	n	33	5	
PP-poor	x	2.44 + 0.88	2.16 + 0.34	.5
Head	n	52	14	
PP-rich	x	1.09 + 0.50	1.01 + 0.37	.6

[a] Number of determinations in that category.
[b] Fractional percent area of insulin-containing beta cells in the pancreatic tissue.

One unexpected and interesting observation was that the relative percent area of the insulin-containing cells was consistently lower in the PP-rich "ventral" part of the head of the pancreas than it was in the *any* of the PP-poor areas – ie, all of the remainder of the organ, the "dorsal" part of the head, the body, and the tail. This discrepancy was observed, without exception, in both the SIDS and control infants (Table 10.4).

Because the relative percent area of beta cells is likely to diminish with increasing age of the infant as the result of disproportionate growth of acinar elements, one would expect the somewhat older *control* infants to have *lower* figures for the percent insulin-containing cells; our data suggest that, in general, this is correct (Table 10.4). The only exception was in the PP-poor areas in the head. Still, the difference between the means for cases and controls was not significant, and both appear to be well within the normal range.

Discussion

Jaffe et al[13] suggested that the normal range for total endocrine cell mass in infants 2 to 8 months of age was 5.1% to 7.7% (mean 6.1%).[13] If that is so, our data for insulin-containing cells, ranging from 1.01% to 2.18%, seem to be low because beta cells in infants comprise 58.8% of the total endocrine cell population[11]; 58.8% of 6.1% is 3.6%. However, our figures correspond to those of Heitz, who reported a mean of 2.4% for total combined cells and 1.4% for beta cells. Jaffe attributed the discrepancy between his own results and those of Heitz (and by inference, ours) to Heitz's use of an automatic image analyzer. Jaffe contends that mesenchymal tissue in infants of this age is an intimate component of the pancreas and that much of the endocrine tissue lies within it; thus, failure to exclude the connective tissue from the calculation leads to underestimation of the relative amount of endocrine tissue. Exclusion can be accomplished only by visual inspection, as Jaffe did, rather than by automatic analyzer. Therefore, it would appear that the insulin-containing cells of infants 2 to 4 months of age comprise roughly 1.8% of total pancreatic tissue and 3.6% of the pancreatic parenchyma.

One other group of investigators has presented data similar to ours, with *specific* reference to insulin containing cells in SIDS infants. Loo et al[16] reported in 1982 that there was no difference in relative area of pancreatic tissue occupied by beta cells in 23 SIDS infants and 38 controls. They used immunohistochemistry for identification of insulin-containing cells. The method they employed for quantitation was ocular micrometry. Their data showed that SIDS and control infants have similar "cell frequency and distribution" and that the incidence of "nesidioblastosis" is similar in the two groups.

Conclusion

The fractional percent area of insulin-containing islet cells in the pancreata of 80 SIDS infants and 17 controls is not significantly different. This confirmed earlier conclusions, some of which were based on determinations of total endocrine cell mass. The absence of hyperplasia of insulin-containing cells in SIDS infants does not necessarily exclude the possibility of hyperinsulinemia, since structure does not necessarily correspond to function. Nevertheless, on the basis of these results, it seems unlikely that significant numbers of crib deaths occur as the result of hypoglycemia secondary to hyperinsulinemia.

Acknowledgments. We are deeply indebted to Dr Alfred Steinschneider of the American SIDS Institute who so kindly arranged our access to the systematic collection of autopsy material at the Office of the Medical Examiner for the State of Maryland in Baltimore; to the late Dr Russel Fisher, then Director of that office; and to forensic pathologists there who performed the necropsies. We thank Dr Chen-Chih J. Sun for painstakingly reviewing every aspect of each of the 97 autopsies for us, and Dr Janet Cassady of the University of Miami for analyzing our data.

Our special gratitude is owed Professor R.D.G. Milner of the Children's Hospital of the University of Sheffield for graciously permitting us to work in his laboratory, and Dr Paul Wirdnam, his research assistant, who helped us immeasurably there.

References

1. Cox JM, Guelpa G, Terrapon M: Islet-cell hyperplasia and sudden infant death. (Letter.) *Lancet* 2:739–740, 1976.
2. Swift PGF, Emery JL: Personal communication.
3. Polak JJ, Wigglesworth JS: Islet-cell hyperplasia and sudden infant death. (Letter.) *Lancet* 2:570–571, 1976.
4. Polak JJ, Aynsley-Green A, Bloom SR, Wigglesworth JS: Nesidioblastosis as a cause of sudden neonatal death. *Scand J Gastroenterol* Suppl 49:143, 1978.
5. Gepts W: Pathologic anatomy of the pancreas in juvenile diabetes. *Diabetes* 14: 619–633, 1965.

6. Van Assche VFA: The foetal endocrine pancreas. A quantitative morphological approach. Ortho Pharmaceutica Thesis, Katholiek Universiteit, Belgium, 1970.
7. Kloppel G, Altenahr E, Menke B: The ultrastructure of focal islet cell adenomatosis in the newborn with hypoglycemia and hyperinsulinism: Contribution to the classification of neonatal insulinomas. *Virch Arch Pathol Anat Histol* 366:223–236, 1975.
8. Sovik O, Vidnes J, Falkmer S: Persistent neonatal hypoglycemia. *Acta Pathol Microbiol Scand* 83A:155–166, 1975.
9. Kissane JM: *Pathology of Infancy and Childhood*. St Louis: Mosby, 1975, p 334.
10. Jaffe R, Hashida Y, Yunis EJ: Pancreatic pathology in hyperinsulinemic hypoglycemia of infancy. *Lab Invest* 42:356–365, 1980.
11. Heitz PJ, Kloppel G, Hachi WH, Polak JJ, Pearse AGE: Nesidioblastosis: The pathologic basis of persistent hyperinsulinemic hypoglycemia in infants. Morphologic and quantitative analysis of seven cases based on immunostaining and electron microscopy. *Diabetes* 26:632–642, 1977.
12. Aynsley-Green A, Polak JJ, Keeling J, Gough MH, Baum JD: Averted sudden neonatal death due to pancreatic nesidioblastosis. (Letter.) *Lancet* 1:550–551, 1978.
13. Jaffe R, Hashida Y, Yunis EJ: The endocrine pancreas of the neonate and the infant. *Perspect Pediatr Pathol* 7:137–165, 1982.
14. Nadji M, Morales AR: *Immunoperoxidase Techniques. A Practical Approach to Tumor Diagnosis*. Chicago: ASCP Press, 1966, pp 3–5.
15. Baetens D, Malisse-Lagae F, Perrelet A, Orci L: Endocrine pancreas. Three dimensional reconstruction shows two types of islets of Langerhans. *Science* 206:1323–1325, 1979.
16. Loo SW, Kozakewich HP, Wald RA, Vawter GF: The sudden infant death syndrome and nesidioblastosis: No evidence for pathologic relationship. Lab Invest 46:10, 1982 (abstract).

11
Cot Death for Real! Families with Repeat SIDS

JOHN L. EMERY

When Enid Barness suggested the title "Cot Death for Real!" to me, I could not but agree. But when I came to look at the title again I wondered. I know what a cot is in England, but in the New World they are called cribs – they are structures made for children and babies to sleep in or on. I think I understand the meaning of the word "death," at least in its pathological sense, but when it comes to the meaning of "for real" I am on soft ground. When it comes to the meaning of reality, I have great sympathy with the great lexicographer Dr Johnson when, in defiance of Bishop Berkley, he kicked the stone and said, "That stone is real." But, even in this materialistic world, I still find myself unable to get round Berkley's concept of subjectivism[1] and cannot get away from the belief that "real" is what all of us believe at any one time.

Thus, I now believe that this world is round but that at the time of Christ the world was certainly equally flat. What it actually is I don't know, but I have no alternative now but to act as if the world is round. I do not know how many of you go along with your own contemporary philosopher David Lewis on the "plurality of worlds."[2] I find him a little difficult to follow at times. But we must not neglect him, as we professional allopaths tend to assume that we alone are concerned with the "real world."

The reason why Enid asked me to speak on this topic was, I suspect, because, when a few years ago she asked me, "What do you think is the cause of SIDS?," my reply was, "I don't believe in SIDS." She looked at me as the typical simple, ignorant limey that I am. Of course an argument has been going on ever since. I take the same line with my old friend Dr Molly Dapena, and she benignly looked down on me as a sort of "flat-earther." What I intend to do is to emulate Dr Johnson and "kick a few stones" related to the reality of the concept SIDS.

It has been my lot to dissect many children who have died, and, over a period of something like nearly 50 years as a full-time pediatric pathologist, I have

From the Wolfson Unit, Department of Paediatrics, University of Sheffield, Sheffield, England.
Presented in honor of Lewis A. Barness, MD, November 11, 1988.

carried out about 5,000 necropsies, including more than 2,000 on children who had presented as unexpected deaths at home, in cribs, in cots, in cars, and so forth—children who, in perhaps 95% of instances, would be called SIDS at the present time and in this country and in many other places. One of the most fascinating aspects of observing morbid anatomy over a long period has been that the grossness of pathology has progressively diminished. This is probably as striking in hospital deaths as in unexpected deaths at home. The gross conditions that we saw in England before and during the last war—empyema, osteomyelitis, really gross bronchopneumonia—are now just not around, although they are to be seen in hospitals serving the black population in South Africa. To some extent the present dilemma among pathologists concerning the so-called pathologies of unexpected death are an extension of this progressive disappearance of what may be called "classic pathology." However, my concern is not to talk about the philosophies of child pathology but to present at a pragmatic clinical level some recent studies that we have been carrying out in England in some of our attempts to grapple with some of the problems of unexpected child deaths.

In Europe we continually react to what happens in the United States. In 1970 the Seattle group created the concept of sudden infant death syndrome,[3] and Steinschneider[4] and others suggested that these deaths were due to apnoea unresponsiveness. They advocated the use of apnea monitors. One of the pediatric journals in the United States suggested that a pediatrician could be considered negligent if he did not prescribe the use of such a device in any child whom he thought to be at risk of unexpected death. Apnea monitors were being widely prescribed and were purchasable by the general public at drug stores. We in the United Kingdom were told about this, particularly by the lay press. Many of us who had read available literature were completely unconvinced by the evidence, not that apnea unresponsiveness does not occur, but that it was related to the majority of children presenting as unexpected deaths, or that apnea monitors could prevent such deaths. So, in July 1979 the British Foundation for the Study of Infant Deaths held a conference on apnea and unexpected child death, inviting speakers concerned with child respiratory physiology and also Albert Steinschneider. At the end of the conference it was agreed that the evidence for the association of apnea with unexpected child death was not there.[5] Steinschneider agreed that the evidence was incomplete, but insisted that from a scientific point of view the situation in the United States was completely out of hand, despite warning by Bergman et al.[6] It would now be impossible to attempt any sort of scientific or controlled study of the possibility that apnea monitors could affect the rate of unexpected child deaths.

Would such a study be possible in the United Kingdom? The logistics of such a study were daunting. The group that had been the target in the United States consisted of families that had had a previous cot death (Sibs of SIDS), but the prevalence of repeat deaths was uncertain.[7] It was thought that the risk was possibly 1 in 160, and this group was the one for which some parents were clamoring for help. Another group was twins, where the risk of cot death was probably greater than in the sibs of SIDS. This was a group in which there was no public call for monitors or particular support. The third possible group was those in which a risk of death had been derived on statistical grounds.[8] However, by that time we realized that we had highlighted many families with immense social problems, families that had such irregular lives that the use of a monitor would be both impractical and uncontrollable. Thus the only practical group was the sibs of SIDS. It was decided to do a pilot study first to see if parents would submit to a controlled trial when they had had a previous cot death. We also needed to explore alternative methods of support for the parents and see later whether it would be possible to ascertain in a controlled way, for the whole country, the advantage of any one system of support. These studies have been carried out over the past 8 years under the direction of Sylvia, Countess of Limerick, the leading lay person related to cot deaths in the United Kingdom; Robert Carpenter, medical statistician; and myself.

The pilot study was carried out using parents who had contacted the Foundation for the Study of Infant Deaths. Mothers were prepared to take part in a controlled trial, and 100 such subsequent births were followed.[9,10]

Parents completed a daily chart of all the symptoms that the child had, symptoms in siblings and the family, and events taking place in the family. The support system was organized through the family doctors and by health visitors who visited the home once a week. These personnel went through the symptom charts with the parents and discussed any problems that arose. As a control, we provided scales in the house for the parents to weigh the child every day. The weights were recorded on charts we had devised following the work by Kristiansson[11] which contained permissible variability lines. These charts had been derived by Carpenter from our long-term studies involving weights and symptoms in Sheffield.

This pilot study showed that parents were equally satisfied with the use of scales as with monitors, although they were able to get more immediate satisfaction with the monitors. There was greater ease in weaning parents from scales than monitors. Although the morbidity requirements for hospital admission were the same in the two groups, the number of symptoms that the parents with the children on monitors observed was lower than in those having scales. It was felt by many of the health visitors that when parents had the monitor there was a tendency for them to focus their attention on the monitor rather than on the child, and this was a probable cause of the difference in symptom reporting.

Having ascertained that a controlled trial was possible, we then tried to determine whether a controlled trial would be feasible throughout the country. A similar regimen was offered to administrative regions. By 1987 10% of the country had been covered, and by this time approximately 600 sibs of SIDS had been surveyed, 300 each with monitor or scales. The general findings regarding increased symptomatology in one group rather than the other and the general satisfaction of both regimens were maintained. There were six instances among these 600 sibs of SIDS in which the surveyed child had died, and these six deaths are reported here.

Case 1

The mother came to the surveillance scheme through the Cot Death Foundation. She was member of a local parent group, having had a girl who died as a cot death at 3 months. Her new pregnancy was normal. The baby boy weighted 3,280 g at term and was randomly allocated an apnea monitor. He was breast-fed for 3 weeks and then placed on bottle feeds, receiving cereal foods by 12 weeks. He attended the family doctor for a throat infection at 5 weeks and a chest infection at 28 weeks, antibiotics being given on both occasions. The apnea monitor was reported to have sounded 158 times during the 28 weeks that the child was on the machine, and on 119 instances the parents reported that the alarm was still ringing when they reached the baby, who was breathing, though shallowly. No mechanical fault in the monitor had been found.

As part of our regimen, the monitor, or scales, was used for 6 months or for 1 month after the age of the previous child's cot death, and so the monitor was withdrawn from this mother and child at 28 weeks, a couple of weeks later than usual because the child had a mild infection. The mother was happy to take the child off the monitor. Four weeks later the child died unexpectedly, and death was registered as "unexpected death in infancy."

When we first heard of this, the first reaction was "If we had left the monitor longer the child would not have died." When we looked into the whole case, the following came to light. First, these parents, aged 21 (mother) and 32 (father), had been drug addicts, and the father had been abused as a child. None of this had been recorded. The mother was a great user of medical facilities, went frequently to the clinic with the baby, but unfortunately not the same clinic of the surveillance health visitor who visited her once a week. She also ignored the advice given her by the clinic. When the baby was reported dead, the health visitor immediately visited her and found the mother's reaction not of grief but of relief. She was completely composed and simply said, "It has happened now." The mother also told the health visitor how happy she was now that she could go out in the evenings, "doing all the things one can't do with a baby," though she said that sometimes she felt a little guilty about feeling so happy. When we explored the period preceding the child's death, the mother said that the baby was "never satisfied," was always hungry, and was requiring too much sleep. Apparently, in the few days prior to death he had slept for a full 12 h, from 11 p.m. to 11 a.m. When we checked the weights from the clinic records, it became apparent that this child had gained no weight during the 14 weeks prior to its death, and its weight at the age of 26 weeks was the same as that at 15 weeks. During this time the health visitors had told the mother to take the baby to the medical officer at the clinic, but the mother had not done so.

We have only the local pathologist's report on the necropsy findings on this child. These were reported as typical of a cot death, but the story prior to the child's death with this excessive sleeping is so like some children that we have seen dying with hypernatremia that we suspect that there must have been a major biochemical upset at the time of death that had not been observed in the routine pathology.

Our research health visitor, interviewing the mother, was very disturbed about the mother's mental state, and an attempt was made to see if the mother could not be seen by a psychiatrist. This has not been possible. The mother's 15-year-old brother lives in the home, and he is deeply into glue sniffing. This boy has apparently been completely rejected by his own parents. The whole home situation of this mother is precarious, with virtually no extended family. Attempts are being made to persuade her not to have any further children. We have a feeling that we are innocent players in a very complicated and precarious home circumstance over which we have no control.

Case 2

These parents, an able seaman and his wife, had lost a little boy at the age of 11½ months, who had been found dead in his cot. No abnormalities were found at necropsy. The mother was very distressed and took an overdose of Valium on the Mothering Sunday following the child's death.

When she became pregnant again she joined our surveillance scheme. Following an apparently normal pregnancy, she was delivered at 40 weeks of a 3,160-g boy. The baby was randomly allocated scales, but at 11 days refused to feed all one day and had what was described as a possible apneic attack. He was admitted to the hospital, where no abnormalities were found, and he was discharged 2 days later. The mother was anxious, and the pediatrician prescribed the use of an apnea monitor. This was started at 5 weeks. At the age of 6 weeks he was readmitted to the hospital because the mother thought he was failing to thrive, although his weight gain plotted on the chart was satisfactory. The child was weaned but the mother remained very anxious, appeared to be in a state of depression, and was prescribed antidepressants.

He was readmitted for the third time at 9 weeks following two possible cyanotic attacks and was discharged after 6 days. When the child was 13 weeks old the father left for sea. Following this the mother's depression increased, and she was put on Valium. One week later the baby died (Fig. 11.1).

The mother said that the child had been well the night before. In the morning she went to him at breakfast and found him pale and unresponsive but still breathing; the apnea monitor was still clicking. She took him into her arms, and while he was in her arms he stopped breathing and the apnea alarm rang. She immediately commenced artificial respiration. The child was taken to the hospital, where resuscitative measures were attempted, but he was proclaimed dead a little later that day. The necropsy on the baby was carried out locally and revealed no abnormality.

A study of the family background of this child revealed that the father's brother was epileptic, the mother's brother was epileptic, and the father had two uncles who were epileptic. Two of this baby's maternal uncles had died in infancy unexpectedly of unknown causes.

This couple have since had another child. This child was taken to London Hospital and submitted to very extensive studies, where he was found to have an

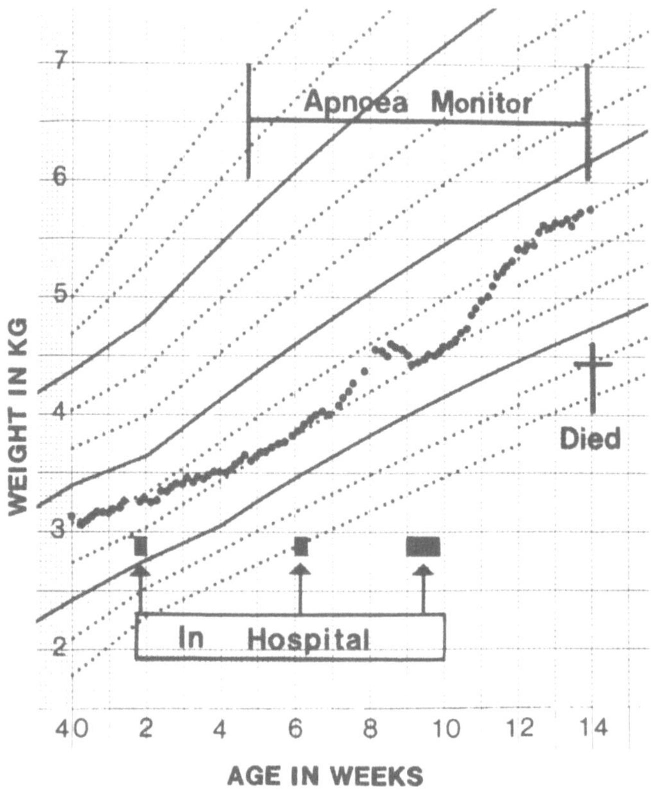

FIGURE 11.1. Weight chart of case 2. Child on both daily weighing and apnea monitor. (Note: in all figures, age in weeks on Sheffield growth charts.)

abnormal EEG. He was reared using an apnea monitor and scales from birth, but also received anticonvulsant therapy. He is now almost 2 years old, and although the EEG is still abnormal, he is progressing satisfactorily.

The necropsies on both of these children were done by general pathologists, and a full survey of tissues to exclude the presence of some type of familial dysplasia was not possible. It seems quite likely that the background of the deaths in this family could well be some type of familial dysplasia, possibly related to tuberosclerosis.

Case 3

This mother had had two cot deaths before she came to us. When she was 19 and unmarried, she had given birth to a healthy baby girl. That child was adopted and remains alive and well. She then married a man who had other children, became pregnant again, and had a baby by Cesarean section for fetal distress at 34 weeks' gestation. Birth weight was 1.82 kg (Fig. 11.2).

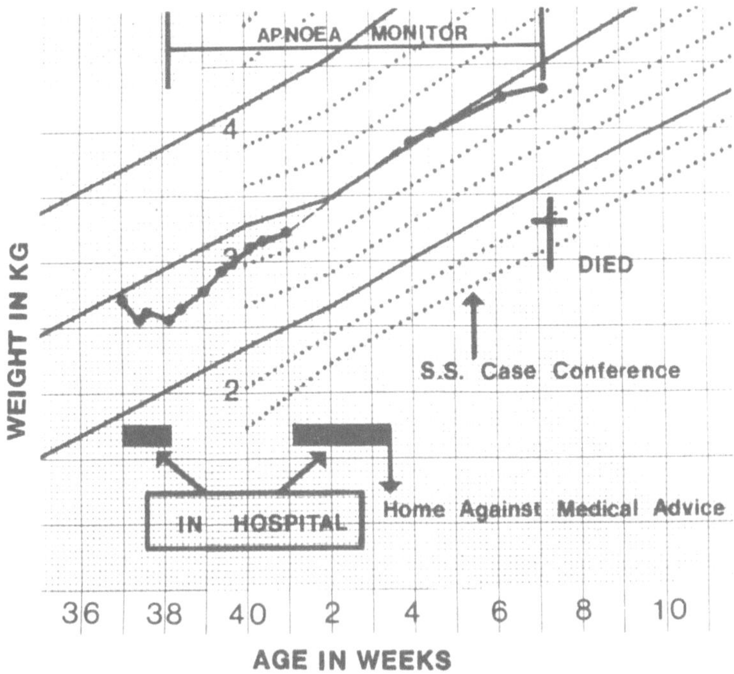

FIGURE 11.2. Weight chart of case 3.

The baby developed mild respiratory distress syndrome but did not need to be put on a ventilator. She was discharged at 4 weeks. At 13 weeks she was admitted for 14 h with a history of poor feeding and vomiting, but nothing abnormal was found. Following this the baby was seen in the hospital several times for afebrile convulsions, for one of which she was admitted. At no time were convulsions witnessed by any of the hospital or attending staff. The baby was found dead at home at the age of 4½ months. Necropsy was carried out by the local forensic pathologist, and a diagnosis of death from epilepsy was given. The comment at necropsy was that the child was thought to have been brain damaged due to prematurity and death was due to natural causes.

The third child was born 9 months later, again delivered by Cesarean section at 34 weeks, weighed 2.12 kg, and required intubation. She did not have respiratory distress but had jaundice requiring phototherapy. She was discharged fit and was apparently developing well until she developed what was described as an "apneic episode" at home at 5 months. This child was examined in great detail. An initial EEG was thought to be abnormal but was later reported as normal. No fits were observed while the child was under my supervision. The child was sent home and was found dead as a cot death at the age of 8 months. This child had been issued an apnea alarm, but it had not been used. Necropsy was carried out by a forensic pathologist of very high standing who found nothing abnormal, and a diagnosis of sudden infant death syndrome was made.

The fourth child was the one that was our concern. This baby was also born by elective Cesarean section at 37 weeks' gestation and weighed 2.7 kg. This child required no initial resuscitation and came under our Sibs of SIDS scheme, being allocated an apnea monitor. When she was about a month old she was admitted to the hospital with a history of a possible apenic attack, and while on the ward an episode occurred in which the apnea alarm rang. All investigations were negative, and the mother took the baby home from the hospital against medical advice. A vast amount of time and care was spent on this family. The weekly health visitor's report from home indicated that the health visitors and social services, as well as a clinical psychologist, were extremely worried.

However, when the baby was 3 months old, the mother said that she responded to an apnea alarm and found the baby dead. The health visitor had examined the child at home half an hour earlier and had thought the child to be well. Again at necropsy by the forensic pathologist, no lesions other than those likely to be associated with terminal asphyxia were found, and this child also was diagnosed as sudden infant death syndrome.

Meanwhile, a further incidence had taken place that was a little disturbing. When this mother was pregnant at 6 months with her most recent child, she was baby-sitting for a friend. While she was baby-sitting, the child died as a cot death. The forensic pathologist's report for this child reads as follows:

> The findings at autopsy are essentially negative. This is entirely in keeping with natural death from Sudden Infant Death Syndrome. But it is impossible entirely to exclude some mechanical means of suffocation. This difficulty is always the case in all cases of Sudden Infant Death and there is no evidence in this baby to suggest that suffocation has in fact taken place.

What would you advise we do about this woman's next baby?

Case 4

Our study case was the fourth pregnancy of a young woman who had had one miscarriage and three live births, with one surviving child of 2 years. She was aged 21 and cohabiting with an unemployed man of 20. She was uncertain of the parentage of her children. The child who had died as a cot death was a boy, who died at the age of 13 weeks.

In the pregnancy leading to the birth of the child we were concerned with, she had had a small antepartum hemorrhage but a normal spontaneous birth of a boy weighing 2.6 kg. There was some difficulty with the child's breathing at birth, and he was in an incubator for 2 days. He was randomly allocated an apnea monitor and was sent home.

At the age of 1 week, he developed thrush which lasted 3 weeks, and at 5 weeks an umbilical hernia was noticed. The parents reported "great difficulties with the monitor, particularly in keeping the sensor attached to the baby." There were frequent alarms associated with mechanical defects. However, no defects could be found by the health visitor and other staff. The mother did not use the monitor consistently and probably discontinued it. At 9 weeks the health visitor thought that the baby was overweight, but the mother would not accept advice about feeding. The baby was found dead in its cot at the age of 14 weeks, not on the monitor. Two weeks prior to this the mother had failed to fill in the symptom chart, and for 4 nights before his death they had called in the emergency medical service because the baby had excessive crying, for which Merbentyl was prescribed.

This mother and child were part of a very well known problem family complex in the inner-city area in which they dwelt. This mother dressed well and presented herself well. Extreme difficulty was experienced in getting an adequate history from this family, as they told completely different stories to different people. For example, while the mother admitted that both she and her cohabitee smoked more than 20 cigarettes a day, she claimed that they did not drink alcohol. The health visitor describes a visit to the mother 2 days after the baby's death as follows:

> When I arrived Tuesday morning I had difficulty in waking them up. Eventually a relative of George's (the co-habitee) answered the door. He and his "wife" had stayed the night because "they were all too drunk to go anywhere else." I was concerned to see this couple. Their 3 children are in care for N.A.I. Mary (the mother) was woken up. . . . She said that she had "drunk rather a lot to get to sleep."

Autopsy on this child revealed no evidence of any violence, and death was ascribed to sudden infant death syndrome, as had been the death of the previous child. The people looking after this family say that this woman attends clinics regularly and goes through all the gestures of conforming, but ignores advice and has what they consider to be an abysmal level of parenting ability. Her one surviving child is apparently being looked after by the grandmother.

Case 5

This was the fourth pregnancy of a woman of 23 and a man of 22 who was unemployed. The woman had had two miscarriages and one live birth. The live-born child had been apparently normal at birth and had died completely unexpectedly at the age of 2 days in the hospital. No cause for death was found, and the child had been diagnosed as a cot death.

The present pregnancy had been complicated by proteinurea, edema, and hypertension. She was found to have twins, both of whom were delivered naturally at 38 weeks, one weighing 2.21 kg and the other 2.68 kg. The twins were binovular, but the placenta of twin 1, the smaller twin, was reported to be "very infarcted." This twin required tube feeding for the first few days but was otherwise normal.

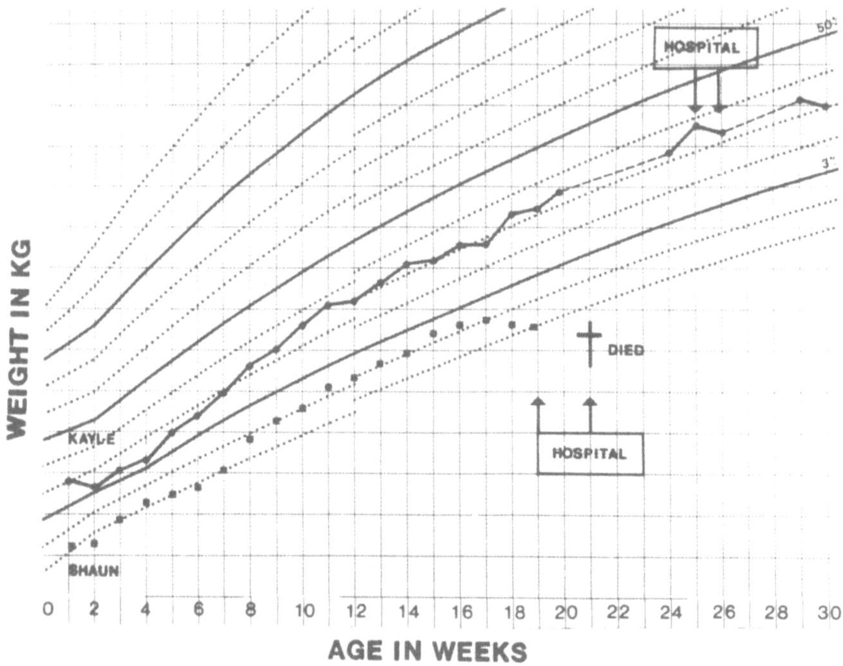

FIGURE 11.3. Simplified weight charts of the twins—case 5.

The twins went home with scales for daily weighing (Fig. 11.3). Both children put on weight fairly consistently, although the father, who did the weighing, was worried if the children did not put on weight every day. Both children had occasional sniffles, coughs, and loose stools, and twin 1, who died, was taken to the hospital with loose stools and diarrhea at the age of 6 weeks but was not admitted. At 8 weeks he had oral and genital thrush which cleared up by week 10 on Nystatin cream. However, in week 12 the thrush returned and the child vomited and had loose stools for 3 days, treated by the family doctor. The occasional vomiting continued during the 12th week, but when he was given a general checkup by the pediatrician in the hospital, he was found to be bright and alert. However, during the 15th week he gained no weight, and there was some abdominal pain, and he was taken to the hospital and admitted on the surgical side as a possible intussusception. He was discharged within a few days, continued to lose weight, and was readmitted on the medical side during his 18th week. He was extremely ill, hypoglycemic, with a large liver, and died 2 weeks later despite very intensive medical care. The clinical presentation of the child was that of a Reye's syndrome. At necropsy an extremely fatty liver was found, and after a number of investigations the diagnosis of a medium-chain amino acid deficiency state was made.

The surviving twin was examined but has continued to grow and develop in a normal fashion. When the previous child death was explored it was found that

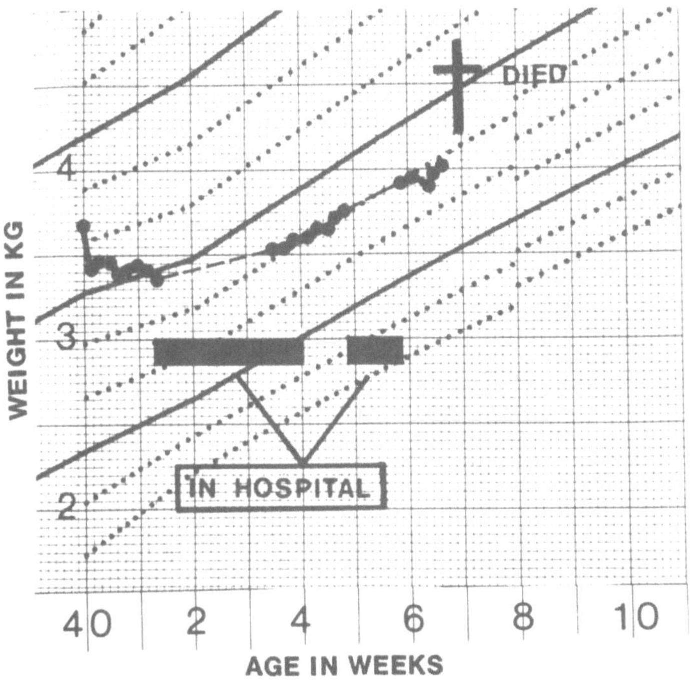

FIGURE 11.4. Weight chart from case 6.

that child had a histological abnormality of the liver which is currently being investigated. The whole background to these cases is that of a hereditary metabolic error.

Case 6

The father of this child was 22 and Chilean and the mother 19 and half Arab. They had had one previous child a year earlier, who died at the age of 3 weeks, having been diagnosed as a SIDS. The family were nonsmokers, the mother did not drink, the father drank occasionally. They were unmarried, and the father was unemployed.

This pregnancy was uncomplicated. An elective Cesarean section was carried out at term, producing a female child weighing 3.68 kg. She was completely normal at birth, required no resuscitation, and had no abnormal symptoms in the neonatal period. She went home on day 5 with scales (Fig. 11.4).

At home she did not thrive and was readmitted to the hospital. The nurses found her extremely difficult to feed, and she occasionally vomited, so she was thought to have a pyloric stenosis. This was not confirmed. Altered pigmentation and lumps had been apparent in the child's skin, and neurofibromatosis had been diagnosed. It was thought that the failure to thrive might have had something to do with her neurofibromatosis. She was given slightly thickened feeds, gained a little weight, and was discharged home on an open-door basis; ie, the mother could bring the child back to the hospital and have her admitted immediately on request.

The mother had no experience whatsoever in handling children and could not cope, and after a week at home the baby was readmitted for about 10 days. In the middle of the 6th week after birth the mother went to the baby at about 9:00 in the morning, found her floppy, and picked her up, obviously dead. This occurred while the husband was running in the local marathon.

Postmortem examination showed an apparently well-cared-for but small child. There were neurofibromata of the skin and over the right psoas muscle, but no lesions were noticed within the viscera, except for a possible area of dysplasia in the cerebellum. As no immediate cause of death could be found, the child was recorded as "unexpected death in infancy," with neurofibromatosis as a possible contributory cause.

Reading the case notes in the ward and those of the health visitor and family doctor, it was obvious that all were worried about this child and all were aware that the child was not thriving, and no one seemed capable of doing anything about it. When interviewed, the mother said that she had killed the child, meaning that she had killed the child by giving it her familial disease. One of the mother's sisters died from a brain tumor associated with neurofibromatosis. She has a living sister with neurofibromatosis, and she herself has neurofibromatosis and has had masses removed from her own back. She had an elder sibling who died in infancy from what was then diagnosed as bronchial pneumonia. This couple have since separated.

When the previous cot death had occurred, the pathologist doing the postmortem had had no history of neurofibromatosis and had not made any particular search for the condition. A review of the sections available from the necropsy revealed no lesions.

Discussion

What do these cases add up to? Here we have the complete repeat death roll from 600 children who have been registered as siblings of SIDS throughout the United Kingdom. They all appear to be different, and not one of them is a "SIDS" in the Beckwithian style. Are these "cot deaths for real?" While too much notice should not be taken of a series of six deaths, it is completely unselected, being all of the repeat cot deaths in 600 families known to their family doctors, their pediatricians, and health visitors as having had a true SIDS, and this in England, where the necropsy rate leading to this diagnosis is still well over 95%.

Could any of these repeat deaths have been prevented? It is possible that the first child, if the weights had been recorded appropriately, would have been admitted to the hospital, and something possibly could have been done about it.

Case 2 is an open question. In the series of deaths that included case 3, if the concept of SIDS had not been so well established that it is virtually impossible to go to a court of law without evidence of massive physical abuse, the situation could have been different. If that woman's child had been taken into care as several had wanted at the case conference a few weeks before death, it is possible that the child would be alive now.

In case 4, the total circumstances of that child's life and death were such that the use of home help or some sort of local assistance could well have prevented that child's death. With cases 5 and 6, the child with probable Reye's syndrome and the family with neurofibromatosis, there are still considerable questions. Had the one child not been on our surveillance scheme, it is extremely likely that it would have died at home unexpectedly. In the neurofibromatosis family, the family history had not come to light at the time of the first cot death.

Before discussing further it is necessary to point out that with the six deaths we have looked at, we are only able to comment on 6 of the 600 families in our study, and these six are of necessity a special group. We cannot comment on the others. There is an increasing literature on repeat cot deaths with as yet no clear pictures.[12,13]

The death rate in our study has been higher than we had expected. We are now bringing this attempt at a controlled trial of the efficacy of apnea monitors for the prevention of cot deaths to a close. We have a death rate of 1 in 100 in these families. Two children died while on apnea monitors, but were they true cot deaths? The pressure to investigate the efficacy of apnea monitors in preventing cot deaths has now virtually disappeared, but the study has left us a little unhappy. Our attempts to prevent baby deaths using monitors is certainly not successful. Could we be doing harm? In a study in France in which apnea monitors were used in many centers involving nearly 1,000 children, the death rate of those on monitors was higher than that in children not on monitors.[14]

We introduced daily home weighing as an alternative to apnea monitors, as we had noticed that some children lost weight before presenting as unexpected deaths. In our current study, in the children being weighed the scales seemed to alert us to the probability that something was wrong. But we see scales as part of general support and in no way confined to children at risk of unexpected death.

Since the notion of SIDS was first introduced and it became a registerable cause of death, there has been a transfer of death registrations from (in particular) acute respiratory tract infection to SIDS in almost all countries in the world. There has been a tendency at the same time, however, for the total number of cases of postperinatal deaths to either flatten out or increase as is shown by the chart from Australia produced by Newman. This can be only partially explained by bringing in other conditions than acute infections.

If we look at the numbers of deaths and rates of deaths in children, we are now seeing continuing falls in baby mortalities in almost all countries in everything except unexpected home death rates and the death rates in children between the ages of 1 month and 1 year. In these we are observing a rise. This rise is only partially explained by the shift of deaths from the perinatal to the postperinatal period. This has been noted in Scandinavia, where they have very low overall rates,[15,16] and also at the opposite end of the world, in New Zealand.[17]

The question I think we need to ask is: "Is the whole idea of SIDS limiting us as we look at the apparently increasing presentation of children as unexpected deaths, and can the concept itself be increasing the numbers?" If, as some of us believe, up to 1 in 10 of children presenting and diagnosed as SIDS[18] is filicide, there is a danger in this group of the SIDS diagnosis being a license to kill. An original reason for the introduction of the term "SIDS" was because too many parents were falsely accused of killing their children. Have we now swung too far the other way?

Consequent upon the use of the diagnosis of SIDS, we are seeing in the United Kingdom and in Europe a tendency toward a reduction of the study in depth of many of these children, with coroners tending to refrain from asking for necropsies. A coroner recently asked, "Why pay a pathologist to find nothing and probably cause the parents the unnecessary disturbance of a necropsy?" In a highly developed country like Holland, necropsies are carried out on only 50% of children presenting as unexpected deaths.[19] If the numbers of unexpected home deaths were falling, perhaps all would be well, but with the evident rise, we need to look at the whole situation closely.

To pretend that, with all the skill in the world, we would be able to explain all unexpected deaths, would be nonsense. There are completely unexplained deaths in all age groups, particularly in the very old and the very young. The question is, what is the best method of study? A recent dramatic article by Carolyn Szybist,[20] a parent of an unexpected child death in Chicago, written on the 21st anniversary of the baby's death, ends with the sentence, "Will there be a coming of age for the Sudden Infant Death Syndrome?" It is to be hoped so. But how?

Perhaps before I stop on this occasion of honoring one of the greatest medical editors of our day, I may venture to discuss the use of one of the words that we use in our trade. In this country, where "SIDS" was invented, when someone dies, a postmortem examination and autopsy are conducted. When I was younger I was instructed on how to carry out a necropsy. The word necropsy means "looking at the dead," but the word autopsy is not quite so simple. My Greek scholar friends tell me that while autopsy can mean, as many pathology books tell us, "to *look* for onself," its chief meaning is that of looking "*at* oneself." It is a truism that we can see only what we know or what our minds allow us to see. Since it is easy to find almost nothing at necropsy, the diagnosis of SIDS at necropsy is perhaps too seductive–or, to make an "abortionable" word, too "autopsive."

Acknowledgments. This study was funded by the Foundation for the Study of Infant Deaths, depending on the active help of health visitors, family doctors, and pediatricians. With the cases reported here we are particularly indebted to Dr K. Dodd, Dr S. Eades, Dr J. Harris, Dr A.C. Hunt, Dr J. Hyde, Dr T. Perham, Mrs Purcel, Dr J. Sills, Dr M. Smith, Dr T. Taylor, Mrs M. Trobridge, Dr S. Variend, and Mrs A. Waite.

References

1. Berkeley G: *The Principles of Human Knowledge*. London: T. Nelson, 1942.
2. Lewis D: *On the Plurality of Worlds*. Oxford, UK: Blackwell, 1986.
3. Beckwith JB: Discussion of terminology and definition of sudden infant death syndrome. In Bergman AB, Beckwith JB, Ray CG (eds): *Proceedings of the Second International Conference on Causes of Sudden Death in Infants*. Seattle: University of Washington Press, 1970.
4. Steinschneider A: Prolonged apnoea and the sudden infant death syndrome: Clinical and laboratory observations. *Pediatrics* 50(4):646–654, 1973.
5. Conference on Apnoea and Unexpected Child Death sponsored by the Foundation for the Study of Infant Deaths, July 15–16, 1979. London: FSID.
6. Bergman AB, Beckwith JB, Ray CG: The apnoea monitor business. *Pediatrics* 56:1–2, 1975.
7. Peterson DR, Chinn NM, Fisher LD: The suddent infant death syndrome—repetition in families. *J Pediatr* 97:265, 1980.
8. Carpenter RG, Gardner A, McWeeny PM, Emery JL: Multistage scoring system for identifying infants at risk of unexpected death. *Arch Dis Child* 52(8):606–612, 1977.
9. Emery JL, Waite AJ, Carpenter RG, Limerick SR, Blake D: Apnoea monitors compared with weighing scales for siblings after cot death. *Arch Dis Child* 60:1053–1060, 1985.
10. Waite AJ: Managing subsequent sibling of cot death victims. *Health Visitor* 61: 244–246, 1988.
11. Kristiansson B: *Low Weight Gain in Infancy and Early Childhood. A Clinical Prospective Study.* Goteborg, Sweden: Department of Paediatrics, University of Goteborg.
12. Beal SM, Blundell HK: Recurrence incidence of sudden infant death syndrome. *Arch Dis Child* 63:924–930, 1988.
13. Emery JL: Families in which two or more cot deaths have occurred. *Lancet* 1:313–315, 1986.
14. Monod N: Personal communication.
15. Norvenius SG: Sudden infant death syndrome in Sweden 1973–1977 and 1979. *Acta Paediatr Scand* (Suppl):333:138, 1987.
16. Norvenius SG: Personal communication, 1988.
17. Hassall IB: Sudden infant death syndrome: A serious New Zealand health problem. *NZ Med J* 99:233–234, 1986.
18. Emery JL, Taylor EM: Investigation of SIDS. (Letter.) *Lancet* 2:1676, 1986.
19. Huber J: Review of 60 cases of sudden and unexpected infant deaths. *Pediatr Pathol* 8:345, 1988.
20. Szybist C: Sudden infant death syndrome revisited. *J Dev Behav Pediatr* 9(1):33–37, 1988.

12
Metabolic Cardiomyopathy of Childhood

ENID GILBERT-BARNESS

Introduction

The cardiomyopathies are a group of disorders characterized by an intrinsic decrease in myocardial contractility. As long as stroke volume is maintained, congestive heart failure does not occur. However, when stroke volume falls, congestive heart failure ensues.[1,2]

Given the work distribution of the mature heart, left ventricular failure predominates, with tachypnea, dyspnea, and pulmonary edema. Hepatomegaly, venous distension, and ascites are relatively late findings. Dysrhythmias are common and are exacerbated by catecholamines, digitalis, electrolyte disturbances, and acidosis. Mural thrombi occur with embolization, especially to the cerebral circulation. The dilated left atrium can compress or collapse the left mainstem or left lower lobe bronchus, with resultant ventilation-perfusion abnormalities. Death due to cardiomyopathy results from congestive cardiac failure, cardiogenic shock, dysrhythmias, thromboembolic phenomena, or pulmonary dysfunction.[3,4]

The World Health Organization has divided congestive cardiomyopathy into two categories: (1) primary, or idiopathic; and (2) secondary, or related to underlying definable systemic disorders.[1]

A list of metabolic disorders that both frequently and predominantly affect the cardiovascular system is shown in Table 12.1. Many metabolic diseases result in myocardial involvement with cardiomyopathy of the three functional types: (1) congestive, as in carnitine deficiency; (2) obstructive, as in Fabry disease; or (3) restrictive, as in Gaucher's disease, or in the glycogen storage diseases, types II to IV, mucolipidoses, sphingolipidoses, and neuronal ceroid lipofuscinosis. In addition, neuromuscular disorders may be associated with congestive cardiomyopathy due to disturbance of the contractility of the myocardium.

From the Departments of Pathology and Pediatrics, University of Wisconsin School of Medicine, Madison, Wisconsin.
Presented in honor of Lewis A. Barness, MD, November 11, 1988.

TABLE 12.1. Metabolic cardiomyopathies.

- Disorders of amino acid metabolism
  - Alkaptonuria
  - Homocystinuria
  - Oxalosis
  - Hyperglycinemia
- Storage diseases
  - Glycogen storage diseases (Types II, III, IV)
  - Mucopolysaccharidoses
  - Mucolipidoses
    - I cell disease
    - Gangliosidioses GM_1 types I and II
      GM_2 types I and II
  - Lipid storage diseases
    - Fabry disease
    - Gaucher disease
    - Neuronal ceroid lipofuscinosis
- Carnitine deficiency
  - Primary
  - Secondary
- Disorders of metal and pigment metabolism
  - Hemosiderosis and hemochromatosis
  - Wilson's disease
  - Menkes' kinky hair syndrome
  - Dubin-Johnson syndrome
- Neuromuscular diseases
  - Duchenne muscular dystrophy
  - Becker's muscular dystrophy
  - Nemaline myopathy
  - Malignant hyperthermia
  - Familial periodic paralysis
  - Friedreich's ataxia
  - Kugelberg-Welander syndrome
  - Myotubular myopathy
  - Kearns-Sayre syndrome
  - Mitochondrial myopathies
- Connective tissue disorders
  - Marfan syndrome
  - Ehlers-Danlos syndrome
  - Osteogenesis imperfecta
  - Pseudo-xanthoma elasticum
- Neonatal effects of maternal disorders
  - Infant of diabetic mother
  - Thyrotoxic cardiomyopathy
- Catecholamine cardiomyopathy

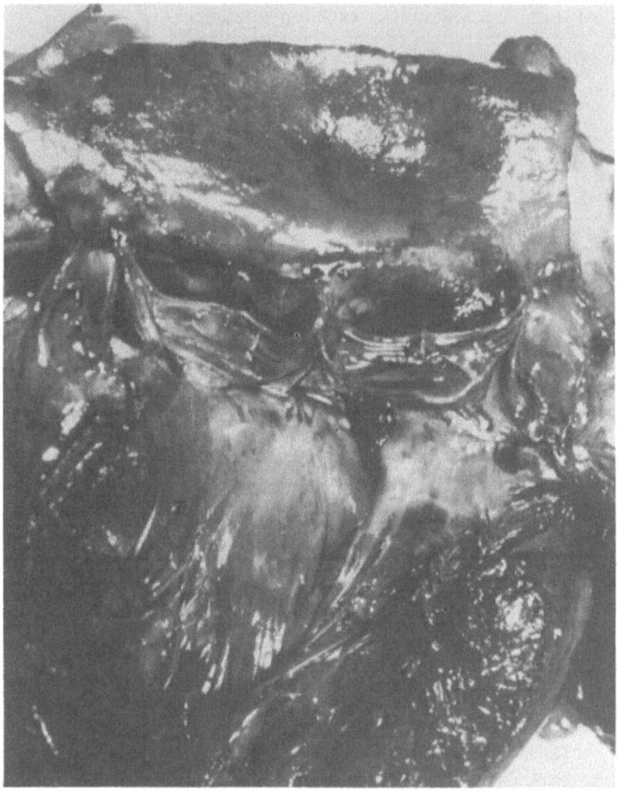

FIGURE 12.1. Gross appearance of the heart in alkaptonuria. The aortic valve cusps and the endocardium are heavily pigmented. From ref. 8, with permission.

Restrictive or congestive forms of cardiomyopathy may occur in patients with metal and pigment metabolic disorders and include iron storage disease, either hemochromatosis or hemosiderosis secondary to multiple transfusions, Wilson's disease, and Menkes' kinky hair syndrome.

Connective tissue disorders such as Marfan syndrome and osteogenesis imperfecta may involve the cardiovascular system, frequently with predominant involvement of the cardiac valves.

Disorders of Amino Acid Metabolism

Alkaptonuria

Alkaptonuria, a recessive trait, results in the deposition of pigment produced by the oxidation and polymerization of homogentisic acid, an intermediate metabolite of tyrosine and phenylalanine.[5,6] Ochronotic pigment is deposited in cartilage, skin, and sclerae as well as the heart valves and valvular annuli, especially

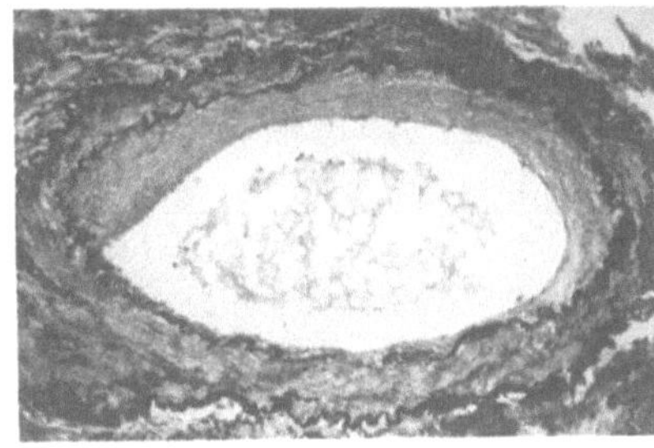

FIGURE 12.2. Cross section of a pulmonary artery showing thick fragmented elastic tissue in homocystinuria. (Elastic van Gieson, mag ×65.)

the mitral and aortic valves, the endocardium, the aorta, and the coronary arteries (Fig. 12.1). The atherosclerotic process is accelerated by the deposition of ochronotic pigment, and a frequent mode of death in patients with alkaptonuria is myocardial infarction from coronary atherosclerosis.[7,8] The melaninlike pigment is deposited both intra- and extracellularly.

Homocystinuria

A defect in the activity of cystathionine synthetase, which converts homocysteine to cystathionine, results in homocystinuria with mental retardation, seizures, skeletal deformities, ectopia lentis similar to that seen in the Marfan syndrome, and occlusive vascular disease. Histologically, the aorta shows intimal thickening and marked fragmentation of elastic fibers.[9] Muscular arteries demonstrate marked fibromuscular intimal thickening, fragmentation of the internal elastic lamina, and medial fibrosis (Fig. 12.2).[9] Thrombosis related to an increase in platelet consumption and a decrease in platelet survival time and pronounced fragility of the endothelium predispose to the formation of platelet thrombi.[9]

Oxalosis

Primary oxalosis, an autosomal-recessive trait, includes two rare disorders of glyoxalate metabolism.[10] It is characterized by nephrocalcinosis and by extrarenal deposits of calcium oxalate.

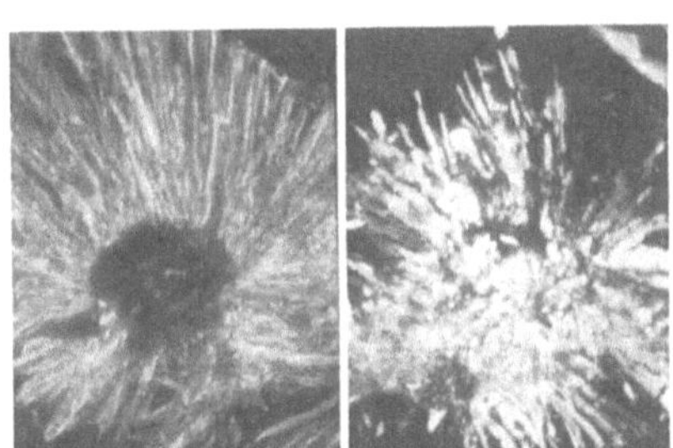

FIGURE 12.3. Oxalate crystals as seen under polarized light in primary oxalosis involving the conduction system of the heart (mag ×260.) From ref. 8, with permission.

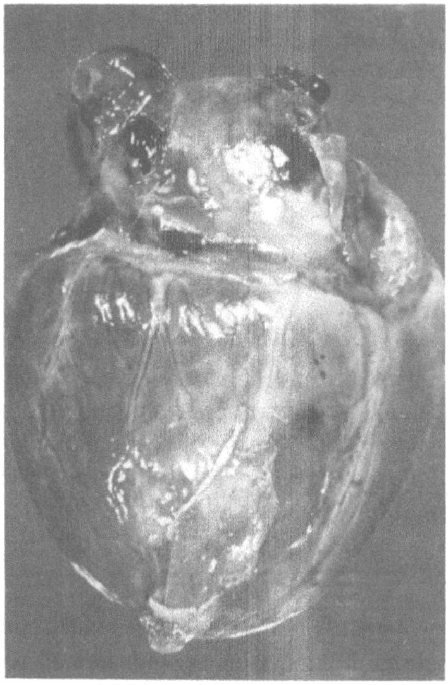

FIGURE 12.4. Large globular heart in glycogen storage disease, type 2 (Pompe's disease). From ref. 8, with permission.

In type I, the most common form of the disease, deficiency of 2-oxoglutarate: glyoxylate carboligase, results in systemic accumulation of glyoxylate and excessive urinary excretion of oxalic, glycolic, and glyoxylic acids. In type II (L-glyceric aciduria), deficiency of D-glyceric dehydrogenase results in accumulation of hydroxypyruvate and excessive urinary excretion of oxalic and glyceric acids. The heart is the site of widespread deposition of oxalate crystals.[11-14] including the conduction system (Fig. 12.3). Oxalate crystals in arterioles and capillaries are often larger than the vessel wall and may extrude from them.

Secondary oxalosis due to ingestion of oxalic acid, oxalates, or ethylene glycol; hyperalimentation or enteric hyperoxaluria occurring in patients with severe disease of the small bowel; and pyridoxine deficiency[10] resulting from chronic renal insufficiency have resulted in oxalate deposition in the heart and blood vessels.[15-17]

Hyperglycinemia

Fatal cardiomyopathy has been reported in an 8-year-old girl with hyperglycinemia due to β-ketothiolase deficiency.[18]

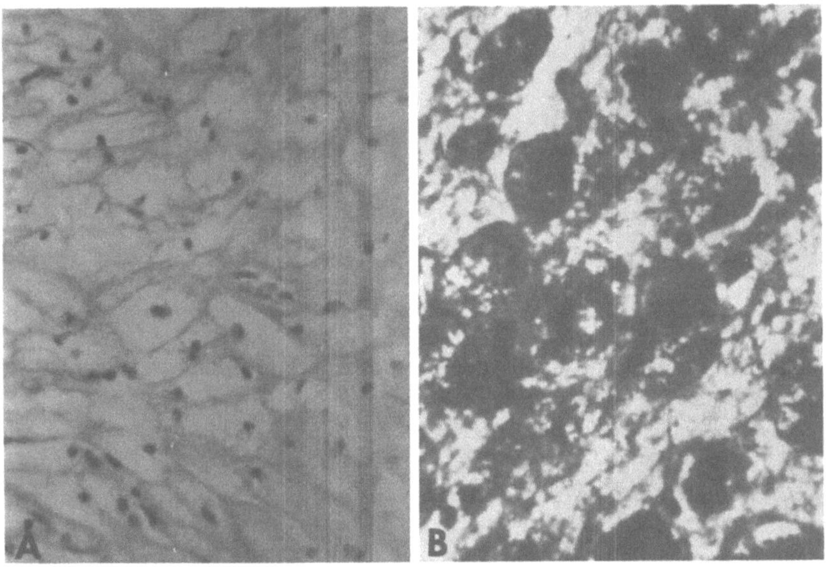

FIGURE 12.5. (A) Glycogen storage disease, type II. Microscopic section of the heart showing vacuolated myocardial fibers filled. (H&E, mag ×100.) (B) PAS stain showing positive reaction in myocardial cells due to glycogen (mag ×100.) From ref. 8, with permission.

Storage Diseases

Glycogen Storage Diseases (GSD)

In type II (Pompe's disease), type III (Cori's disease), and type IV GSD (Andersen's disease), cardiac involvement may occur,[9] resulting in accumulation of glycogen in the heart and blood vessels.

In Pompe's disease, the heart is grossly enlarged (Fig. 12.4) and the walls of all chambers are thickened, especially the left ventricular free wall and the papillary muscles.[19-22]

Fibroelastic thickening of the endocardium occurs in about 20% of patients with Pompe's disease.[23] The cardiac muscle cells show massive glycogen deposits (Fig. 12.5) that are also present in vascular smooth muscle and endothelium.[24,25] The myocardial glycogen content is increased[26,27] up to 9% of wet tissue weight (normal, 0.77%).[28]

Cardiac involvement in type III and type IV glycogen storage diseases is less common.

Two other, milder forms of GSD type II, the juvenile and the adult types, show predominantly skeletal muscle involvement simulating muscular dystrophy.

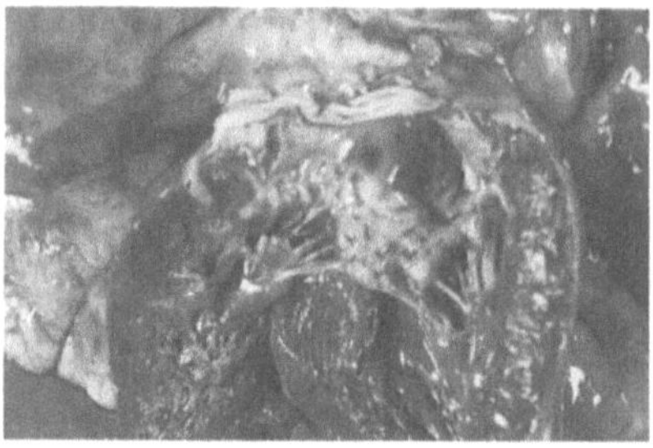

FIGURE 12.6. Gross appearance of the heart in mucopolysaccharidosis, type I, showing hypertrophy of the heart. The mitral valve is greatly thickened and distorted.

Fatal infantile cardiomyopathy due to phosphorylase β-kinase deficiency has been reported.[29-31]

Mucopolysaccharidoses (MPS)

Mucopolysaccharidoses are characterized by deficiencies in lysosomal enzymes involved in the degradation of various glycosaminoglycans. Severe cardiac involvement occurs in MPS I, Hurler's syndrome, MPS I-H (Scheie syndrome), MPS I-HS (Hurler-Scheie syndrome), MPS II (Hunter syndrome) and MPS III A-D (Sanfilippo syndrome).

Cardiovascular lesions involve the valves, endocardium, myocardium, coronary arteries, and large systemic arteries. The valves are thickened, and chordae tendineae of the atrioventricular valves are moderately shortened and thickened (Fig. 12.6). The large extramural coronary arteries are rigid and thickened, and their lumina are severely narrowed. The aorta and large systemic arteries have raised intimal plaques. Lipid and acid mucopolysaccharide accumulate in the cardiac muscle cells, and the coronary arteries and the heart valves also contain deposits of glycolipid. In contrast, the lesions in peripheral arteries resemble fibrous atherosclerotic plaques.[32] In these disorders death usually results from cardiac failure.

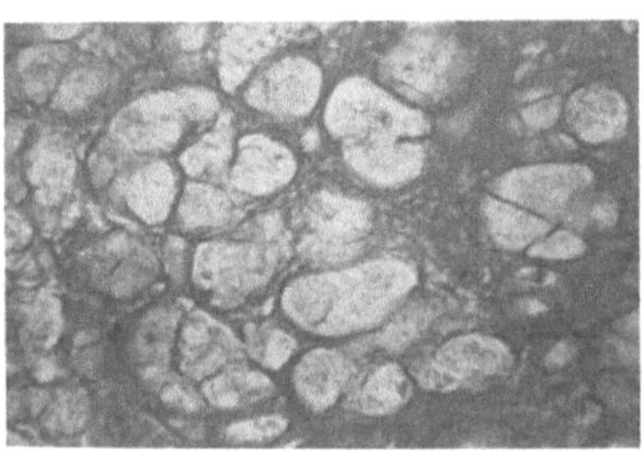

FIGURE 12.7. Microscopic section of the myocardium in I cell disease. The cells are distended and vacuolated, and contain granular material. (PAS, mag ×165.)

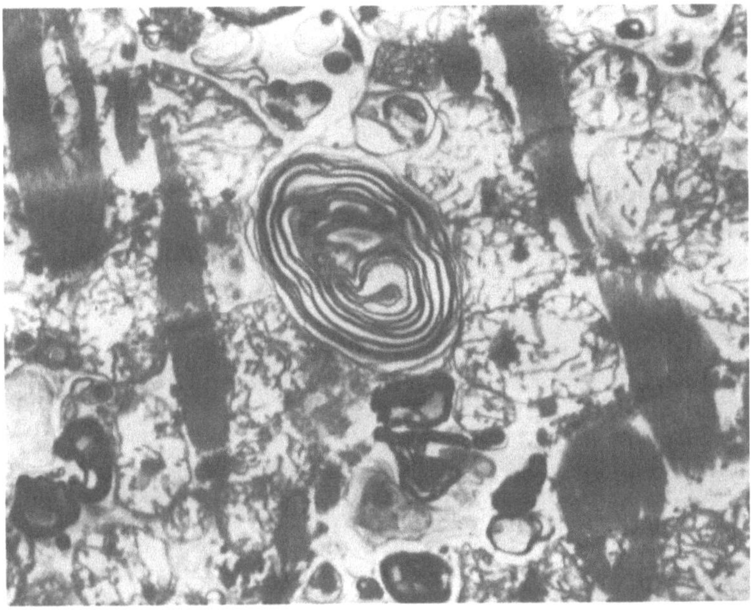

FIGURE 12.8. Electron micrograph of the heart in GM_1 gagliosidosis showing myocardial cell with concentric membranous body. (Uranyl acetate and lead citrate, mag ×7,550.) From ref. 8, with permission.

Mucolipidoses

Mucolipidosis II

In mucolipidosis II (I cell disease), an autosomal-recessive trait, there is a deficiency of multiple lysosomal hydrolases active in the degradation of lipids and mucopolysaccharides. The changes in the cardiovascular systems are similar to those seen in the mucopolysaccharidoses (Fig. 12.7). Myocardial involvement is prominent and death usually results from congestive heart failure.[33-37] Ultrastructural studies show membrane-bound lysosomes with vacuoles containing pleomorphic inclusions with concentric membranous arrays (Fig. 12.8) and membranogranular material.[38]

Fabry Disease

Fabry disease, caused by a deficiency of lysosomal α-galactosidase A (ceramide trihexosidase), is an X-linked recessive disorder manifested by skin lesions (angiokeratomas), pain and paresthesias in the extremities, and progressive renal and cardiovascular disease. Cardiac hypertrophy and dilatation, congestive heart failure, anginal pain, and hypertension are related to the presence of deposits of

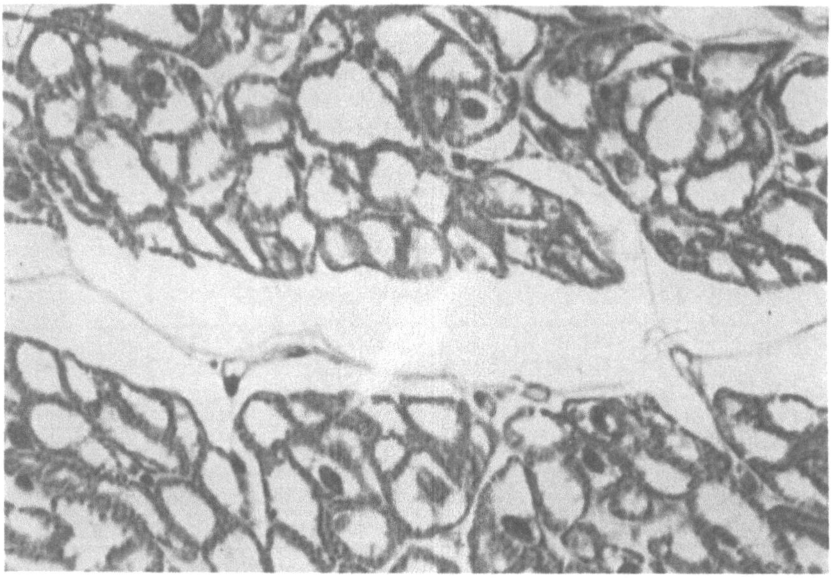

FIGURE 12.9. Microscopic section of heart showing vacuolated myocardial cells in Fabry's disease. (H&E, mag ×165.) Thick section showing osmiophilic deposits.

ceramide trihexoside in lyososomes in endothelial and smooth muscle cells throughout the vascular system, especially in the coronary arteries, as well as in renal glomeruli and tubules, cardiac muscle cells, specialized tissues of the atrioventricular conduction system, and valvular tissue. Myocardial infarction at an early age has been reported in several patients with Fabry disease,[39-41] and hypertrophic obstructive cardiomyopathy may occur.[42] Cardiac valvular lesions have been described in some patients with Fabry disease and include mitral stenosis,[43] aortic regurgitation,[44] and pulmonary regurgitation.[45]

Deposits of ceramide trihexoside appear as vacuoles in frozen sections; they are sudanophilic, periodic acid-Schiff (PAS)-positive, and strongly birefringent. In cardiac muscle cells these deposits result in a lacework pattern (Fig. 12.9) similar to that seen in type II glycogenosis. By electron microscopy the ceramide trihexoside deposits form intralysosomal aggregates of concentric or parallel lamellae spaced 4 to 5.5 nm apart (Fig. 12.10).[46-50] The lamellar structures of the deposits are best seen on freeze-fractured preparations.[50]

Gaucher Disease

In the adult form of Gaucher disease (glucosyl ceramide lipidosis, caused by deficiency of a lysosomal glucocerebrosidase), pulmonary hypertension or cor pulmonale due to occlusion of alveolar capillaries by Gaucher cells may occur.[51] Constrictive calcific pericarditis may result from intrapericardial hemorrhage due to a bleeding diathesis that is frequent in Gaucher disease.[52,53]

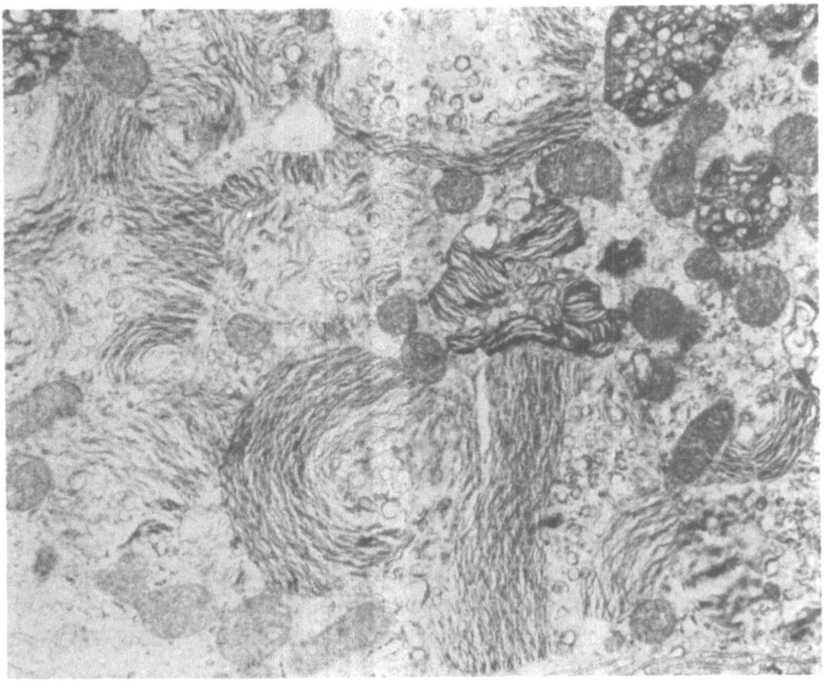

FIGURE 12.10. Electron microscopic appearance of the pleomorphic lipid profiles in Fabry's disease. Electron-dense deposits, lamellar arrays, and stacked membranes are present. (Uranyl acetate and lead citrate, mag ×7,650.) From ref. 8, with permission.

Gangliosidosis

In type I and type II generalized GM_1 gangliosidosis cardiovascular lesions include cardiomegaly and diffuse, nodular thickening of the mitral and tricuspid valves. Microscopically, swollen histiocytes containing PAS and Alcian Blue–positive cytoplasmic granules are seen. Similar cells have been found in the aortic valve, which is usually only slightly thickened.[54,55]

On ultrastructural study, these cells are filled with two types of deposits: concentric, electron-dense lamellae, and membrane-bound vacuoles containing reticulogranular material.[56]

Two types of GM_2 gangliosidosis include Tay-Sachs disease (type I) with deficiency of hexosaminidase A, and Sandhoff disease (type II) with deficiency of β-N-acetylhexosaminidase. Patients with Tay-Sachs disease have no clinical manifestations of cardiovascular disease but show nonspecific electrocardiographic changes and accumulations in heart tissue of a GM_2 ganglioside similar to that found in excessive amounts in the brain.[57]

Cardiomegaly and mitral regurgitation in Sandhoff disease[58-61] occur, similar to the changes seen in GM_1 gangliosidosis.

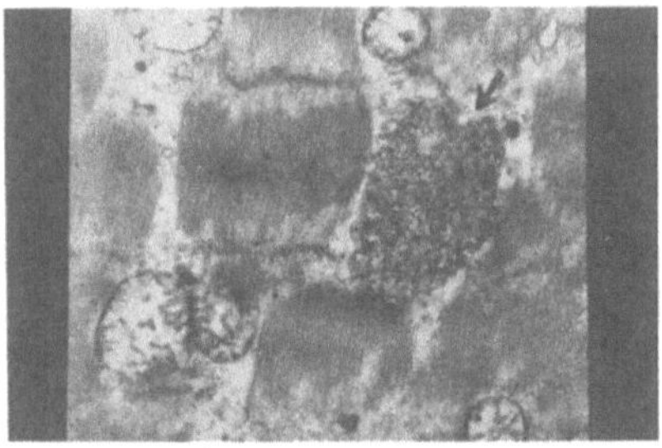

FIGURE 12.11. Electron micrograph of the myocardium in neuronal ceroid lipofuscinosis showing the presence of curvilinear bodies (arrow). (Uranylacetate and lead citrate, mag ×26,775.) (Courtesy of Dr M. Daria Haust.) From ref. 8, with permission.

Neuronal Ceroid Lipofuscinosis (NCL) (Batten-Spielmeyer-Vogt Syndrome)

This is characterized clinically by progressive loss of intellect and vision, appearance of seizures, and, pathologically, by the accumulation of lipopigment in neural and other tissues.[62] In the late infantile and juvenile forms, the heart is large and hypertrophied, and the valvular tissue is thickened. By light microscopy, the myocardial fibers are vacuolated owing to the lipid storage material. By electron microscopy, curvilinear bodies (Fig. 12.11) that seem to be specific for this disorder as well as fingerprint patterns and electron-dense deposits of lipofuscin are seen.

The storage material stains positively for PAS and acid phosphatase and is autofluorescent, giving peak emission when stimulated at around 500 Å.[63] The storage material is far more abundant in neurons, but it can also be found in virtually all tissues. In skin[64-70] the inclusions are most readily seen in capillary endothelial cells.

Carnitine Deficiency

Carnitine is an essential cofactor in the transfer of long-chain fatty acids across the inner mitochondrial membrane. Carnitine deficiency results in the accumulation of neutral lipid within type I skeletal muscle fibers, the myocardium, and the liver.

Skeletal muscle weakness, episodic hypoglycemia, encephalopathy, congestive and hypertrophic cardiomyopathies, and bradydysrhythmic cardiac arrests are

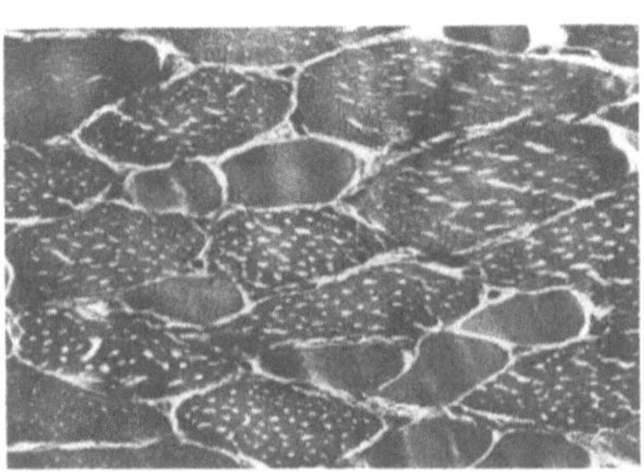

FIGURE 12.12. Microscopic section of the skeletal muscle in carnitine deficiency showing accumulation of granular material at the periphery of the cells (ragged red fibers). (Gomori trichrome stain, mag ×160.) (From Gilbert[76] with permission.)

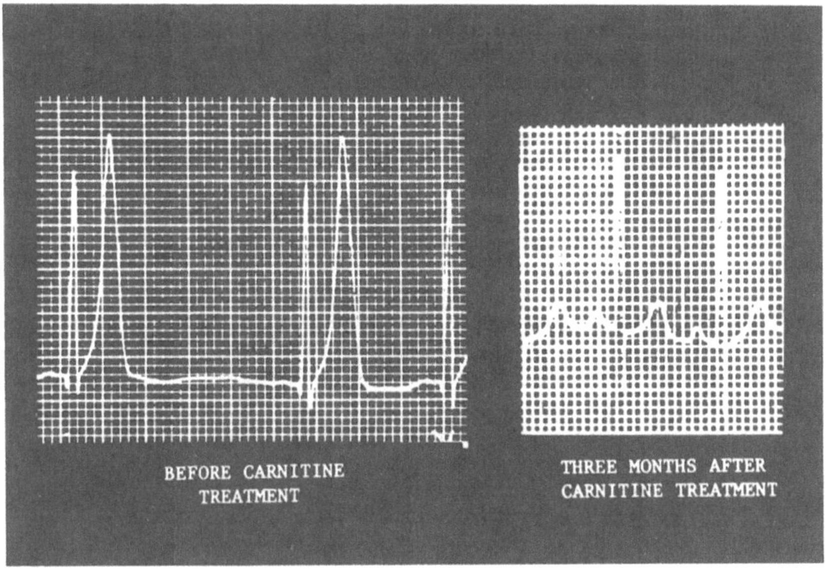

FIGURE 12.13. Electrocardiogram in carnitine deficiency showing high peaked T waves before carnitine treatment reverting to normal after carnitine treatment.

common in carnitine deficiency.[71,72] The disease is diagnosed by muscle biopsy and by the direct measurement of carnitine concentrations in plasma.

Systemic carnitine deficiency is generally diagnosed early in life. Two clinical subtypes are recognized: (1) that associated with multiple episodes of acute encephalopathy which resemble Reye syndrome,[73-75] and (2) that associated with cardiomyopathy characterized by cardiomegaly and congestive failure at an early age[71] with striking T-wave changes in the EKG (Fig. 12.12).

The heart is large and globular. The endocardium may show mild endocardial fibrosis. The skeletal muscle contains a myriad of small vacuoles in type I fibers (Fig. 12.13), and with the modified Gomori stain there are large subsarcolemmal accumulations of mitochondria that are red and granular (ragged red fibers). Ultrastructurally, myofibrils are disrupted, and there is an accumulation of large aggregates of mitochondria and lipid deposits within the skeletal muscle and myocardium.

The clinical response to L-carnitine may be dramatic. Determination of plasma carnitine and skeletal muscle biopsy seems justified in all patients with familial cardiomyopathy.

Secondary carnitine deficiency may be due to genetic defects of intermediary metabolism, particularly those with acidosis, following hemodialysis and other conditions (Table 12.2).[76]

Other inherited disorders of neutral and phospholipid storage may manifest with cardiac dysfunction including abetalipoproteinemia and phytanic acid storage disease (Refsum disease). Endocardial fibroelastosis has been reported in phos-

Table 12.2. Secondary carnitine deficiency.

Defects of intermediary metabolism
Carnitine octanoyltransferase deficiency
Cytochrome c oxidase deficiency
Fatty acyl-coenzyme A dehydrogenase deficiencies
Long-chain deficiency
Medium-chain deficiency
Multiple deficiencies associated with ornithine transcarbamylase deficiency
Isovaleric acidemia
Methylenetetrahydrofolate reductase deficiency
Methylmalonyl-coenzyme A apomutase deficiency
Mitochondrial adenosine triphosphatase deficiency
Nicotinamide adenine dinucleotide-ubiquinone reductase deficiency
Propionyl-coenzyme A carboxylase deficiency
Secondary to other conditions
Chronic renal failure treated with hemodialysis
Total parenteral nutrition in premature infants
Myxedema, hypopituitarism, and adrenal insufficiency
Valproate-induced Reye's syndrome
Hyperammonemia associated with valproic acid therapy
Kwashiorkor
Renal Fanconi syndrome
Chronic severe myopathies
Cirrhosis with cachexia
Pregnancy

Source: Gilbert,[76] with permission.

phorylceramidosis (Niemann-Pick disease), and disseminated lipogranulomatosis (Farber's disease) may be associated with cardiomyopathy and arrhythmia.

Disorders of Metal and Pigment Metabolism

Hemosiderosis and Hemochromatosis

Cardiac iron deposits occur in hemochromatosis as well as in hemosiderosis, secondary to iron overloading. The amount of iron in the heart correlates with the presence and severity of congestive heart failure, which has been reported in one third of patients with hemochromatosis.[77] Supraventricular arrhythmias correlate with the extent of iron deposition in the atrial myocardium.[78] The heart has a rusty-brown discoloration with hypertrophy and dilatation. The coronary arteries and heart valves are not involved.[79-81] Cardiac muscle has a greater affinity for iron than does skeletal or smooth muscle (Fig. 12.14). The iron deposits are localized in lysosomes that contain electron-dense particles, 6 nm in diameter. Deposits are readily identified by histochemical staining and by energy-dispersive ray microanalysis.

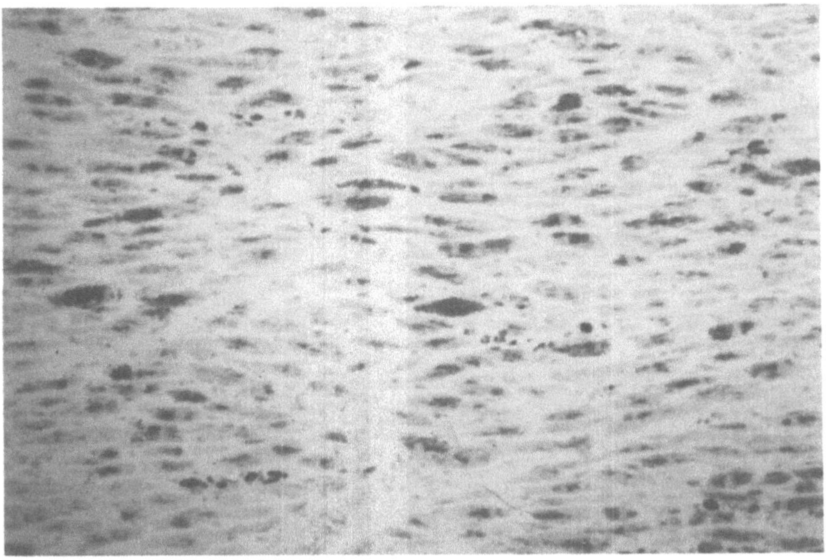

FIGURE 12.14. Microscopic section of the heart in hemosiderosis showing deposits of iron in the myocardial cells. (Prussian Blue stain, mag ×65.) From ref. 8, with permission.

Wilson's Disease

Wilson's disease (hepatolenticular degeneration) is an autosomal-recessive trait characterized by cirrhosis of the liver, degenerative changes in the brain (especially in the basal ganglia), Kayser-Fleischer corneal rings, low serum copper concentrations, decreased serum ceruloplasmin levels, increased urinary copper, and deposition of copper in various tissues. Cardiac hypertrophy and increased copper concentrations in the heart have been described.[82,83]

Menkes' Kinky Hair Syndrome

This is a sex-linked, recessively transmitted copper deficiency state related to impaired absorption of copper from the gastrointestinal tract.[84] Copper is a cofactor for the enzyme responsible for the formation of cross-links between lysine residues in elastin and collagen. The heart in Menkes' syndrome is normal, but superficial vessels often appear tortuous or dilated,[85] and aneurysm formation often involves major arteries and veins. In the arterial wall there are fragmentation, splitting, and reduplication of the internal elastic lamina (Fig. 12.15). Vascular lumina often are compromised and occasionally are obliterated.[86,87] Ultrastructural study of the aorta shows elastic lamellae composed of clumps of elastin surrounded by large numbers of connective tissue microfibrils.[9]

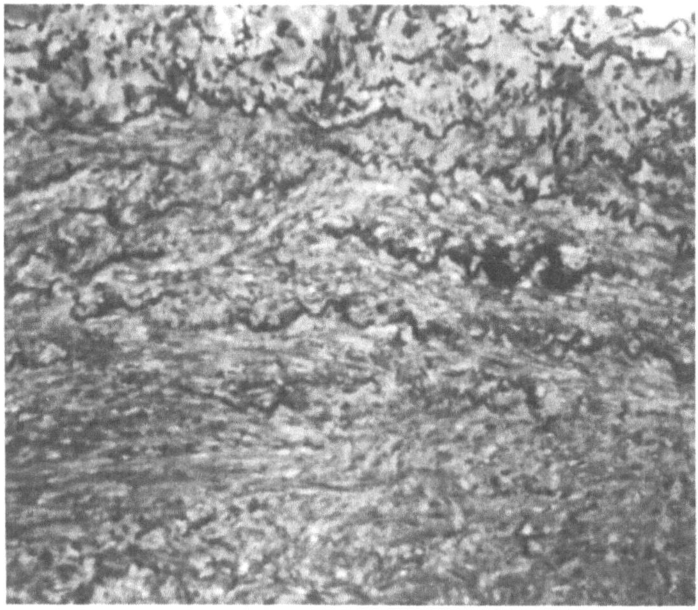

FIGURE 12.15. Microscopic section of the aorta in Menkes' kinky hair syndrome showing fragmentation of the elastica. (Elastic Van Gieson stain, mag ×80.) From ref. 8, with permission.

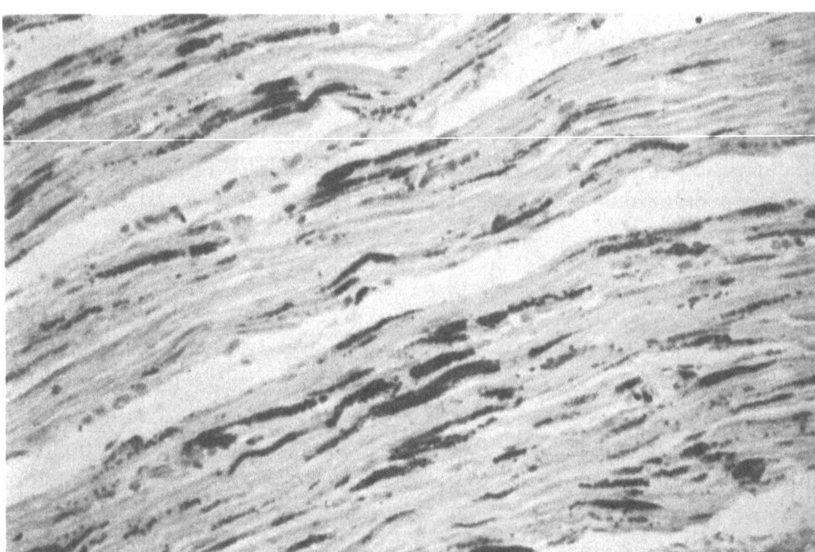

FIGURE 12.16. Microscopic section of the myocardium in Dubin-Johnson syndrome. The myocardial fibers contain an abundanc of melaninlike pigment. (H&E, mag ×62.) From ref. 8, with permission.

Dubin-Johnson Syndrome

Dubin-Johnson syndrome is a familial condition characterized by chronic, benign, intermittent jaundice with conjugated hyperbilirubinemia and bilirubinuria.[88-90] The liver cells contain a brown pigment that is histochemically similar to melanin.[91]

Studies of families suggest autosomal-dominant inheritance with considerable variability of expression.[92] The heart may show extensive deposition of pigment within the myocardial cells (Fig. 12.16). This does not appear to interfere with cardiac function.[9]

Neuromuscular Diseases

The Muscular Dystrophies

In the rapid progressive form of Duchenne muscular dystrophy, an X-linked recessive disorder, cardiomegaly is usually present, with dilatation, hypertrophy, and fibrosis within the ventricular myocardium.[93-95] Endocardial fibrous thickening has also been reported.[96] The large extramural coronary arteries are normal, although the small intramural coronary arteries show luminal narrowing due to fibromuscular intimal proliferation, especially the arteries to the SA and AV nodes.[97,98] By electron microscopy, the myocardium shows myofibrillar lysis, with loss of actin and myosin filaments, disorganization of Z-band material, and preservation of the structure of the transverse tubular system.[99]

Papillary muscle involvement with mitral prolapse and insufficiency is common. Ventricular compliance may be decreased. Arrhythmias and respiratory embarrassment are frequent complications. Response to medical therapy is temporary.[100,101]

Cardiac involvement in the milder X-linked Becker's type of muscular dystrophy is less common and less severe.[102]

Cardiac involvement in Steinert's myotonic dystrophy, an autosomal-dominant disorder characterized by myotonia and contractures, is frequently manifested as conduction abnormalities or dysrhythmias. Congestive heart failure may occur late in the course of the disease.[103] Electrocardiographic abnormalities and arrhythmias are also common in congenitally myotonic infants born to dystrophic mothers.[104]

Cardiac involvement is rare and clinically unimportant in the facioscapulohumeral dystrophy of Landouzy-Dejerine. Conduction disturbances may occur in the Erb type of limb girdle dystrophy. Pathological studies of the heart in these two diseases, although not reported in detail, do not appear to reveal any significant abnormalities.[98]

Nemaline myopathy has been reported with fatal cardiomyopathy, and in some cases, cardiorespiratory distress has been common.[105] Electronmicroscopy of skeletal muscle demonstrates the characteristic nemaline rods (Fig. 12.17) and is diagnostic.

The majority of patients with myotubular myopathy die of cardiorespiratory failure and arrhythmias in the first decade.[106]

Given the frequency of coincident cardiac and skeletal muscle disorders, histologic examination of skeletal muscle in patients with cardiomyopathy may be helpful in the diagnostic evaluation.

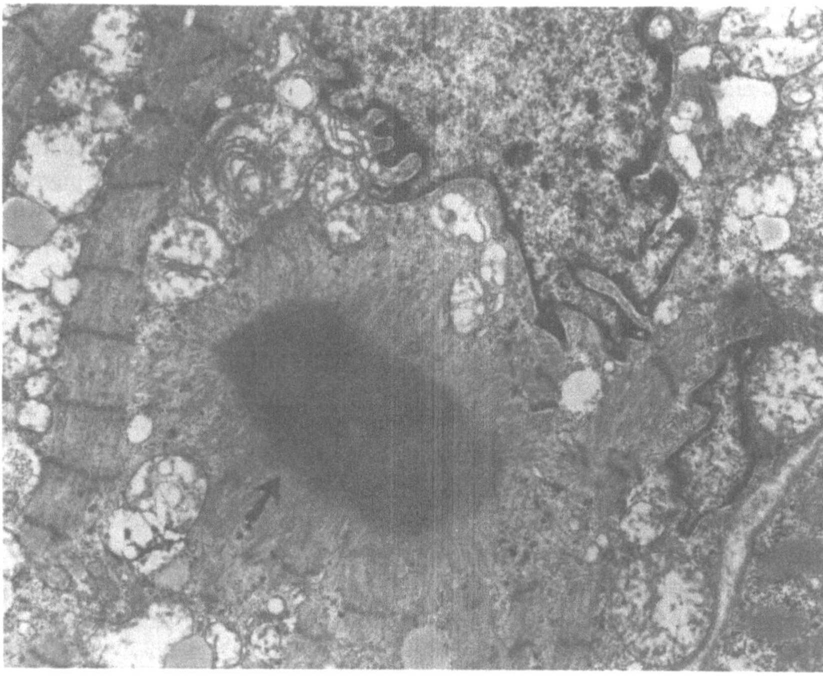

FIGURE 12.17. Electron micrograph of skeletal muscle in nemaline myopathy. Nemaline rod is shown by arrow. (Uranyl acetate and lead citrate, mag ×26,775.)

Cardiac failure and dysrhythmias may also occur in *malignant hyperthermia* and *familial periodic paralysis*.[107,108]

Friedreich's ataxia chiefly involves the spinocerebellar and pyramidal tracts and dorsal columns. One third of patients have physical signs and symptoms of heart disease (progressive heart failure and precordial pain), 90% eventually develop ECG abnormalities, and 100% show cardiac involvement at autopsy.[109] Cardiomegaly, patchy or diffuse interstitial fibrosis, and, less frequently, endocardial thickening and mural thrombosis[110-112] may occur, with a high incidence of hypertrophic cardiomyopathy with asymmetrical hypertrophy of the ventricular septum.[113-116] Small intramural coronary arteries are frequently the site of marked intimal thickening, which may be occlusive.[117]

Kugelberg-Welander syndrome (the juvenile form of progressive spinal muscular atrophy) is associated with atrial arrhythmias, AV conduction disturbances, and congestive heart failure. Cardiomegaly is usually present. Loss of myosin filaments and mitochondrial and Z-band alterations have been described.

The majority of patients with *myotubular myopathy* die of cardiorespiratory failure and arrhythmias in the first decade.[118]

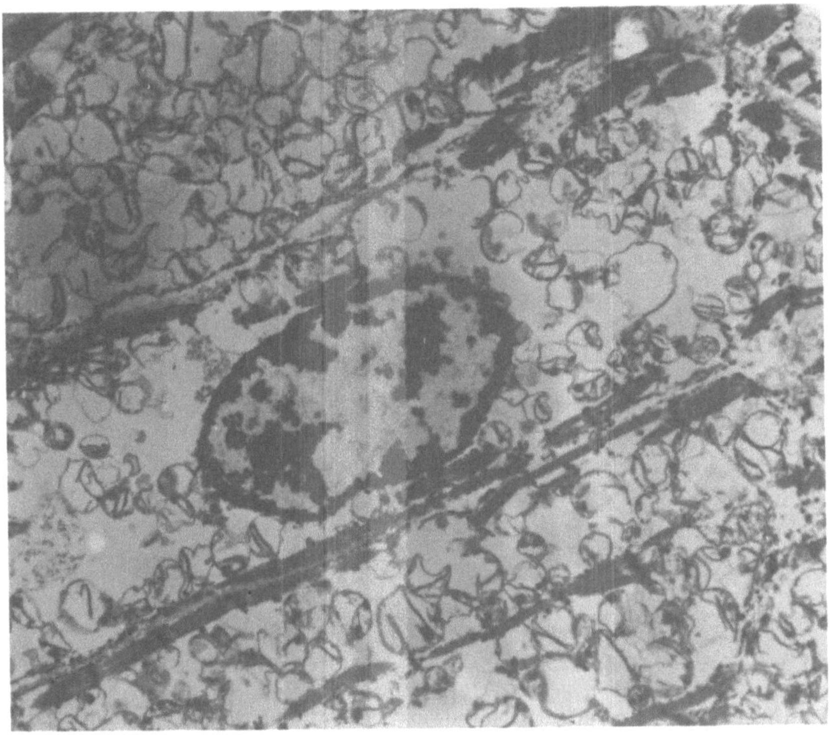

FIGURE 12.18. Electron micrograph of myocardium in mitochondrial myopathy. The mitochondria are large with disrupted cristae and intramitochondrial dense bodies. (Uranyl acetate and lead citrate, mag ×32,000.) (Courtesy of Dr N. Gould.)

Mitochondrial Disorders

Heart function relies predominantly on mitochondrial energy production, and nearly 30% of total myocardial volume consists of these organelles.[119] In mitochondrial disorders myocardial biopsy demonstrates an absolute increase in the number and size of mitochondria, while the activity of mitochondrial enzymes is decreased.[120]

Mitochondrial disorders may present with a slowly progressive skeletal myopathy and cardiomyopathy with congestive heart failure. Kearns-Sayres syndrome includes ophthalmoplegia, degenerative retinopathy, renal tubular dysfunction, delayed growth, short stature, and slow mental and neurologic deterioration with progressive heart block.[121,122]

Morphological abnormalities of mitochondria are generalized. Biopsies of skeletal muscle stained by a modified Gomori's trichrome stain show intracellular aggregates of coarse, red, granular material predominantly involving the aerobic type I fibers—so-called ragged red fibers. By electron microscopy these aggregates consist of masses of abnormally large mitochondria with bizarre morphological features (Fig. 12.18). This morphology is not specific and occurs in

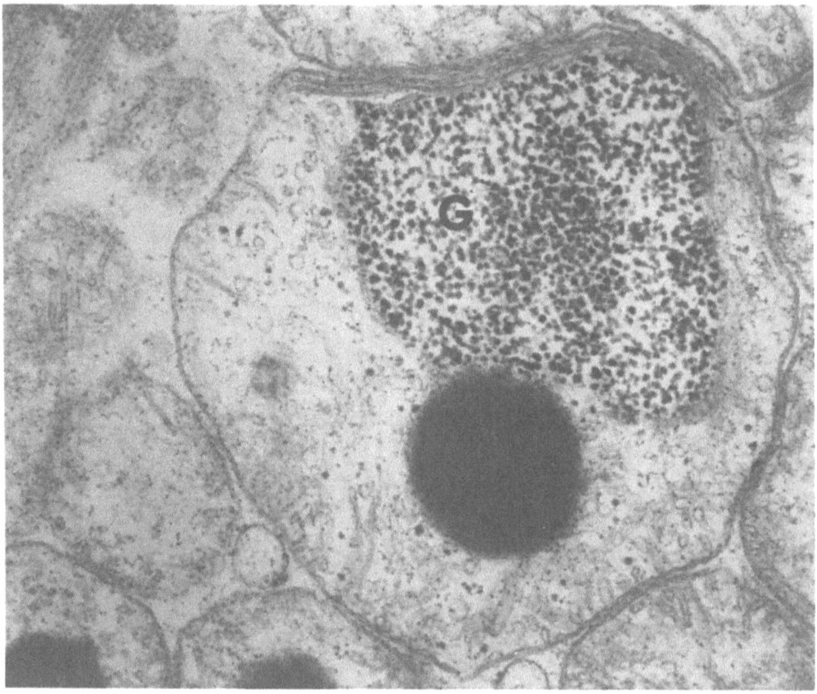

FIGURE 12.19. Electron micrograph showing abnormal mitochondria in the myocardial cells in X-linked recessive cardiomyopathy. Note glycogen particles (*G*) and dense body in mitochondrion. (Uranyl acetate and lead citrate, mag ×83,500.) (Courtesy of Dr Beverly Dahms.)

most mitochondrial disorders. Vacuolization with lipid, glycogen, or other amorphous materials may be seen.

An X-linked form of mitochondrial myopathy has been described (Fig. 12.19)[123] Since then other cases have been described with neutropenia[124,125] and short stature. Two patients reported by Ino et al[125] had abnormalities in carnitine metabolism with dramatic response to L-carnitine therapy. There is a high degree of variable penetrance; Egger and Wilson[126] noted that of the 130 siblings in 21 sibships with mitochondrial myopathy, 88 (68%) were known to be affected.

Connective Tissue Disorders

Marfan Syndrome

Marfan syndrome is transmitted as an autosomal-dominant trait and is characterized by musculoskeletal abnormalities, ectopia lentis, and cardiovascular lesions, the most striking of which are dilatation of the aortic root and mitral and aortic

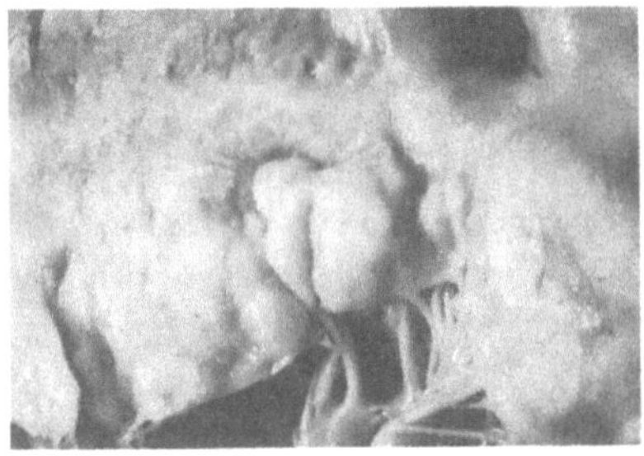

FIGURE 12.20. Gross appearance of a floppy mitral valve in Marfan's syndrome. The mitral valve leaflets are thick and redundant. From ref. 8, with permission.

regurgitation, saccular aneurysms of the ascending aorta, dissection of the entire aorta, and mitral valve prolapse (Fig. 12.20). Aneurysms in Marfan syndrome have been reported in the descending, thoracic, and abdominal aorta[127-129]; pulmonary artery[130]; cerebral vessels[131]; ductus arteriosus[132]; and coronary arteries.[129,133] Walls of the vessels show severe fragmentation, atrophy, and loss of elastic fibers; an increase in collagen; and a marked increase in acid mucopolysaccharide material which forms pools between the remaining elastic lamellae (Fig. 12.21)[134-136] Elastic fibers have a moth-eaten appearance; their amorphous component shows by electron microscopy an increase in electron density and frequently masses of dark granules.[9]

Aortic lesions in the Marfan syndrome are more common in adults; mitral lesions are more common in children.[137,138] Papillary muscle dysfunction can also occur.[139] In the floppy mitral valve, mucoid material is mainly present in the spongiosa.[140,141] Cardiac hypertrophy may result from the aortic and mitral valve lesions. Congenital heart malformations have been observed in association with the Marfan syndrome, including coarctation of the aorta and atrial septal defect.[130,142,143]

Ehlers-Danlos Syndrome

Ehlers-Danlos syndrome is a heterogeneous group of at least 13 genetically distinct disorders of connective tissue synthesis.[144] Cardiovascular lesions have been described in types I to IV. Dissection of the aorta and tears in peripheral arteries

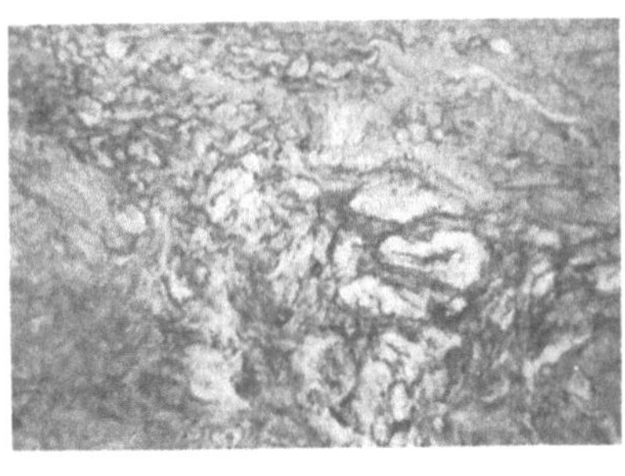

FIGURE 12.21. Microscopic section of the aortic wall showing cystic medionecrosis in Marfan's syndrome. The cystic spaces are filled with mucopolysaccharide. (Alcian Blue, ×160.) From ref. 8, with permission.

have been reported in type I, the gravis form.[145] In type II, the mitis form, atrial septal defect, congenital AV block, aneurysm of the ascending aorta,[146] and aneurysms of the brachial artery and the abdominal aorta have been described.[147] Mitral valve prolapse occurs in type III.[148] Major vascular complications are most common in type IV – the ecchymotic, arterial, or Sack type.[149-153] Sudden death from rupture of the aorta or other major arteries or veins may occur. Histologically, there is thinning of the walls of the vessels with a diffuse decrease in elastic tissue in the media, deposition of acid mucopolysaccharide between the medial elastic lamellae, and a decrease in adventitial and medial collagen.

Osteogenesis Imperfecta

Osteogenesis imperfecta is a generalized disorder of connective tissue. There are at least four well-defined forms of the disorder[154,155] and a number of presently unclassified examples. There appears to be a marked heterogeneity of these defects, but principally they involve the synthesis of the pro-alpha chains of procollagen monomers.[155-157]

The most common valvular lesion is aortic regurgitation; less common is mitral regurgitation.[158-165] Dilatation of the aortic root and deformity of the valvular leaflets result from an abnormally dilated mitral annulus; the mitral leaflets are attenuated and redundant, and tend to prolapse; and the chordae tendineae may rupture.

In lethal perinatal osteogenesis imperfecta (0I type II), the chordae tendineae are short and fragile; both the atrioventricular valves and the chordae tendineae are hypercellular. By electron microscopy little organized collagen in the chordae tendineae is seen in fetuses with a marked decrease in the adventitial and intramural collagen of the intramyocardial arteries and great vessels.[166]

Pseudo-Xanthoma Elasticum

Pseudo-xanthoma elasticum (PXE) is a recessive disorder manifested by cutaneous lesions, retinal angioid streaks, gastrointestinal hemorrhages, and fragmentation and calcification of elastic fibers. Cardiovascular manifestations result from enlargement and calcification of elastic fibers in the intima and media of peripheral muscular arteries.[167] Endocardial plaques composed of degenerated, calcified elastic fibers are located in deeper areas of the endocardium,[168,169] principally involving the atria.

Neonatal Effects of Maternal Disease

Cardiomyopathy in the Infant of a Diabetic Mother (IDM)

In cardiomyopathy of IDM, hypertrophy and hyperplasia of myocardial cells occur with cardiomegaly.[170] There frequently are marked thickness of the interventricular septum (IVS) and decreased left ventricular function. Some infants

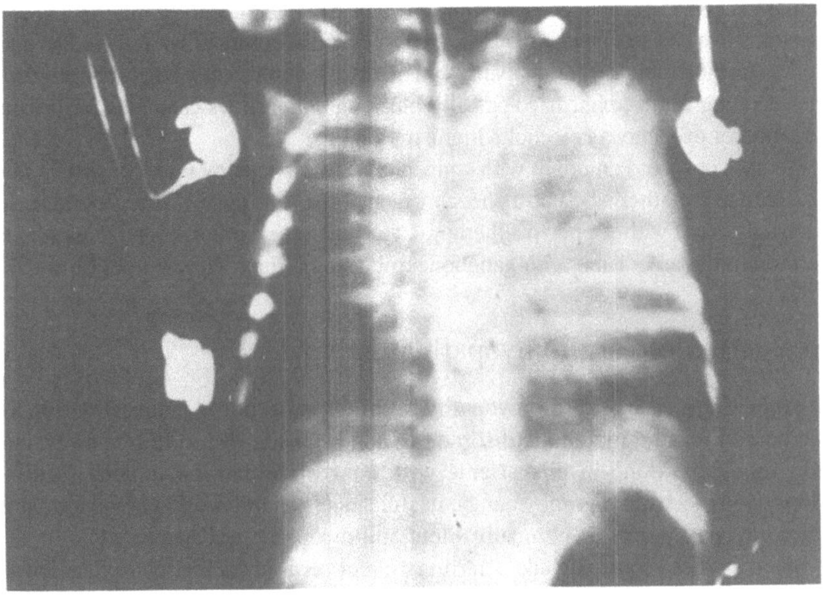

FIGURE 12.22. Chest X-ray in a newborn infant with thyrotoxic cardiomyopathy. The heart is massively enlarged.

may develop obstructive cardiomyopathy with features of obstructive asymmetric hypertrophy[171] of the interventricular septum. There may be excessive accumulation of glycogen in the myocardial cells. Idiopathic cardiac enlargement in IDM usually resolves within the first few months of life.[172]

Thyrotoxic Cardiomyopathy

In hyperthyroidism, excessive thyroid hormone partially uncouples oxidative metabolism, with production of high-energy phosphate bonds. Cardiac inefficiency may occur. Arrhythmias and congestive heart failure may result.[173]

The myxedematous heart is large and poorly contractile with bradydysrhythmias. Massive pericardial effusion with or without tamponade may overshadow decreases in myocardial contractility. In both hyperthyroidism and hypothyroidism, control of thyroid status usually reverses cardiac dysfunction.[173] We have observed a neonate with fatal thyrotoxic cardiomyopathy with massive cardiomegaly (Fig. 12.22) born to a mother with thyrotoxicosis treated with propylthiouracil.

Catecholamine Cardiomyopathy

Catecholamine cardiomyopathy results in excessive myocardial oxygen demand and decreased myocardial efficiency caused by endocrine or pharmacologic catecholamine excess. Catechol-secreting tumors such as pheochromocytoma and neuroblastoma can be associated with decreased myocardial contractility and cardiac dilation. Catecholamine cardiomyopathy can be reversed in its early stages by resecting the secreting tumor, pharmacologically blocking endogenous catechols, or discontinuation of exogenous catechol administration.[174]

We have observed an infant with congenital cardiomyopathy with congestive failure, born to a mother who had a pheochromocytoma. The condition regressed in the neonatal period with supportive therapy. Catecholamine cardiomyopathy appears to be more often associated with ganglioneuroblastoma than with neuroblastoma.

Evaluation of Cardiomyopathy

In evaluating a case of cardiomyopathy in childhood a thorough investigation for the possibility of a metabolic disorder should be made. Neuromuscular evaluation should be done in all patients with congestive cardiomyopathy. Muscle biopsy and electromyography can be useful since skeletal muscle involvement in cardiomyopathy may be clinically silent and myopathy not suspected.

Blood studies should include determination of serum iron and phosphate levels, muscle enzymes (especially lactate dehydrogenase and creatine phosphokinase with their isozymes), thyroid hormones, and plasma carnitine. Trace metals and urinary amino acids, organic acids, and catecholamines should be measured.

Recent studies have demonstrated that coronary sinus flow studies and substrate extraction may define metabolic abnormalities in the cardiomyopathic heart.[175,176] Endomyocardial biopsy affords a measure of direct assessment of cardiac tissue in characterizing cardiomyopathy.[177,178]

Management of Cardiomyopathy

It is of primary importance that the underlying cause of myocardial dysfunction be defined. If secondary cardiomyopathy is present, such as in carnitine deficiency, pheochromocytoma, or hemosiderosis, specific therapy should be instituted. Routine therapy for congestive heart failure is relatively ineffective in primary metabolic disorders,[179] and the inotropic effects of digitalis may be negligible.[180]

Major complications of congestive cardiomyopathy are dysrhythmias and thromboembolism. The progressive atrioventricular block of Kearns-Sayre syndrome is pathognomonic for this disorder. Cautious, specific drug therapy and timely implantation of cardiac pacemakers may avoid sudden and unexpected death in children with dysrhythmias. Patients with atrial fibrillation or atrial standstill, with known mural thrombi, or with a definite or probable history of thromboembolus should be given anticoagulants.[181]

Intercurrent infections should be treated with appropriate antibiotics, antipyretics, bed rest, and oxygen. Decompensation is frequently triggered by an infectious process.

It is important to recognize that the majority of patients with metabolic disease with cardiac involvement die from cardiomyopathy and/or its complications.

References

1. Brandenburg RO, Chazov E, Cherian G, et al: Report of the WHO/ISFC task force on definition and classification of cardiomyopathies. *Circulation* 64:437A, 1981.
2. Goodwin JF: Prospects and predictions for the cardiomyopathies. *Circulation* 50: 210, 1974.
3. Hastreiter AR, Fisher EA: Endocardial fibroelastosis. In Moss AJ, Adams FH, Emmanouilides GC (eds): *Heart Disease in Infants, Children and Adolescents.* Baltimore: Williams and Williams, 1977, pp 496–505.
4. Greenwood RD, Nadas AS, Fyler DC: The clinical course of primary myocardial disease in infants and children. *Am Heart J* 92:549, 1976.
5. Galdston M, Steele JM, Dobriner K: Alcaptonuria and ochronosis. With a report of three patients and metabolic studies in two. *Am J Med* 13:432, 1952.
6. O'Brien WM, LaDu BN, Bunim JJ: Biochemical, pathologic, and clinical aspects of alcaptonuria, ochronosis and ochronotic arthropathy. *Am J Med* 34:813, 1963.
7. Abreo K, Oberley TD, Gilbert EF, Opitz JM, Updike J: Clinicopathological conference: A 29-year-old man with recurrent episodes of fever, abdominal pain, and vomiting. *Am J Genet* 18:264, 1984.
8. Gilbert EF: The effects of metabolic diseases on the cardiovascular system. *Am J Cardiovasc Pathol* 1:189, 1987.
9. Ferrans VJ, Boyce SW: Metabolic and familial diseases. In Silver MD (ed): *Cardiovascular Pathology.* New York: Churchill Livingstone, 1983, pp 945–1004.
10. Chaplin AJ: Histopathological occurrence and characterization of calcium oxalate: A review. *J Clin Pathol* 30:800, 1977.
11. Beil E, Seibel K, Riecker G: Herzerkrankug bei primarer Oxalose. *Klin Wochenschr* 47:513, 1969.
12. Coltart DJ, Hudson REB: Primary oxalosis of the heart: A cause of heart block. *Br Heart J* 33:315, 1971.
13. Tonkin AM, Mond HG, Mathew TH, Solman JG: Primary oxalosis with myocardial involvement and heart block. *Med J Aust* 1:873, 1976.
14. West RR, Salyer WR, Hutchins GM: Adult-onset primary oxalosis with complete heart block. *Johns Hopkins Med J* 133:195, 1973.
15. Blackburn WE, McRoberts JW, Bhathena D, Vazquez M, Luke RG: Severe vascular complications in oxalosis after bilateral nephrectomy. *Ann Intern Med* 82:44, 1975.
16. Fayemi AO, Ali M, Braun EV: Oxalosis in hemodialysis patients. A pathologic study of 80 cases. *Arch Pathol Lab Med* 103:58, 1979.
17. Hahlweg G, Orf G: Sog fibroplastische myocarditis bei oxalose. *Pathol Microbiol* 29:1, 1966.
18. Henry CG, Strauss AW, Keating JP, et al: Congestive cardiomyopathy associated with β-ketothiolase deficiency. *J Pediatr* 99:754–757, 1981.
19. Ehlers KH, Hagstrom JWC, Lukas DS, Redo SF, Engle MA: Glycogen-storage disease of the myocardium with obstruction to left ventricular outflow. *Circulation* 25:96, 1962.
20. Rees A, Elbl F, Minhas K, Solinger R: Echocardiographic evidence of outflow tract obstruction in Pompe's disease (glycogen storage disease of the heart). *Am J Cardiol* 37:1103, 1976.
21. Bordiuk JM, Legato MJ, Lovelace RE, Blumenthal S: Pompe's disease. Electromyographic, electron microscopic and cardiovascular aspects. *Arch Neurol* 23: 113, 1970.

22. Hohn AR, Lowe CU, Sokal JE, Lambert EC: Cardiac problems in the glycogenoses with specific reference to Pompe's disease. *Pediatrics* 35:313, 1965.
23. Dincsoy MY, Dincsoy HP, Kessler AD, Jackson MA, Sidbury JB Jr: Generalized glycogenosis and associated endocardial fibroelastosis. Report of 3 cases with biochemical studies. *J Pediatr* 67:728, 1965.
24. Hers HG, De Barsy T: Type II glycogenosis (acid maltase deficiency). In Hers HG, Van Hoff F (eds): *Lysosomes and Storage Disorders*. New York: Academic Press, 1973, p 197.
25. Engel AG, Gomez MR, Seybold ME, Lambert EH: The spectrum and diagnosis of acid maltase deficiency. *Neurology (Minneapolis)* 23:95, 1973.
26. Caddell JL, Whittemore R: Observations on generalized glycogenosis with emphasis on electrocardiographic changes. *Pediatrics* 29:743, 1962.
27. Garancis JC: Type II% glycogenosis. Biochemical and electron microscopic study. *Am J Med* 44:289, 1968.
28. Ehlers KH, Hagstrom JWC, Lukas DS, Redo SF, Engle MA: Glycogen-storage disease of the myocardium with obstruction to left ventricular outflow. *Circulation* 25: 96, 1962.
29. Besley GTN. Phosphorylase β kinase deficiency in glycogenosis type VIII: differentiation of different phenotypes and heterozygotes by erthrocyte enzyme assay. *J Inherited Metab Dis* 10:115–118, 1987.
30. Mizuta K, Kashimoto E, Tsutou A, et al: A new type of glycogen storage disease caused by deficiency of cardiac phosphorylase kinase. *Biochem Biophys Res Commun* 119:582–587, 1984.
31. Servidei S, Metlay LA, Chodosh J, DiMauro S: Fatal infantile cardiomyopathy caused by phosphorylase β kinase deficiency. *J Pediatr* 113:82–85, 1988.
32. Goldfischer S, Coltoff-Schiller B, Biempica L, Wolinsky H: Lysosomes and the sclerotic arterial lesion in Hurler's disease. *Hum Pathol* 6:633, 1975.
33. Blank E, Linder D: I-cell disease (mucolipidosis II): A lysosomopathy. *Pediatrics* 54:797, 1974.
34. Gilbert EF, Dawson G, ZuRhein GM, Opitz JM, Spranger JW: I-cell disease, mucolipidosis II. Pathological, histochemical, ultrastructural and biochemical observations in four cases. *Z Kinderheilk* 114:259, 1973.
35. Glaser JH, McAlister WH, Sly WS: Genetic heterogeneity in multiple lysosomal hydrolase deficiency. *J Pediatr* 85:192, 1974.
36. Nagashima K, Sakakibara K, Endo H, et al: I-cell disease (mucolipidosis II). Pathological and biochemical studies of an autopsy case. *Acta Pathol Jpn* 27:251, 1977.
37. Patriquin HB, Kaplan P, Kind HP, Giedion A: Neonatal mucolipidosis II (I-cell disease): Clinical and radiologic features in three cases. *AJR* 129:37, 1977.
38. Herd JK, Subramanian S, Robinson H: Type III mucopolysaccharidosis: Report of a case with severe mitral valve involvement. *J Pediatr* 82:101, 1973.
39. Falck I: Angiokeratoma corporis dissusum Fabry mit vasorenalem Symptomenkomplex. *Samml Selt Klin Falle* 9:20, 1955.
40. Parkinson JE, Sunshine A: Angiokeratoma corporis diffusum universale (Fabry) presenting as suspected myocardial infarction and pulmonary infarcts. *Am J Med* 31:951, 1961.
41. Wise D, Wallace HJ, Jellinek EH: Angiokeratoma corporis diffusum. A clinical study of eight affected families. *Q J Med* 31:177, 1962.
42. Fritz P, Schneider H, Heimburg P, Wegner G: Sekundare hypertrophe obstruktive Kardiomyopathic bei Morbus Fabry. *Med Welt* 29:1851, 1978.

43. Leder AA, Bosworth WC: Angiokeratoma corporis diffusum universale (Fabry's disease) with mitral stenosis. *Am J Med* 38:814, 1965.
44. Dubach UC, Gloor F: Fabry-Krankheit (Angiokeratoma corporis diffusum universale). Phosphatidspeicherkrankheit bei zwei Familien. *Dtsch Med Wochenschr* 91: 241, 1966.
45. Matsui S, Murakami E, Takekoshi N, et al: Cardiac manifestations of Fabry's disease. Report of a case with pulmonary regurgitation diagnosed on the basis of endomyocardial biopsy findings. *Jpn Circ J* 41:1023, 1977.
46. Becker AE, Schorl R, Balk AG, Van der Heide RM: Cardiac manifestations of Fabry's disease. Report of a case with mitral insufficiency and electrocardiographic evidence of myocardial infarction. *Am J Cardiol* 36:829, 1975.
47. Desnick RJ, Blieden LC, Sharp HL, Hofschire PJ, Moller JH: Cardiac valvular anomalies in Fabry disease. Clinical, morphologic and biochemical studies. *Circulation* 54:818, 1976.
48. Duncan C, McLeon GM: Angiokeratoma corporis diffusum universale (Fabry's disease): A case with gross myocardial involvement. *Aust NZ J Med* 1:58, 1970.
49. Ferrans VJ, Hibbs RG, Burda CD: The heart in Fabry's disease. A histochemical and electron microscopic study. *Am J Cardiol* 24:95, 1969.
50. Roth J, Roth H: Elektronenmikroskopische Befunde an inneren Organen bei Morgus Fabry. *Virchows Arch (Pathol Anat)* 378:75, 1978.
51. Roberts WC, Fredrickson DS: Gaucher's disease of the lung causing severe pulmonary hypertension with associated acute recurrent pericarditis. *Circulation* 35:783, 1967.
52. Benbassat J, Bassan H, Milwidski H, Sacks M, Groen JJ: Constrictive pericarditis in Gaucher's disease. *Am J Med* 44:647, 1968.
53. Harvey PKP, Jones MC, Anderson EG: Pericardial abnormalities in Gaucher's disease. *Br Heart J* 31:603, 1969.
54. Gonatas NK, Gonatas J: Ultrastructural and biochemical observations on a case of systemic late infantile lipidosis and its relationship to Tay-Sachs disease and gargoylism. *J Neuropathol Exp Neurol* 24:318, 1965.
55. Hadley RN, Hagstrom JWC: Cardiac lesions in a patient with familial neurovisceral lipidosis (generalized gangliosidosis). *Am J Clin Pathol* 55:237, 1971.
56. Gilbert EF, Varakis J, Opitz JM, et al: Generalized gangliosidosis type II (juvenile GM gangliosidosis). A pathological, histochemical and ultrastructural study. *Z Kinderheilk* 120:151, 1975.
57. Rodriquez-Torres R, Schneck L, Kleinberg W: Electrocardiographic and biochemical abnormalities in Tay-Sachs disease. *Bull NY Acad Med* 47:717, 1971.
58. Haust MD, Gordon BA, Hong R, et al: Clinicopathologic conference: An adolescent girl with severe mental impairment and mucopolysaccharidosis. *Am J Med* 22:1, 1985.
59. Blieden LC, Desnick RJ, Carter JB, Krivit W, Moller JH, Sharp HL: Cardiac involvement in Sandhoff's disease. Inborn error of glycosphingolipid metabolism. *Am J Cardiol* 34:83, 1974.
60. Dolman CL, Chang E, Duke RJ: Pathologic findings in Sandhoff disease. *Arch Pathol* 96:272, 1973.
61. Krivit W, Desnick RJ, Lee J, et al: Generalized accumulation of neutral glycosphingolipids with GM_2 ganglioside accumulation in the brain. Sandhoff's disease (variant of Tay-Sachs disease). *Am J Med* 52:763, 1972.
62. Zeman W, Donahue S, Dyken P, et al: The neuronal ceroid lipofuscinosis (Batten-

Vogt syndrome). In Vinken PJ, Bruyn GW (eds): *Handbook of Clinical Neurology*, Vol 10. Amsterdam: North Holland, 1970, pp 588–679.
63. Miley CE III, Gilbert EF, France TD, O'Brien JF, Chun RWM: Clinical and extraneural histologic diagnosis of neuronal ceroid-lipofuscinosis. *Neurology* 28:1008, 1978.
64. Carpenter S, Karpaty G, Andermann F: Specific involvement of muscle, nerve, and skin in late infantile and juvenile amaurotic idiocy. *Neurology* 22:170–186, 1972.
65. Dolman C, Change EP: Visceral lesions in amaurotic familial idiocy with curvilinear bodies. *Arch Pathol* 94:425–430, 1972.
66. Martin JJ, Jacobs K: Skin biopsy as a contribution to diagnosis in late infantile amaurotic idiocy with curvililinear bodies. *Eur Neurol* 10:281–291, 1973.
67. Dolman CL, MacLeod PM, Chang E: Skin punch biopsies and lymphocytes in the diagnosis of lipidoses. *Can J Neurol Sci* 2:67–73, 1975.
68. Arsenio-Nunes ML, Goutieres F: An ultramicroscopic study of the skin in the diagnosis of the infantile and late infantile types of ceroid-lipofuscinosis. *J Neurol Neurosurg Psychiatry* 38:994–999, 1975.
69. O'Brien JS, Bernett J, Veath ML, et al: Lysosomal storage disorders: Diagnosis by ultrastructural examination of skin biopsy specimens. *Arch Neurol* 32:592–599, 1975.
70. Farrell DF, Sumi SM: Skin punch biopsy in the diagnosis of juvenile neuronal ceroid-lipofuscinosis: A comparison with leukocyte peroxidase assay. *Arch Neurol* 34:39–44, 1977.
71. Tripp ME, Katcher ML, Gilbert EF, et al: Systemic carnitine deficiency presenting as familial endocardial fibroelastosis. *N Engl J Med* 305:385–390, 1981.
72. Waber LJ et al: Carnitine deficiency presenting as familial cardiomyopathy: A treatable defect in carnitine transport. *J Pediatr* 101:700–705, 1982.
73. Danks BM, Campbell PE, Stevens BJ, Mayne V, Cartwright E: Menkes' kinky hair syndrome. An inherited defect in copper absorption with widespread effects. *Pediatrics* 50:188, 1972.
74. Karpati G, Carpenter S, Engel AG, et al: The syndrome of systemic carnitine deficiency: Clinical, morphologic, biochemical and pathophysiologic features. *Neurology* 25:16–24, 1975.
75. Engel AG, Rebouche CJ: Pathogenetic mechanisms in human carnitine deficiency syndromes. In Schotland DL (ed): *Disorders of the Motor Unit*. New York: Wiley, 1982, pp 643–656.
76. Gilbert EF: Carnitine deficiency. *Pathology* 17:161–169, 1985.
77. Finch SC, Finch CA: Idiopathic hemochromatosis, an iron storage disease. *Medicine (Baltimore)* 34:381, 1955.
78. Buja LM, Roberts WC: Iron in the heart. Etiology and clinical significance. *Am J Med* 52:209, 1971.
79. Lewis HP: Cardiac involvement in hemochromatosis. *Am J Med Sci* 227:544, 1954.
80. Swan WGA, Dewar HA: The heart in hemochromatosis. *Br Heart J* 14:117, 1952.
81. Tucker HS Jr, Moss LF, Williams JP: Hemochromatosis with death from heart failure. *Am Heart J* 35:993, 1948.
82. Bottiger LE, Mollerberg H: Increased copper content of hypertrophic myocardium. *Acta Med Scand* 165:413, 1959.
83. Azevedo EM, Scaff M, Barbosa ER, Gouveia Neto AE, Canelas HM: Heart involvement in hepatolenticular degeneration. *Acta Neurol Scand* 58:296, 1978.
84. Danks BM, Campbell PE, Stevens BJ, Mayne V, Cartwright E: Menkes' kinky hair

syndrome. An inherited defect in copper absorption with widespread effects. *Pediatrics* 50:188, 1972.
85. Uno H, Arya S, Laxova R, Gilbert EF: Menkes' syndrome with vascular and adrenergic nerve abnormalities. *Arch Pathol Lab Med* 107:286, 1983.
86. Martin JJ, Flament-Durand J, Farriaux JP, Buyssen N, Ketelbant-Balasse P, Jansen C: Menkes' kinky hair disease. A report on its pathology. *Acta Neuropathol (Berl)* 42:25, 1978.
87. Wheeler EM, Roberts PF: Menkes' steely hair syndrome. *Arch Dis Child* 51:269, 1976.
88. Dubin IN: Chronic idiopathic jaundice. A review of fifty cases. *Am J Med* 24:268, 1958.
89. Dubin IN, Johnson FB: Chronic idiopathic jaundice with unidentified pigment in the liver cells: A new clinicopathological entity with a report of twelve cases. *Medicine* 33:155, 1954.
90. Sprinz H, Nelson RS: Persistent nonhemolytic hyperbilirubinemia associated with lipochrome-like pigment in liver cells: Report of four cases. *Ann Intern Med* 14:952, 1954.
91. Wegmann R, Rangier M, Eteve J, et al: Melanose hepato-splenique avec ictere chronique a bilirubine directe: Maladie de Dubin-Johnson? histochimique et Spectrographique du pigment abnormal. *Sem Hop Paris* 36:1761, 1960.
92. Butt HR, Anderson VE, Faulk WT, et al: Studies of chronic idiopathic jaundice (Dubin-Johnson syndrome). II. Evaluation of a large family with the trait. *Gastroenterology* 51:619, 1966.
93. Frankel KA, Rosser RJ: The pathology of the heart in progressive muscular dystrophy: Epimyocardial fibrosis. *Hum Pathol* 7:375, 1976.
94. Matsuda M, Akatsuka N, Yamaguchi T, et al: Systolic time intervals in patients with progressive muscular dystrophy of the Duchenne type. *Jpn Heart J* 18:638, 1977.
95. Rubler S, Perloff JK, Roberts WC: Duchenne's muscular dystrophy. *Am Heart J* 94:776, 1977.
96. Storstein O: The heart in progressive muscular dystrophy. *Exp Med Surg* 22:13, 1964.
97. James TN: Observations on the cardiovascular involvement, including the cardiac conduction system, in progressive muscular dystrophy. *Am Heart J* 63:48, 1962.
98. Perloff JK, Roberts WC, DeLeon AC Jr, O'Doherty D: The distinctive electrocardiogram of Duchenne's progressive muscular dystrophy. *Am J Med* 42:179, 1967.
99. Sanyal SK, Johnson WW, Thapar MK, Pitner SE: An ultrastructural basis for electrocardiographic alterations associated with Duchenne's progressive muscular dystrophy. *Circulation* 57:1122, 1978.
100. Sanyal SK, Johnson WW, Dische MR, et al: Dystrophic degeneration of papillary muscle and ventricular myocardium: A basis for mitral valve prolapse in Duchenne's muscular dystrophy. *Circulation* 62:430–438, 1980.
101. Biddison JH, Dembo DH, Spalt H, et al: Familial occurrence of mitral valve prolapse in X-linked muscular dystrophy. *Circulation* 59:1299–1304, 1979.
102. Kuhn E. Fiehn W, Schroder JM, et al: Early myocardial disease and cramping myalgia in Becker-type muscular dystrophy: A kindred. *Neurology* 29:1144–1149, 1979.
103. Prystowsky EN, Pritchett ELC, Roses AD, et al: The natural history of conduction system disease in myotonic muscular dystrophy as determined by serial electrophysiologic studies. *Circulation* 60:1360–1365, 1979.

104. Sarnat HB, O'Connor T, Byrne PA: Clinical effects of myotonic dystrophy on pregnancy and the neonate. *Arch Neurol* 33:459–465, 1976.
105. Meier C et al: Nemaline myopathy presenting as cardiomyopathy. *N Engl J Med* 308:1536, 1983.
106. Pearson CM: Myotubular myopathy. In Bergsma D (ed): *Birth Defects Compendium*. New York: National Foundation, 1979.
107. Huckell VR, Staniloff HM, Britt BA, et al: Cardiac manifestations of malignant hyperthermia susceptibility. *Circulation* 58:916–925, 1978.
108. Kramer LD et al: Cardiac dysfunction in a patient with familial hypokalemic periodic paralysis. *Chest* 75:189–192, 1979.
109. Perloff JK: The myocardial disease of heredofamilial neuromyopathies. In Fowler NO (ed): *Myocardial Disease*. New York: Grune and Stratton, 1973, p 319.
110. Hewer RL: The heart in Friedrich's ataxia. *Br Heart J* 31:5, 1969.
111. Ivemark B, Thoren C: The pathology of the heart in Friedreich's ataxia. Changes in coronary arteries and myocardium. *Acta Med Scand* 175:227, 1964.
112. Schilero AJ, Antzia E, Dunn J: Friedriech's ataxia and its cardiac manifestations. *Am Heart J* 44:805, 1952.
113. Barrillon A, Bensaid J, Coirault R, Scebat L, Maurice P, Gerbaux A: Myocardiopathie obstructive et maladie de Friedreich. *Arch Mal Coeur* 66:1525, 1973.
114. Gach JV, Andriange M, Franck G: Hypertrophic obstructive cardiomyopathy and Friedreich's ataxia. Report of a case and review of literature. *Am J Cardiol* 27:436, 1971.
115. Pernot C: La Myocardiopathie de la maladie de Friedreich. A propos d'une serie de 17 observations. *Arch Fr Pediatr* 36:11, 1979.
116. Smith ER, Sangalang VE, Hoffernan LP, Welch JP, Flemington CS: Hypertrophic cardiomyopathy: The heart disease of Friedreich's ataxia. *Am Heart J* 94:428, 1977.
117. James TN, Fisch C: Observations on the cardiovascular involvement in Friedreich's ataxia. *Am Heart J* 66:164, 1964.
118. Pearson CM: Myotubular myopathy. In Bergsma D (ed): *Birth Defects Compendium*. New York: National Foundation, 1979.
119. Page E, Polimeni PI, Zak R, et al: Myofibrillar mass in rat and rabbit heart muscle. *Circ Res* 30:430–439, 1972.
120. Peters TJ, Wells G, Oakley CM, et al: Enzymic analysis of endomyocardial biopsy specimens from patients with cardiomyopathies. *Br Heart J* 39:1333–1339, 1977.
121. Carafoli E: Mitochondria and disease. *Mol Aspects Med* 3:295–429, 1980.
122. Egger J, Lake BD, Wilson J: Mitochondrial cytopathy: A multisystem disorder with ragged red fibers on muscle biopsy. *Arch Dis Child* 56:741–752, 1981.
123. Neustein HB, Lurie PR, Dahms B, Takahashi M: An X-linked recessive cardiomyopathy with abnormal mitochondria. *Pediatrics* 64:24, 1979.
124. Barth TG, Scholete HR, Derden JA, et al: An X-linked mitochondrial disease affecting cardiac muscle, skeletal muscle and neutrophil leukocytes. *J Neurol Sci* 62:237, 1983.
125. Ino T, Sherwood WJ, Cutz E, Benson L, Rose V, Freedom RM: Dilated cardiomyopathy with neutropenia, short stature, and abnormal carnitine metabolism. *J Pediatr* 113:511, 1988.
126. Egger J, Wilson J: Mitochondria inheritance in a mitochondrially mediated disease. *N Engl J Med* 303:142–146, 1983.
127. Goertz K, Diehl AM, Vaseenon T, Mattioli L: A catastrophic complication. Acute dissection of an aortic aneurysm in a child with Marfan's syndrome. *J Kans Med Soc* 79:115, 1978.

128. Houston HE: Abdominal aortic aneurysm in Marfan's syndrome. *J Ky Med Assoc* 76:492, 1978.
129. Thilenius OG, Bharati S, Arcilla RA, Lev M: Cardiac pathology of Marfan's syndrome: Can dissection and rupture of aortic aneurysms be prevented? *Cardiology* 65:193, 1980.
130. McKusick VA: The cardiovascular aspects of Marfan's syndrome: A heritable disorder of connective tissue. *Circulation* 11:321, 1955.
131. Julien J, De Boucaud D: Aneurysme dans le systeme de la veine de Galien et syndrome de Marfan. *Bordeaux Med* 11:3245, 1971.
132. Crisfield RJ: Spontaneous aneurysm of the ductus arteriosus in a patient with Marfan's syndrome. *J Thorac Cardiovasc Surg* 62:243, 1971.
133. Fournier C: Les lesions cardio-vasculaires due syndrome de Marfan. *Coeur Med Interne* 16:331, 1977.
134. Bolande RP: The nature of the connective tissue abiotrophy in the Marfan syndrome. *Lab Invest* 12:1087, 1963.
135. Saruk M, Eisenstein R: Aortic lesion in Marfan syndrome. The ultrastructure of cystic medial degeneration. *Arch Pathol Lab Med* 101:74, 1977.
136. Takebayashi S, Kubota I, Takagi T: Ultrastructural and histochemical slides of vascular lesions in Marfan's syndrome, with report of 4 autopsy cases. *Acta Pathol Jpn* 23:847, 1973.
137. Roberts WC: Congenital cardiovascular abnormalities usually "silent" until adulthood: Morphologic features of the floppy mitral valve, valvular aortic stenosis, discrete subvalvular aortic stenosis, hypertrophic cardiomyopathy, sinus of Valsalva aneurysm, and the Marfan syndrome. In Roberts WC (ed): *Congenital Heart Disease in Adults*. Philadelphia: Davis, 1979, p 407.
138. Phornphutkul C, Rosenthal A, Nadas AS: Cardiac manifestations of Marfan syndrome in infancy and childhood. *Circulation* 57:587, 1973.
139. Simpson JW, Nord JJ, McNamara DG: Marfan's syndrome and mitral valve disease: Acute surgical emergencies. *Am Heart J* 77:96, 1969.
140. Olinger GN, Korns ME, Bonchek LI: Acute aortic valvular insufficiency due to isolated myxomatous degeneration. *Ann Intern Med* 88:807, 1978.
141. Jortner R, Shihin W, Eshkol D, Gueron M, Levy MJ: Cardiovascular manifestations and surgery for Marfan's syndrome. *Chest* 56:24, 1969.
142. Eldridge R: Coarctation in the Marfan syndrome. *Arch Intern Med* 113:342, 1964.
143. Marvel RJ, Genoves PD: Cardiovascular disease in Marfan's syndrome. *Am Heart J* 42:814, 1951.
144. McKusick VA, Neufeld EF: The mucopolysaccharide storage disease. In Stanbury JB et al (eds): *The Metabolic Basis of Inherited Disease*, 5th Ed, vol 36. New York: McGraw-Hill, 1983, pp 751–777.
145. Beighton P: Lethal complications of the Ehlers-Danlos syndrome. *Br Med J* 3:656, 1968.
146. Rotberg T, Sanagustin MT, Salinas L, Macias R: Sindrome de Ehlers-Danlos asociado a communicacion interauricular, bloqueo A-V completo, aneurisma de aorta y crecimento del ventriculo izquierdo (miocardiopatia). *Arch Inst Cardiol Mex* 47:462, 1977.
147. Burnett HF, Bledsoe JH, Char F, Williams GD: Abdominal aortic aneurysmectomy in a 17-year-old patient with Ehlers-Danlos syndrome: Case report and review of the literature. *Surgery* 74:617, 1973.
148. Caheen WR Jr, Reza MJ, Kovick RB, Stern MS: Mitral valve prolapse and conduction defects in Ehlers-Danlos syndrome. *Arch Intern Med* 137:1227, 1977.

149. Scully RE, Galdabini JJ, McNeely BU: Case 3-1979, presentation of case (case records of the Massachusetts General Hospital). *N Engl J Med* 300:129, 1979.
150. Beighton P: Lethal complications of the Ehlers-Danlos syndrome. *Br Med J* 3:656, 1968.
151. Barabas AP: Vascular complications in the Ehlers-Danlos syndrome. With special reference to the "arterial type" or "Sack's syndrome." *J Cardiovasc Surg* 13:160, 1972.
152. Schoolman A, Kepes JJ: Bilateral spontaneous carotid cavernous fistulae in Ehlers-Danlos syndrome. Case report. *J Neurosurg* 26:82, 1967.
153. Umlas J: Spontaneous rupture of the subclavian artery in the Ehlers-Danlos syndrome. *Hum Pathol* 3:121, 1972.
154. Sillence DO, Senn A, Danks DM: Genetic heterogeneity in osteogenesis imperfecta. *J Med Genet* 16:101, 1979.
155. Sillence DO, Barlow KK, Garber AP, Hall JG, Rimoin DL: Osteogenesis imperfecta type II delineation of the phenotype with reference to genetic heterogeneity. *Am J Med Genet* 17:407–423, 1984.
156. Steinmann B, Rao VH, Vogel A, Bruckner P, Gitzelmann B, Byers PH: Cysteine in the triple-helical domain of one allelic product of the alpha 1 (I) gene of type I collagen produces a lethal form of osteogenesis imperfecta. *J Biol Chem* 259:11129–11138, 1984.
157. Spranger J, Cremin B, Beighton P: Osteogenesis imperfecta congenita. *Pediatr Radiol* 12:21, 1982.
158. Cohen IM, Vieweg WVR, Alpert JS, Kaufman JA, Hagan AD: Osteogenesis imperfecta tarda. Cardiovascular pathology. *West J Med* 126:228, 1977.
159. De los Arcos E, Urguia M, Torrano E, et al: Osteogenesis imperfecta e insuficiencia aortica. Rev Clin Esp 133:531, 1974.
160. Heckman BA, Steinberg I: Congenital heart disease (mitral regurgitation) in osteogenesis imperfecta. *AJR* 103:601, 1968.
161. Melamed R, Aygen MM, Lowenstein A: Osteogenesis imperfecta with mitral insufficiency due to ballooning of the mitral valve. A case report. *Isr J Med Sci* 12:1325, 1976.
162. Pijoan de Beristain C: Asociacion de insuficiencia aortica con osteogenesis imperfecta, en dos sujetos de la misma familia. *Rev Esp Cardiol* 26:405, 1973.
163. Remigio PA, Grinvalsky HT: Ostegenesis imperfecta congenita. Association with conspicious extraskeletal connective tissue dysplasia. *Am J Dis Child* 119:524, 1970.
164. Siggers DC: Osteogenesis imperfecta with aortic valve replacement. *BDOAS* 10:495, 1974.
165. Stein D, Kloster FE: Valvular heart disease in osteogenesis imperfecta. *Am Heart J* 94:1172, 1977.
166. Wheeler VR, Cooley NR, Blackburn WR: Cardiovascular pathology in osteogenesis imperfecta type IIA with a review of the literature. *Pediatr Pathol* 8:55–64, 1988.
167. Goodman RM, Smith EW, Paton D, et al: Pseudoxanthoma elasticum: A clinical and histopathological study. *Medicine* 42:297, 1963.
168. Mendelsohn G, Bulkley BH, Hutchins GM: Cardiovascular manifestations of pseudoxanthoma elasticum. *Arch Pathol Lab Med* 102:298, 1978.
169. Schachner L, Young D: Pseudoxanthoma elasticum with severe cardiovascular disease in a child. *Am J Dis Child* 127:571, 1974.
170. Haust MD: Maternal diabetes mellitus–Effects on the fetus and placenta. In Naeye RL, Kissane JM, Kaufman N (eds): *Perinatal Pathology*. Baltimore: Williams and Wilkins, 1981, p 20 (Chapter 8).

171. Gutgesell HP, Mullins CE, Gillette PC, Speer M, Rudolph AJ, McNamara DG: Transient hypertrophic subaortic stenosis. *J Pediatr* 89:120–125, 1976.
172. Miller HC: Cardiac hypertrophy and extramedullary erythropoiesis in newborn infants of prediabetic mothers. *Am J Med Sci* 209:447, 1945.
173. Symons C: Thyroid heart disease. *Br Heart J* 41:257–262, 1979.
174. Schaffer MS, Zuberbuhler P, Wilson G, et al: Catecholamine cardiomyopathy: An unusual presentation of pheochromocytoma in children. *J Pediatr* 99:276–279, 1981.
175. Baim D, Rothman M, Harrison D: Improved catheter for regional sinus flow and metabolic studies. *Am J Cardiol* 45:997–1000, 1980.
176. Baim D, Rothman M, Harrison D: Simultaneous measurement of coronary venous blood flow and oxygen saturation during transient alterations in myocardial oxygen supply and demand. *Am J Cardiol* 49:743–752, 1982.
177. Kober G, Kunkel B, Becker HJ, et al: Technical aspects, experiences and complications of right and left ventricular endomyocardial biopsy. In Kaltenbach M, Loogen F, Olsen EGT (eds): *Cardiomyopathy and Myocardial Biopsy.* New York: Springer-Verlag, 1978.
178. Fujita M, Neustein HB, Lurie PR: Transvascular endomyocardial biopsy in infants and small children: Myocardial findings in 10 cases of cardiomyopoathy. *Hum Pathol* 10:15, 1979.
179. Tripp ME: *Congestive Cardiomyopathy of Childhood.* Chicago: Year Book, 1984, pp 179–202.
180. Gruhzit CC, Farah AE: A comparison of the positive inotropic effects of ouabain and epinephrine in heart failure induced in the dog heart-lung preparation by sodium pentobarbital, dinitrophenol, sodium cyanide and sodium azide. *J Pharmacol Exp Ther* 114:334–342, 1959.
181. Daly K et al: Significant incidence of mural thrombi in acute myocarditis–indication for early anticoagulation. *J Am Coll Cardiol* 1:584, 1983.

13
Hypoplastic Myenteric (Auerbach) Plexus of Small Intestine and Colon of Premature Infants with Bronchopulmonary Dysplasia Who Had Nissen Fundoplication for Gastroesophageal Reflux

DANIEL A. GALVIS, THEADIS R. WELLS, FRANK SINATRA,
BENJAMIN H. LANDING, MASOUD SHAMSZADEH

Introduction

Gastroesophageal reflux (GER) is well documented in premature infants with bronchopulmonary dysplasia (BPD).[1-3] When medical management is inadequate or no longer effective in improving reflux, Nissen fundoplication is the therapy most often used.[4] However, it has been our experience that these patients often continue to have gastrointestinal (GI) motility problems after surgery, and a variety of sequelae of fundoplication possibly related to abnormal intestinal motility, including persistent retching[5] and dumping syndrome,[6,7] have been reported in such patients. Whether gastric overdistension severe enough to cause gastric or visceral infarction occurs in the absence of other causes of intestinal obstruction such as adhesions[8] or volvulus[9] in infants who have had fundoplication is not known. This study demonstrates by a microdissection flat-mount preparation technique the structural abnormalities of the MEP of the small intestine and colon of premature infants with BPD who had gastroesophageal reflux treated by Nissen fundoplication. The abnormalities may explain continuing gastrointestinal tract dysmotility in such patients.

Presented as a poster presentation at the meeting of the Society for Pediatric Pathology, Feb. 27–28, 1988, Washington, DC.[1]
From the Departments of Pathology and Laboratory Medicine and the Gastroenterology Division of the Department of Pediatrics, Children's Hospital of Los Angeles, and the University of Southern California School of Medicine, Los Angeles, California.
Submitted by Dr Landing in honor of Lewis A. Barness, MD, November 1988.

Materials and Methods

Eight premature infants from the autopsy files of the Anatomic Pathology Division, Department of Laboratories, Childrens Hospital of Los Angeles, with pathological diagnosis of BPD who had GER requiring a Nissen fundoplication were compared to seven premature infants with BPD who had not had a Nissen fundoplication procedure, and to seven premature newborns. Formalin-fixed portions of esophagus, small intestine, and colon were macerated in concentrated hydrochloric acid at 55°C under an alkaline acid trap for 65 to 75 min.[10] Macerated specimens were microdissected by a previously described technique.[11] Photographs of the microdissected preparations were taken with a dissecting microscope, using Polaroid type 665 positive/negative film at magnification 20×. Point count analysis of the print negatives was used to study the relative mass of neural tissue in the plane of the myenteric (Auerbach) plexus (MEP). Control populations to establish normal values for plexus mass of esophagus, small intestine, and colon against gestational age consisted of infants with no genetic or GI tract disease. Statistical analysis of the differences between the study groups was done by Student's t- test. To check for possible cytomegalovirus (CMV) plexitis, sections of paraffin-embedded esophagus, small intestine, and colon from the fundoplication patients were stained for inclusions in ganglion cells using the Histo-Gen PAP-AB prediluted antibody and immunostaining system kit and examined by light microscopy.

Results

Tables 13.1, 13.2, and 13.3 list the patients in the study and give height, age, sex, gestational age for each of the infants studied, and the fraction of neural tissue in the plane of the MEP for esophagus, small intestine, and colon. Specimens from premature newborns (Table 13.1) showed a normal pattern ("circuit diagram") of the MEP and a normal mass of the plexus for all the levels of gastrointestinal tract studied (Figs. 13.1–13.3). For the premature newborns with BPD (Table 13.2) who had not had Nissen fundoplication, the specimens showed a normal pattern of the plexus at all levels and a normal relative fraction of neural tissue for esophagus and colon, but a low value for small intestine (Figs. 13.1–13.3). Specimens from patients who had had a Nissen fundoplication showed a normal pattern and mass of the Auerbach plexus for esophagus (Figs. 13.1, 13.4, 13.5). For the small intestine, however, the specimens showed an abnormal pattern of long, thin interganglionic fibers ("loose net"), and a relative fraction of neural tissue in the plane of the plexus below the normal mean value for height (mean fraction 0.156 ± 0.036, $p < .001$, $N = 8$) (Figs. 13.2, 13.6, 13.7). For colon, a less abnormal plexus patternwas found, and the relative fraction of neural tissue in the plexus was less low compared to normal than the values for small intestine (normal mean value $= 0.259 \pm 0.048, p < .01, N = 7$) (Figs. 13.3, 13.8, 13.9).

TABLE 13.1. Data for newborn infants.

Patient No.	Ht (cm)	Age (days)	Sex	Gestational age (wk)	Fraction of neural tissue in Auerbach plexus: Esophagus	Small intestine	Colon
1	33	3	M	26.5	0.29	0.41	–
2	34	1	M	26	0.36	0.35	0.38
3	35	NB	F	28	0.25	0.29	0.27
4	35	1	M	28	–	0.35	0.30
5	36	1	M	24–26	–	0.33	–
6	36	3	F	29	–	–	0.49
7	48	1	F	37	0.27	0.22	0.25

TABLE 13.2. Data for premature infants with bronchopulmonary dysplasia who had not had Nissen fundoplication.

Patient No.	Ht (cm)	Age (mo)	Sex	Gestational age (wk)	Fraction of neural tissue in plane of Auerbach plexus: Esophagus	Small intestine	Colon
1	31	¼	F	26	–	0.31	–
2	35	¼	M	28–30	0.35	–	0.44
3	36	¼	M	27–28	–	–	0.30
4	38	1	F	27	0.19	0.23	0.43
5	42	1½	F	28	0.26	0.18	0.31
6	42	2	M	27	0.25	0.26	0.36
7	44	¼	M	31–32	–	0.24	0.34

TABLE 13.3. Data on premature babies with bronchopulmonary dysplasia and gastroesophageal reflux who had Nissen fundoplication.

Patient No.	Ht (cm)	Age (mo)	Sex	Gestational age (wk)	Fraction of neural tissue in plane of Auerbach plexus: Esophagus	Small intestine	Colon
1	49	9	F	26–27	0.30	0.14	0.33
2	58	4	M	37	0.32	0.10	0.23
3	62	9	M	22	0.33	0.18	0.22
4	69	18	F	–	0.30	0.17	–
5	71	12	M	36	0.33	0.22	0.21
6	81	15	M	36	0.31	0.15	0.32
7	81	32	M	32–34	0.19	0.16	0.24
8	85	19	M	34	0.38	0.13	0.25

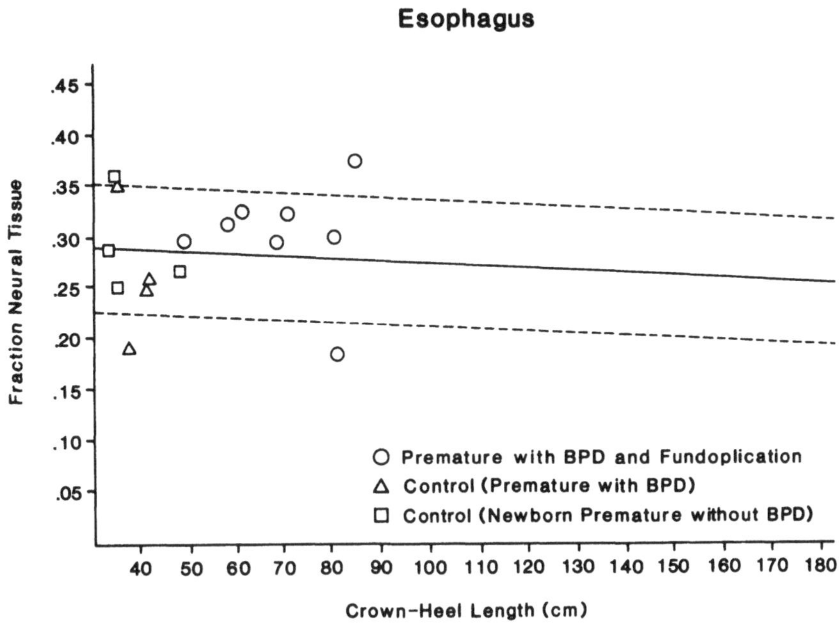

FIGURE 13.1. Fraction of neural tissue in the plane of the Auerbach plexus of the esophagus for the infants studied. The solid line shows the normal mean value of this fraction for infants of differing crown-heel lengths and gestational ages. The dotted lines show the values for 1 SD from the mean. The graph shows that the mean age of the newborn prematures was less than that of the premature infants who had developed bronchopulmonary dysplasia but who had not had a Nissen fundoplication, and that the infants who had had a fundoplication had the greatest mean age of the three groups studied.

CMV marker stain results were negative for viral inclusions in the ganglion cells at all levels of the gastrointestinal tract of all patients.

Discussion

Premature infants who develop BPD and symptomatic GER after receiving a Nissen fundoplication operation for the reflux often still have gastrointestinal motility problems. The results of this study, demonstrating reduced mass (hypoplasia) of the Auerbach plexus of the small intestine and colon of such patients, suggest that this abnormality is an acquired lesion rather than one intrinsic to prematurity. The data show that, for the three groups of patients studied, premature newborns, older premature infants with bronchopulmonary dysplasia, and still older premature infants with BPD who had had Nissen

FIGURE 13.2. Fraction of neural tissue in the plane of the Auerbach plexus of the small intestine of the infants studied. The graph shows that the mass of the plexus of the small intestine in the plane of the plexus normally falls with growth through infancy and childhood more than does the value for esophagus. The values for premature newborns are predominantly (5 of 6) within the normal range, whereas those for premature infants who had developed bronchopulmonary dysplasia but who had not had a Nissen fundoplication are predominantly (4 of 5) below the normal band, and those for all eight patients who had fundoplication are below the normal band.

►

►

FIGURE 13.3. Fraction of neural tissue in the plane of the Auerbach plexus of the colon for the infants studied. The graph shows that the mass of the plexus in the plane of the plexus normally falls with size and age through infancy and childhood. Mean values for the colonic plexus, for premature newborns who had bronchopulmonary dysplasia but who had not had a Nissen fundoplication, were within normal range. Whether "catch-up" growth of the colonic plexus occurs later (80 cm = 31 in.), or whether colonic growth "catches up" to the low plexus mass seen in three of the four post-Nissen patients smaller than 80-cm crown-heel length cannot be stated.

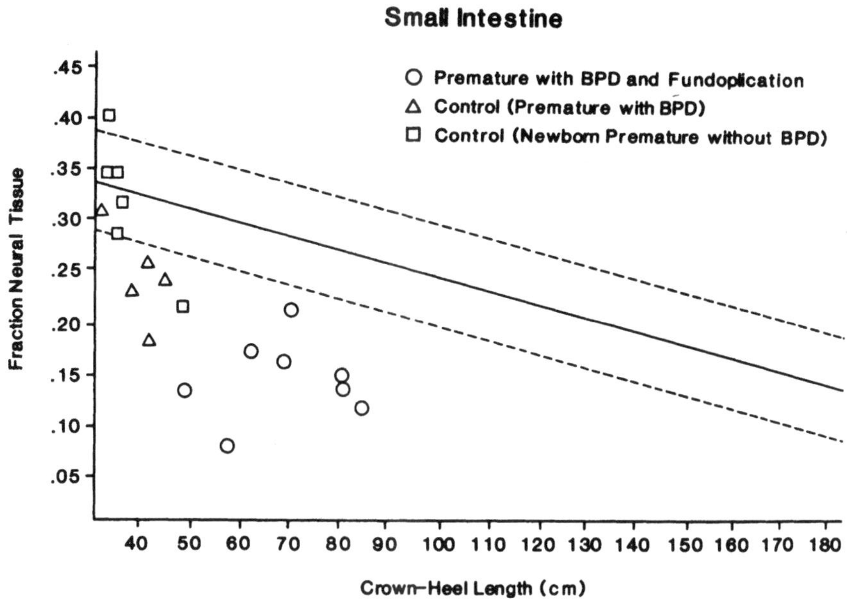
Small Intestine
Premature with BPD and Fundoplication
Control (Premature with BPD)
Control (Newborn Premature without BPD)
Fraction Neural Tissue
.45
.40
.35
.30
.25
.20
.15
.10
.05
40 50 60 70 80 90 100 110 120 130 140 150 160 170 180
Crown-Heel Length (cm)

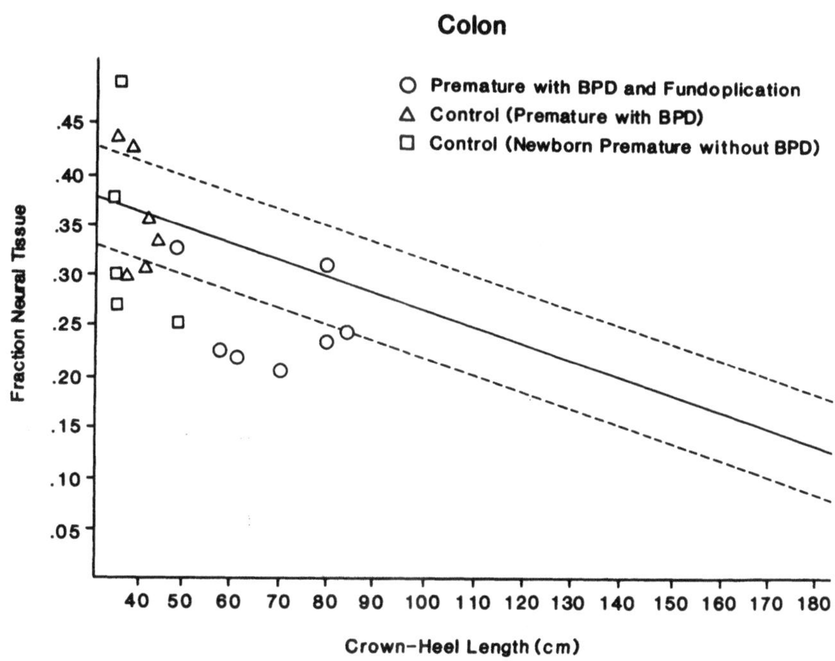
Colon
Premature with BPD and Fundoplication
Control (Premature with BPD)
Control (Newborn Premature without BPD)
Fraction Neural Tissue
.45
.40
.35
.30
.25
.20
.15
.10
.05
40 50 60 70 80 90 100 110 120 130 140 150 160 170 180
Crown-Heel Length (cm)

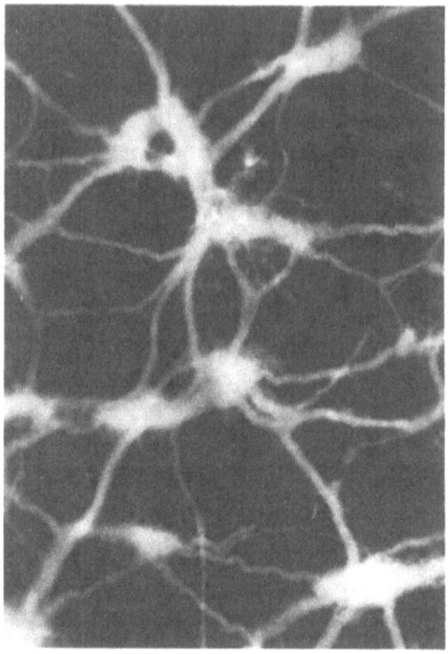

FIGURE 13.4. Normal Auerbach plexus of esophagus of control newborn premature patient (×20), showing the normally discrete and well-demarcated ganglia of the esophageal plexus[11] and the normal pattern of the plexus.

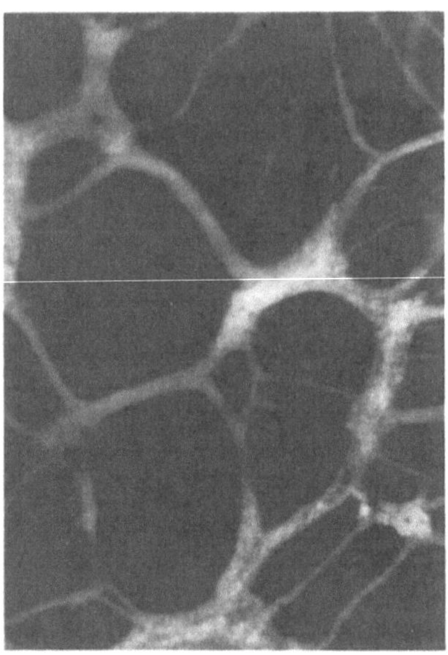

FIGURE 13.5. Auerbach plexus of esophagus of premature infant with bronchopulmonary dysplasia who had had a Nissen fundoplication. The fraction of neural tissue in the plane of the plexus is normal (×20).

fundoplication for gastroesophageal reflux, the MEP of small intestine and colon becomes more abnormal as the patients grow older. There are several possible explanations for this apparently acquired lesion of reduced "growth" (hypoplasia) of the plexus in patients who had received a fundoplication. These patients usually received less oral feeding and were more dependent on parenteral nutri-

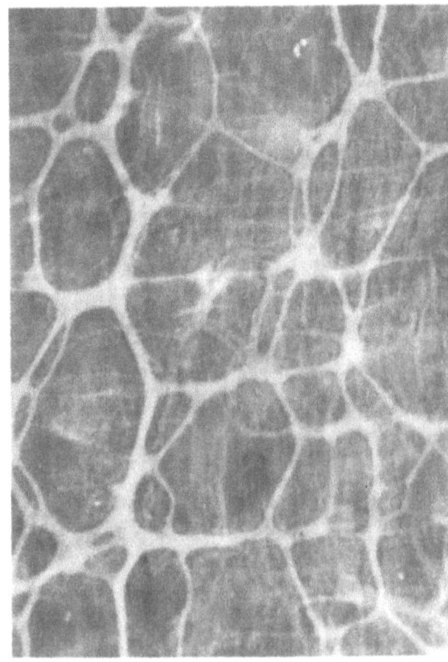

FIGURE 13.6. Normal Auerbach plexus of small intestine of control premature newborn infant, showing slender interganglionic fiber typical of this level of the gastrointestinal tract (×20).

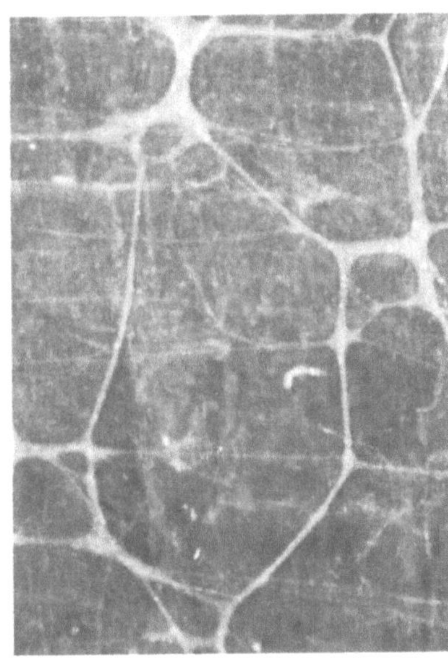

FIGURE 13.7. Auerbach plexus of small intestine of premature infant with BPD and fundoplication, showing reduced fraction of neural tissue in the plane of the plexus resulting from reduced number, reduced size, and wider spacing of the fibers (×20).

tion than the patients in the other two groups. Total parenteral nutrition is reported to result in reduced growth of stomach, small intestine, and colon in experimental animals,[12,13] but whether there is disproportionate retardation of the growth of the MEP in this circumstance has not been studied. If this does occur, the reduced gastrointestinal tract content may result in reduced work of

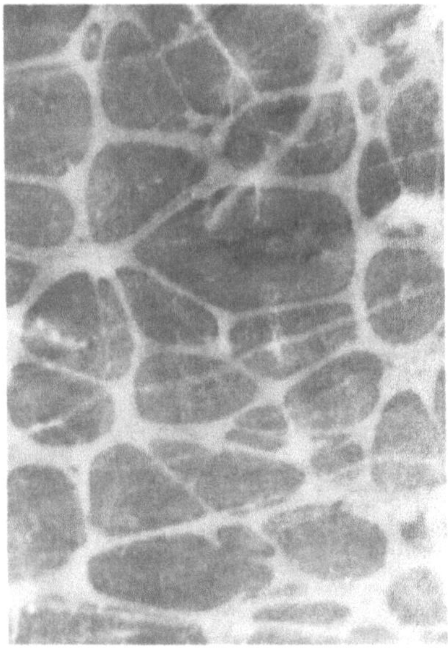

FIGURE 13.8. Normal Auerbach plexus of colon of control newborn premature infant, showing normally thicker interganglionic fibers than are seen in the small intestine (×20).

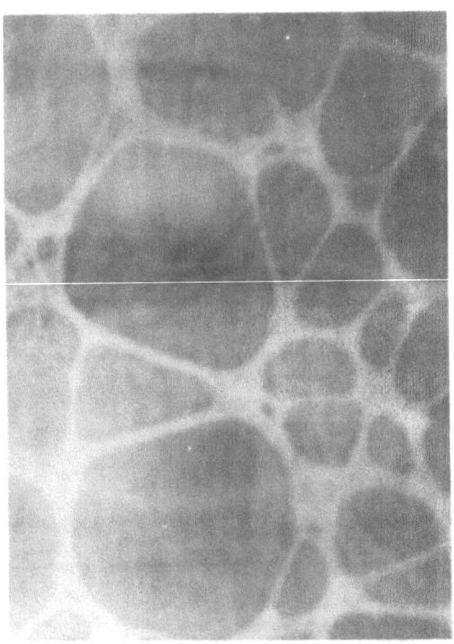

FIGURE 13.9. Auerbach plexus of colon of premature infant with BPD and fundoplication, showing reduced fraction of neural tissue in the plane of the plexus resulting from wider spacing of the fibers of the plexus net (×20).

the neuromuscular system of the GI tract; alternatively, it may be that growth of the plexus depends in part on nutrients directly from the lumen of the bowel rather than delivered by the bloodstream, or on specific chemicals produced by the bacterial flora of the bowel.

Whether episodes of GI tract ischemia not severe enough to lead to necrotizing enterocolitis can adversely affect the growth of the plexus in premature infants in the absence or reduction of oral feedings is also not known. Inadvertent partial vagotomy as a complication of the surgical procedure, although known to cause GI tract dysfunction in some patients and proposed as a possible cause of dumping syndrome following the Nissen procedure,[8,9] appears not to be a likely explanation for our findings, since, at least for the small intestine, MEP hypoplasia was found in premature infants with bronchopulmonary dysplasia who had not had Nissen fundoplication surgery.

Although premature infants are at high risk for developing CMV infection during hospitalization,[14] the findings of this study suggest that CMV plexitis is not the cause of the MEP hypoplasia found in premature infants with bronchopulmonary dysplasia in this study. Appropriate physiologic and functional studies of the kinds of infants analyzed in this study would be of interest as regards a possible effect of enterogastric reflux[15] on gastric emptying, although gastroesophageal reflux has been reported to occur both in patients with decreased rate of gastric emptying and in those with an increased rate.[5] Malagelada[16] says, in discussing neural feedback control of gastric emptying, "These mechanisms are poorly understood." The present study may improve insight into pathogenetic mechanisms underlying such functional disturbances.

References

1. Galvis DA, Wells TR, Sinatra F, Landing BH, Shamszadeh M: Hypoplastic myenteric (Auerbach) plexus of small intestine and colon of premature infants with bronchopulmonary dysplasia who had Nissen fundoplication for gastroesophageal reflux. *Lab Invest* 19:4, 1988 (abstract).
2. Hrabovsky EE, Mallett MD: Gastroesophageal reflux and the premature infant. *J Pediatr Surg* 21:583–587, 1986.
3. Giuffre RM, Rubin S, Mitchell I: Antireflux surgery in infants with bronchopulmonary dysplasia. *Am J Dis Child* 141:648–651, 1987.
4. Leape LL, Ramenolfsky ML: Surgical treatment of gastroesophageal reflux in children. *Am J Dis Child* 134:935–938, 1980.
5. Jolley SG, Tunell WP, Leonard JC, Hoelzer DJ, Smith EI: Gastric emptying in children with gastroesophageal reflux. 2. The relationship to retching symptoms following anti-reflux surgery. *J Pediatr Surg* 22:927–930, 1987.
6. Meyer S, Deckelbaum RJ, Lax E, Schilles M: Infant dumping syndrome after gastroesophageal reflux surgery. *J Pediatr* 99:235–237, 1981.
7. Hirsig J, Baals H, Tuchschmid P, Spitz L, Stauffer UG: Dumping syndrome following Nissen's fundoplication: A cause for refusal to feed. *J Pediatr Surg* 19:155–157, 1984.

8. Glick PL, Harrison MR, Adzick NS, Webb HW, DeLorimier AA: Gastric infarction secondary to small bowel obstruction: A preventable complication after Nissen fundoplication. *J Pediatr Surg* 22:941–943, 1987.
9. Idowu J, Razzouk AJ, Georgeson K: Visceral ischemia secondary to gastric dilatation: A rare complication of Nissen fundoplication. *J Pediatr Surg* 22:939–940, 1987.
10. Wells TR: A rapid method of maceration for microdissection. *Am J Clin Pathol* 47:349–350, 1967.
11. Wells TR, Landing BH, Ariel I, Nadorra R, Garcia C: Normal anatomy of the myenteric plexus of infants and children: Demonstration by flat-mount (circuit diagram) preparation. *Perspect Pediatr Pathol* 11:152–175, 1987.
12. Goldstein RM, Hebiguchi T, Luk GD, et al: The effects of total parenteral nutrition on gastrointestinal growth and development. *J Pediatr Surg* 20:785–791, 1985.
13. Morgan W, Yardley J, Luk G, Niemiec P, Dudgeon D: Total parenteral nutrition and intestinal development: A neonatal model. *J Pediatr Surg* 22:541–545, 1987.
14. Sawyer MH, Edwards DK, Spector SA: Cytomegalovirus infection and bronchopulmonary dysplasia in premature infants. *Am J Dis Child* 141:303–305, 1987.
15. Fisher RS: Pyloric sphincter dysfunction and the consequences of enterogastric reflux. In Dubvis A, Castell DO (eds): *Esophageal and Gastric Emptying*. Boca Raton, FL: CRC Press, 1984, pp 129–143.
16. Malagelada JR: Delayed gastric emptying: Pathophysiology, diagnosis and therapy. In Dubvis A, Castell DO (eds): *Esophageal and Gastric Emptying*. Boca Raton, FL: CRC Press, 1984, pp 95–107.

14
Studies on Early Embryonic Nutrition

ROBERT L. BRENT

In the late 1950s, we initiated an investigative program that appeared to be completely unrelated to placental transport, yolk sac dysfunction, or teratogenesis. We were interested in the changing pattern of tissue antigens throughout embryonic development and especially in the importance of cell surface macromolecules in embryonic development. As a part of that project, we raised numerous heterologous antisera against embryonic and adult rat tissues. During localization studies with these antisera in pregnant rats, we discovered that rabbit anti-rat kidney serum was a potent teratogenic agent (Fig. 14.1).[1] Kidney antiserum produced teratogenesis, growth retardation, and embryonic death during the entire period of early organogenesis. The higher the dose, the greater the effect (Table 14.1).

Characterization of Teratogenic Antisera

A series of experiments followed that identified IgG as the serum component that was teratogenic.[2] Early experiments indicated that an immunoglobulin was the teratogen, or at least some protein, since oral administration of the antiserum was ineffective as a reproductive toxin (Table 14.2) and that intravenous and intraperitoneal administration was the most effective means of producing teratogenesis. The teratogenic immunoglobulin did not need complement to function, was not inhibited by pretreatment with cortisone or antihistamines, localized in the visceral and parietal yolk sac (but not the embryo) (Figs. 14.2, 14.3), and was primarily directed against the visceral yolk sac (VYS).[3-13] The surprising localization of heterologous antiserum against rat kidney in the rat VYS and parietal yolk sac prompted us to prepare antisera against whole yolk sac as well as visceral and parietal yolk sac (Fig. 14.3; Table 14.3). It became clear that the teratogenic

From the Department of Pediatrics, Thomas Jefferson University College of Medicine, Philadelphia, Pennsylvania, and the A.I. duPont Institute and Children's Hospital, Wilmington, Delaware.
Presented in part at the Teratology Society Yolk Sac Symposium, June 1987.
Presented in honor of Lewis A. Barness, MD, November 11, 1988.

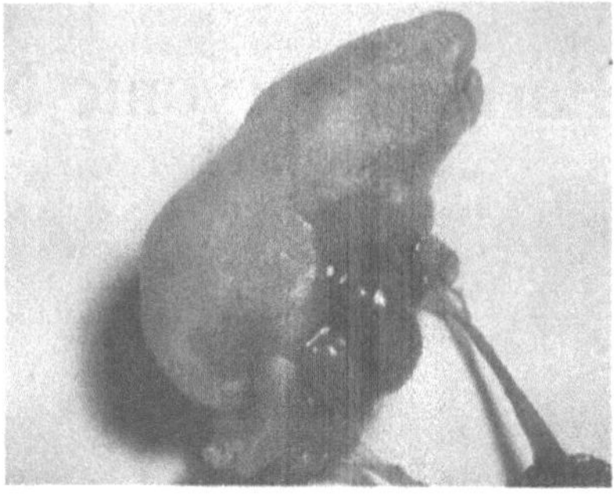

FIGURE 14.1. Serious malformations of all organ systems were produced by rabbit anti-rat kidney sera on the 9th through 12th day of development. This severely malformed term fetus is anencephalic, with no head development above the maxillary processes, and has a large omphalocele, many visceral malformations, and severe limb malformations. The antisera were administered on the 9th day of rat development, and the fetus was examined at term.

TABLE 14.1. Growth-retarding and lethal effects of rabbit anti-rat kidney antiserum and normal rabbit serum on rat embryos on the 8th, 9th 10th, and 11th days of gestation.

Getational age (days)	Dose (ml) per 100-g pregnant rat: Normal rabbit serum	Dose (ml) per 100-g pregnant rat: Rabbit anti-rat kidney antiserum	Numbers of embryos (preinjection)	Term fetuses: Mortality (%)	Term fetuses: No.	Term fetuses: Weight ± SD	Overall percent fetuses malformed
9- and 10-day operative controls	0	0	97	8.2	89	4.80 ± 0.31	1.7
8	2.0	0	49	6.1	46	4.89 ± 0.64	2.2
10	2.0	0	57	7.5	53	4.62 ± 0.71	1.9
11	2.0	0	41	9.7	37	4.91 ± 0.44	0.0
8	0	0.25	73	13.7	63	4.39 ± 0.26	25.4
		0.50	66	45.5	36	3.99 ± 0.90	38.9
		0.75	71	77.5	16	3.83 ± 0.63	81.4
		1.00	52	98.1	1	2.81	100.0
9	0	0.25	68	19.0	55	4.06 ± 0.17	85.6
	0	0.50	87	49.4	44	4.04 ± 0.21	79.6
		0.75	68	97.1	2	1.55	100.0
		1.00	71	100.0	0		
10	0	0.25	102	11.8	90	4.36 ± 0.60	34.4
		0.50	87	38.0	54	4.11 ± 0.74	55.6
		0.75	97	100.0	0		
11	0	0.25	93	7.5	86	4.46 ± 0.80	14.0
		0.50	80	13.6	69	3.80 ± 0.67	42.0
		0.75	72	91.7	6	3.32 ± 0.33	100.0

TABLE 14.2. Teratogenic, lethal, and growth-retarding effects of rabbit anti-rat kidney serum when administered by the intravenous, intraperitoneal, subcutaneous, or oral route to rats on the 9th day of pregnancy.

Route of administration	Dose (ml) per 100-g pregnant rat	No. of embryos (preinjection)	Mortality (%)	Term fetuses		Malformed fetuses (%)
				No.	Wt ± SD	
Intravenous	0.125	58	10.5	52	4.51 ± 0.37	42.3
	0.25	65	24.2	52	4.15 ± 0.52	75.0
	0.50	80	48.9	41	4.19 ± 0.67	95.2
Intraperitoneal	0.25	68	19.0	55	4.06 ± 0.17	85.6
	0.50	87	49.4	44	4.04 ± 0.21	79.6
	0.75	68	97.1	2	1.55	100.0
	1.0	71	100.0	0	–	–
Subcutaneous	0.25	79	5.1	75	5.21 ± 0.502	5.3
	–	–	–	–	–	–
	0.75	68	20.5	53	4.12 ± 0.60	81.2
	1.00	63	31.8	43	3.87 ± 0.62	86.3
Oral	1.00	74	0.0	74	4.44 ± 0.36	0.0
	2.00	59	5.1	56	4.93 ± 0.41	1.9
	3.00	24	4.1	23	5.05 ± 0.31	0.0
Control	–	97	8.2	89	4.80 ± 0.31	1.7

antibody produced malformations only if the antisera localized in the VYS (Figs. 14.4–14.6).[12]

We had developed a model for producing isolated VYS dysfunction. Using the technique of embryo culture, we demonstrated that teratogenic antiserum can affect the development of the yolk sac and embryo directly (Fig. 14.7). Injections of concentrated antisera (IgG) had no effect on the developing embryo when they came in direct contact with the embryo but did not interact with the VYS.[14]

Other laboratories confirmed that certain tissue antisera can be potent teratogens, but did not pursue the matter beyond their original reports.[15-21]

Attempts to isolate the teratogenic stimulating antigens have been reported by Jensen et al,[22] Leung,[23] Freeman and Brown,[24] and Sahali et al.[25] In our laboratory, isoelectric focusing of VYS proteins revealed numerous bands that could produce teratogenic antisera, and these antigens had a wide range of molecular weights. The other three investigators indicated that they had identified the specific teratogenic-stimulating antigen, but all three antigens had different molecular weights. It thus appears that there may be several sites on the VYS plasma membrane that can stimulate the production of teratogenic antibodies, or that a larger protein, containing a teratogenic-stimulating epitope can be broken down into several different-size components.

The teratogenic effect of Trypan Blue had previously been reported by Gillman et al,[26] but we did not see the relationship between their report and our research. They did not pursue the mechanism of teratogenesis except to point out that Trypan Blue stained the yolk sac heavily but not the embryo. They also suggested

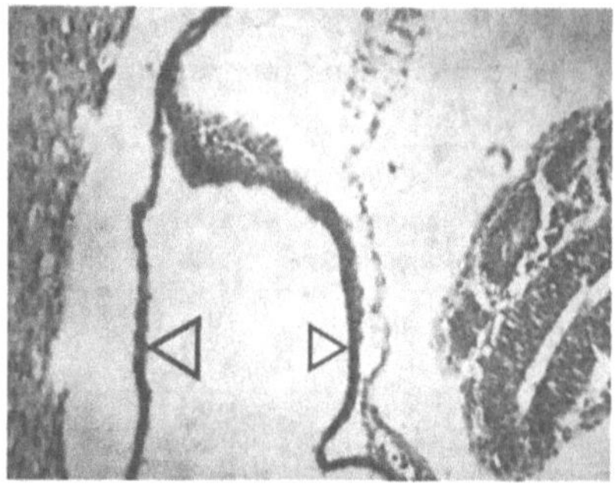

FIGURE 14.2. Embryonic site obtained on the 11th day following injection of the rat 48 h before sacrifice with ^{125}I-labeled sheep anti-rat kidney gamma globulin. Autoradiographs were prepared and stained with hematoxylin and eosin. There is a heavy concentration of silver grains in the parietal (large arrow) and visceral yolk sac (small arrow). The embryo and placenta have a background concentration of silver grains[7].

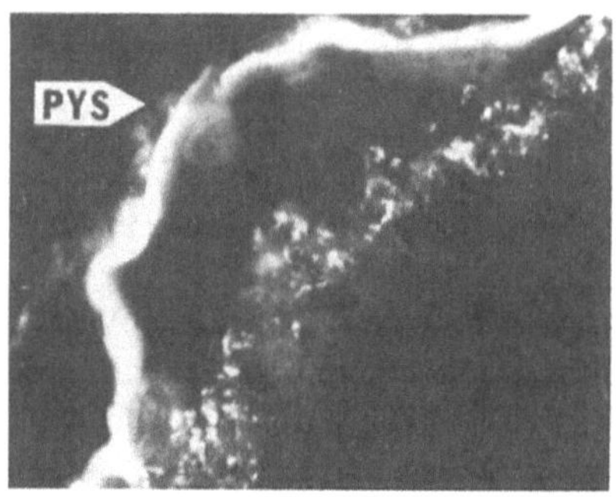

FIGURE 14.3. Frozen section of a 12-day, 4-h-old rat embryo obtained from a pregnant rat injected with sheep anti- yolk sac serum on the 9th day of pregnancy. Localization is heaviest in the parietal yolk sac (RM) (PYS). Visceral yolk sac cells are also outlined by specific fluorescence. Control (nonteratogenic) sheep serum is not present in either the parietal or visceral yolk sac 48 h after injection.

TABLE 14.3. Comparison of the embryopathic effects of antiserum prepared against (1) 14-day-old (15th day) RM, (2) adult rat kidney, and (3) absorbed term whole-rat VYS.

Tissue antiserum injected on the 9th day of pregnancy	Dose (mg/kg)	No. of pregnant rats	Total No. of embryos on 9th day	Total No. of embryos at term	Resorptions (%)	Term fetal weight (g)	Malformations (%)
Control sheep serum	350	9	94	84	10.6	4.68	1.2
RM	50	2	22	22	0.0	4.91	0.0
RM	70–100	6	65	49	24.6	4.26	0.0
RM	110–150	14	169	91	46.1	4.19	0.0
RM	160–200	9	105	20	81.0	3.12	<10
RM	240–600	2	24	0	100.0	–	–
Whole kidney	175	4	50	20	60	3.89	80
Term VYS	100	5	65	47	27.6	3.90	91.4
Term VYS adsorbed with 15th-day RM	70–100	3	34	30	12.3	4.02	100.0
Term VYS adsorbed with 15th-day RM	125	5	58	20	41.2	3.35	100.0
Term VYS adsorbed with 15th-day RM	140	2	30	7	70.0	2.16	100.0
Term VYS adsorbed with 15th-day YS	100–120	3	34	29	14.7	4.89	0.0
Term VYS adsorbed with 15th-day YS	140	2	23	18	21.7	4.37	0.0
Term VYS adsorbed with 15th-day YS	160	2	26	8	69.2	4.12	0.0

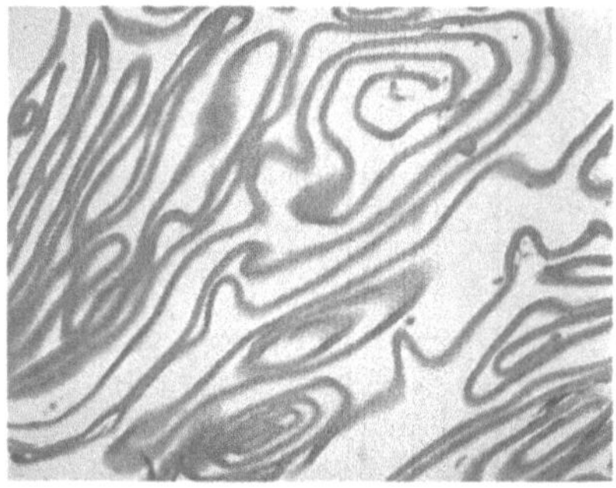

FIGURE 14.4. Reichert's membrane was dissected free on the 14th day of gestation after the embryonic site was frozen at −60°C for at least 24 h. A pure preparation of Reichert's membrane was obtained with this simple procedure.[12]

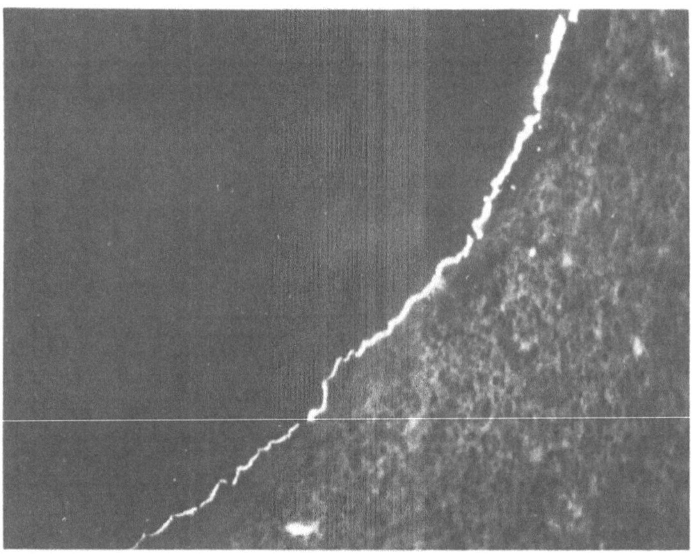

FIGURE 14.5. Frozen section of 11th-day embryonic site from a rat injected with rabbit anti-rat RM serum on the 9th day of gestation and stained with FITC-labeled goat anti-rabbit IgG. Note that the VYS is unstained and therefore not visible. Only RM fluoresces, having localized RM antisera. ×50. This antiserum was not teratogenic.

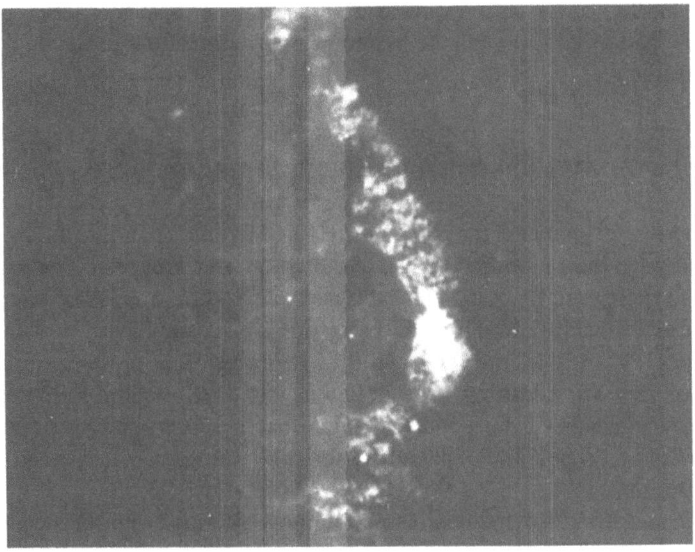

FIGURE 14.6. Four-micrometer frozen section of 11th-day embryonic site from a pregnant rat injected with antiserum on the 9th day of pregnancy. The antiserum injected was teratogenic sheep anti-rat VYS serum adsorbed with RM. The indirect fluorescent technique was utilized in this preparation. Only the cytoplasm of the VYS cells stains with the VYS antiserum adsorbed with RM, yet this adsorbed antiserum is still teratogenic. ×210.

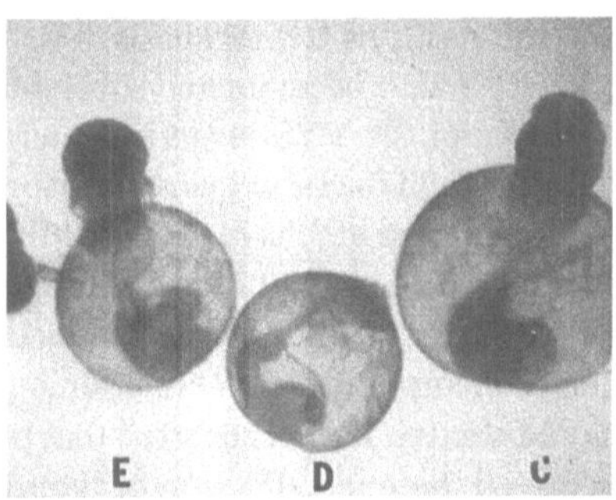

FIGURE 14.7. Rat embryos explanted at 9.5 days of gestation and grown for 24 h. C: Control grown in rat serum. E: Embryo grown in anti-yolk serum at a concentration of 0.1 mg/ml. D: Embryos grown in anti-yolk sac serum at a concentration of 1 mg/ml of antiserum. Embryos grown in anti-yolk sac serum at a concentration of 10 mg/ml of antiserum did not survive. The antiserum used was the gamma globulin fraction. Note that the ectoplacental cone continues to grow normally even in the highest concentration of yolk sac antiserum. Yolk sac development was affected even with the lowest concentration of antiserum.[14]

that the mechanism of action was due to alterations of maternal serum proteins by the Trypan Blue. Although the hypothesis was wrong, it touched on the truth conceptually.

Early Embryonic Nutrition (during organogenesis)

Beck and Lloyd[27] pursued the mechanism of action of Trypan Blue in the 1960s, which focused their attention on the YS. In 1966, our group[4] and their group[24] published reviews in the same journal issue, and neither group was aware of the intimate relationship between our investigations. Beck and Lloyd[27] first hypothesized that Trypan Blue interfered with the degradation of proteins in the lysosomes of the YS, resulting in a deficiency of histiotrophic nutrition. Our laboratory pursued an independent course that led us to consider embryonic malnutrition as a possible explanation for the teratogenic mechanism of yolk sac antiserum.

Kobrin and Brent[28] demonstrated that teratogenic antiserum reduced the concentration of free leucine in the visceral yolk sac and embryo. This suggested that the transport of macromolecules containing leucine was reduced following the administration of teratogenic yolk sac antiserum. It occurred to Lloyd that it was unlikely that Trypan Blue could completely suppress the hydrolase activity in the lysosomes, and he therefore initiated studies to quantitate the endocytosis of macromolecules by the VYS. These studies culminated in demonstrating that Trypan Blue had markedly reduced the endocytosis of macromolecules and that it was this effect of Trypan Blue that explained the reduction in histiotrophic embryonic nutrition and the resulting teratogenesis.[29,30]

Williams and co-workers[31,32] have accumulated substantial circumstantial evidence for the nutritional role of the VYS involving internalization of proteins, their intralysosomal digestion, and the subsequent release of amino acids into the embryonic circulation. Freeman et al[33] have provided direct experimental evidence that radiolabeled amino acid present in protein in the medium is taken up by the VYS of the cultured embryo and digested intracellularly to free amino acids which are eventually incorporated into embryonic protein in vitro. Rowe and Kalaizis,[34] utilizing radioactive serine, reported that proteins synthesized by the VYS and embryo derived the major fraction of their precursor serine from maternal serum proteins and not from free serine in maternal serum.

Role of "Malnutrition" in Embryonic Maldevelopment

It is extremely difficult to study the impact of embryonic malnutrition on the developing human embryo. We know that a large proportion of human malformations has no known etiology[35] and that maternal disease states (diabetes, alcoholism, phenylketonuria, collagen disease, endocrinopathies, etc) are associated with some malformations and embryolethality. Smith[36,37] initially reported the intrauterine impact of famine on the Dutch population to be primarily infertility, growth retardation, and spontaneous abortion. A more recent analysis of the data[38] revealed that prenatal exposure to famine early in gestation increased prenatal and neonatal mortality and increased the incidence of central nervous system abnormalities (spina bifida and hydrocephalus), prematurity, and death from meningitis later in life. Exposure to famine late in gestation resulted in intrauterine growth retardation. It has been estimated that 5% of all live births in the United States and 10% in underdeveloped countries are affected by fetal undernutrition or malnutrition.[39]

Most nutritional studies have not dealt with the period of organogenesis and the relevance of nutritional alterations to major malformations. We have carried these studies further.[40,41] Utilizing radioactive leucine in free and protein-bound form, we have demonstrated that 99% of the leucine utilized by the embryo and YS for protein synthesis is derived from protein-bound leucine and that polyclonal teratogenic VYS antibody markedly inhibits this process. It was further demonstrated that specificity of an antiserum for the yolk sac did not guarantee that it would result in teratogenesis.[42] In fact, we now have demonstrated that many yolk sac localizing antibodies are not teratogenic. The only antisera that are teratogenic are those that localize in the VYS and reduce pinocytosis, thereby decreasing the uptake of proteins by the VYS and depriving the embryo and VYS of an adequate supply of amino acids for embryonic and VYS protein synthesis.

While Brent's early experiments clearly indicated that the teratogenic agent was IgG,[6] the localization studies only provided circumstantial evidence that teratogenic antisera produced yolk sac dysfunction. The studies of New and Brent[14] indicated that the visceral yolk sac was more vulnerable to teratogenic antibodies than was the embryo or chorioplacenta (Fig. 14.7). Furthermore, direct injection of teratogenic antibody into the amniotic cavity or yolk sac cavity did not harm the cultured embryo. This indicated that the antibody had to reach the surface of the endodermal cells of the VYS in order to damage the embryo.

Role of the Primate Yolk Sac

In 1972, Brent et al[43] indicated that it was important to understand the functions of the primate yolk sac (YS) because of its potential role in human teratogenesis. The title of this publication was "The Death of Another Vestigial Organ." In that same year, Gitlin et al[44] published their work dealing with the production of α- fetoprotein by the human YS. Actually, there were prior indications that the primate YS had important functions and played a role in human embryopathology. Arey[45] reported in 1923 an abnormal human embryo without a YS that had spontaneously aborted. Crooij et al[46] reported an abnormal human embryo with spina bifida and an absent YS at the 9th week of gestation. There are some excellent studies dealing with normal human and primate YS development.[47-56] These studies revealed that the human YS continues to grow until the 10th or 11th week of gestation and that it may reach 3 to 4 mm in diameter in early organogenesis.

There have been far fewer functional and morphologic studies dealing with the human and primate YS than those concerned with the rodent YS.[57] Yet, the human YS is a source of hematopoietic cells[58,59] and produces albumin, prealbumin, α-fetoprotein, α_1-antitrypsin, transferrin, and apolipoproteins.[52,60,61] Just as important as these functional studies is the evidence that the human YS and the primate YS have an ultrastructure similar to that of the rodent YS.[56] In fact, there are interesting features with regard to the structure of the microvilli on the endodermal and mesothelial surfaces that by themselves warrant more intensive investigation of the human and primate YS. One other important advance that will accelerate the study of the human YS is the utilization of ultrasonography to locate and describe the YS and to make it possible to determine the extent of the material that may be available for examination and use.[46,62,63] Thus, these recent developments in human and primate YS morphology, function, and availability, along with our laboratories' ability to isolate a spectrum of YS antigens, perform endocytic studies, and prepare monoclonal antibodies, should provide information that will increase our understanding of YS function and dysfunction in the human.

Possible Role of Yolk Sac Immunology in Contraception or Pregnancy Control

The WHO has had a committee looking at immunologic means for pregnancy control and has collected monoclonal antibodies (MCAs) against trophoblast and sperm antigens in an effort to "identify candidate antigens for the development of birth control vaccines."[64] They note that the vast majority of the MCAs cross-react with other tissues. It is interesting that the YS antigens have never been examined by this group even though our own studies indicate that there is less cross- specificity of many YS antigens with adult tissues than with trophoblast and sperm antigens.

Teratogenic Monoclonal Yolk Sac Antibodies

The production of MCAs against various YS antigens has been an important development[65-69] We now have prepared a series of MCAs against VYS antigens that produce congenital malformations, fetal growth retardation, and embryonic death in a dose-related incidence. Having potent, purified teratogenic and non-teratogenic MCAs against VYS antigens presents an opportunity to use MCAs as carriers of macromolecules or drugs to the embryo, to study YS plasma membrane synthesis, to study the effect of varying fluid-phase and receptor-mediated endocytosis on embryonic nutrition and development; to compare yolk sac function among different species, and to determine the cross-specificity of yolk sac antigens with other embryonic and adult tissues. These MCAs also quantitatively suppress pinocytosis of the VYS. Thus, varying degrees of amino acid deprivation can be produced in the growing embryo during organogenesis without interfering with the status of the mother's well-being or nutritional state.

These MCAs provide a unique opportunity to study early embryonic nutrition and to study the relative importance of various amino acids during organogenesis. They also offer us the opportunity to determine the "relative value" of various serum proteins in optimally supporting embryonic growth and development.

Thus, the preparation of monoclonal teratogenic antibodies that suppress VYS pinocytosis has provided us with a powerful new tool to study embryonic nutrition during organogenesis. This aids in establishing a quantitative floor and ceiling for individual amino acids which will permit normal development and determine whether the embryo is more vulnerable to deficiencies or excesses of certain amino acids.

Acknowledgments. This study was supported in part by NIHHD18396. Thanks go to DA Beckman, M Jensen, C Leung, JB Lloyd, and TR Koszaeka for their assistance.

References

1. Brent RL, Averich E, Drapiewski VA: Production of congenital malformations using tissue antibodies. I. Kidney antisera. *Proc Soc Exp Biol* 106:523–526, 1961.
2. Brent RL: The production of congenital malformations using tissue antisera. II. The spectrum and incidence of malformations following the administration of kidney antiserum to pregnant rats. *Am J Anat* 115:525–542, 1964.
3. Brent RL: Effects of proteins, antibodies, and autoimmune phenomena upon conception and embryogenesis. In Wilson JG, Warkany J (eds): *Teratology.* Chicago: University of Chicago Press, 1965, pp 215–233.
4. Brent RL: Immunologic aspects of developmental biology. In Woolam DHM (ed): *Advances in Teratology,* Vol 1. London: Logo Press, 1966, p 82–129.
5. Brent RL: The production of congenital malformations using tissue antiserum. IV. Evaluation of the mechanism of teratogenesis by varying the route and time of administration of anti-rat kidney antiserum. *Am J Anat* 199:555–562, 1966.
6. Brent RL: Some biologic properties of teratogenic antisera. *Official Journal of the Congenital Anomalies Research Association of Japan* 6:12–14, 1966.
7. Brent RL: The effect of immune reactions on fetal development. *Adv Biosci* 6:422–455, 1971.
8. Brent RL, Bragonier JB, Frank MM: Production of congenital malformations using tissue antisera. IX. Effectiveness of structurally modified antikidney antibodies. *Teratology* 3:198, 1970.
9. Brent RL, Johnson AJ, Jensen M: The production of congenital malformations using tissue antisera. VII. Yolk sac antiserum. *Teratology* 4:255–276, 1971.
10. Bragonier JR, Frank MM, Brent RL: Production of congenital malformations using tissue antisera. VIII. Effectiveness of reduced, alkylated, and digested anti-kidney antibodies. *J Immunol* 105:1175–1180, 1970.
11. Slotnick V, Brent RL: The production of congenital malformations using tissue antisera. V. Fluorescent localization of teratogenic antisera in the maternal and fetal tissue of the rat. *J Immunol* 96:606–610, 1966.
12. Jensen M, Koszalka TR, Brent RL: Production of congenital malformations using tissue antisera. XV. Reichert's membrane and visceral yolk sac antisera. *Dev Biol* 42:1–12, 1975.

13. Brent RL, Jensen M: Immunologic aspects of development. In Wilson JG, Fraser FC (eds): *Handbook of Teratology*. New York: Plenum Press, Vol 4, 1978, pp 339–396.
14. New DAT, Brent RL: Effect of yolk-sac antibody on rat embryos grown in culture. *J Embryol Exp Morphol* 27:543–553, 1972.
15. Barrow MV, Taylor WJ: The production of congenital defects in rats using antisera. *J Exp Zool* 176:41–60, 1971.
16. David G, Mercier-Parot L, Tuchmann-Duplessis H: Action teratogne d'heteroanticorps tissulaires. I. Production de malformations chez le rat par action d'un serum antirein. *C R Seances Soc Biol* 157:939, 1963.
17. Eyquem A, Gutman G, Bisson J, Mercier-Parot L, David G, Tuchmann-Duplessis H: Etude en immunofluorescence et cytotoxicite des immunserums teratogenes. *Ann Inst Pasteur* 115:841–854, 1968.
18. Gebhardt DOE, Baart de la Faille-Kuyper EH, Nagel J: The embryolethality and localization of anti-kidney serum in the pregnant mouse. *Teratology* 3:143–152, 1970.
19. Mercier-Parot L, David G, Tuchmann-Duplessis H: Action teratogene d'heteroanticorps tissulaires. II. Etude de l'action teratogene chez la souris de serums anti–rein. *C R Seances Soc Biol* 157:974, 1963.
20. Mikailov VM: Pathogenic action of nephrocytotoxic serum on embryonic development of albino rats. *Biull Eksp Biol Med* 63:97–100, 1976.
21. Vaillancourt P, McCallion DJ: Inhibitory effects of nephrotoxic antisera on the growth of rat fetuses. *J Obstet Gynecol* 114:225–231, 1972.
22. Jensen M, Koszalka TR, Vega P, Brent RL: The purification of rat visceral yolk sac antigens which produce teratogenic antiserum by means of isoelectric focusing. *Pediatr Res* 16:270A, 1982.
23. Leung CCW: Isolation, partial characterization, and localization of a rat renal tubular glycoprotein antigen. Antibody-induced birth defects. *J Exp Med* 156:372–384, 1982.
24. Freeman SJ, Brown NA: An in vitro study of teratogenicity in the rat due to antibody-induced yolk sac dysfunction. Identification of the yolk sac antigen involved. *Roux's Arch Dev Biol* 195:236–242, 1986.
25. Sahali D, Mulliez N, Chatelet F, Dupuis R, Ronco P, Verroust P: Characterization of a 280-kD protein restricted to the coated pits of the renal brush border and the epithelial cells of the yolk sac. *J Exp Med* 167:213–218, 1988.
26. Gillman J, Gilbert C, Gillman T, Spence I: A preliminary report on hydrocephalus, spina bifida, and other congenital anomalies in the rat produced by trypan blue: The significance of the results in the interpretation of congenital malformations following maternal rubella. *S Afr J Med Sci* 13:47–90, 1948.
27. Beck F, Lloyd JB: The teratogenic effects of azodyes. In Woolan DHM (ed): *Advances in Teratology*, Vol 1. London: Logo Press, 1966, pp 131–193.
28. Kobrin LE, Brent RL: Effect of yolk sac antiserum on embryonic parameters of free and bound ^{14}C-leucine. *Teratology* 7:A-21, 1973.
29. Williams KE, Kidston ME, Beck F, Lloyd JB: Quantitative studies of pinocytosis. II. Kinetics of protein uptake and digestion by rat yolk sac cultured in vitro. *J Cell Biol* 64:123–134, 1975.
30. Pratten MK, Duncan R, Lloyd JB: Adsorptive and passive pinocytic uptake. In Okkleford CD, Whiye A (eds): *Coated Vesicles*. London: Cambridge University Press, 1980, pp 179–218.
31. Williams KE, Kidston ME, Beck F, Lloyd JB: Quantitative studies of pinocytosis. I. Kinetics of uptake of [^{125}I] polyvinylpyrrolidone by rat yolk sac cultured in vitro. *J Cell Biol* 64:113–122, 1975.

32. Williams KE, Roberts G, Kidston ME, Beck F, Lloyd JB: Inhibition of pinocytosis in rat yolk sac by Trypan Blue. *Teratology* 14:343–354, 1976.
33. Freeman SJ, Beck F, Lloyd JB: The role of the visceral yolk sac in mediating protein utilization of rat embryos cultured in vitro. *J Embryol Exp Morphol* 66:223–234, 1981.
34. Rowe PB, Kalaizis A: Serine metabolism in rat embryos undergoing organogenesis. *J Embryol Exp Morph* 87:137–144, 1985.
35. Brent RL: The complexities of solving the problem of human malformations. In Brent RL, Beckman DA (eds): *Clinics in Perinatology*, Vol 13. Philadelphia: WB Saunders, 1986, pp 491–503.
36. Smith C: The effect of wartime starvation in Holland upon pregnancy and its product. *Am J Obstet Gynecol* 53:599–608, 1947.
37. Smith C: Effects of maternal undernutrition upon the newborn infant in Holland (1944–1945). *J Pediatrics* 30:229–243, 1947.
38. Stein Z, Susser M, Saeger G, Marolla F: *Famine and Human Development. The Dutch Hunger Winter of 1944/45*. New York: Oxford University Press, 1975.
39. Metcoff J: Maternal leukocyte metabolism in fetal malnutrition. In Roche AF, Falkner F (eds): *Advances in Experimental Medicine and Biology: Nutrition and Malnutrition*, Vol 49. New York: Plenum Press, 1974, p 49.
40. Beckman DA, Pugarelli J, Koszalka TR, Jensen M, Lloyd JB, Brent RL: Serum proteins versus free amino acids as a source of amino acids for protein synthesis by cultured rat embryos. *Teratology* 33:83–84C, 1986.
41. Beckman DA, Pugarelli JE, Koszalka TR, Jensen M, Lloyd JB, Brent RL: The effects of teratogenic antisera on protein synthesis and degradation by cultured rat conceptus. *Teratology* 35:70A, 1987.
42. Lerman S, Koszalka TR, Jensen M, Andrew CL, Beckman DA, Brent RL: In vitro studies on the effect of yolk sac antisera on functions of the visceral yolk sac: I. Pinocytosis and transport of small molecules. *Teratology* 34:335–341, 1986.
43. Brent RL, Leung C, London W, Wittingham D: The demise of another vestigial organ. *Teratology* 5:251, 1972.
44. Gitlin D, Pericelli A, Gitlin GM: Synthesis of α_1-foetoprotein, by liver, yolk sac, and gastrointestinal tract of the human conceptus. *Cancer Res*, 32:979–982, 1972.
45. Arcy LB: Two embryologically important specimens of tubal twins. *Obstet Gynecol Surv* 36:407–414, 1923.
46. Crooij MJ, Westhuis M, Schoemaker J, Exalto N: Ultrasonographic measurement of the yolk sac. *Brit J Obstet Gynaecol* 89:931–934, 1982.
47. O'Rahilly R: Developmental States in Human Embryos. *Carnegie Inst Publ* 613:65–68, 1973.
48. Gonzalez-Crussi F, Roth LM: The human yolk sac and yolk sac carcinoma. An ultrastructural study. *Human Pathol* 7:675–691, 1976.
49. Luckett WP: Origin and differentiation of the yolk sac and extraembryonic mesoderm in presomite human and Rhesus monkey embryos. *Am J Anat* 152:59–98, 1970.
50. Hesseldahl H, Larsen JF: Hemopoiesis and blood vessels in human yolk sac. *Acta Anat* 78:274–294, 1971.
51. Hoyes AD: The human fetal yolk sac. An ultrastructural study of four specimens. *Z Zellforsch* 99:469–490, 1969.
52. King BF, Wilson JM: A fine structural and cytochemical study of the Rhesus Monkey yolk sac: endoderm and mesothelium. *Anat Rec* 205:143–158, 1983.
53. Pope CF, Pope VZ, Beck LR: Development of Baboon preimplantation embryos to post-implantation stages in vitro. *Biol Reprod* 27:915–923, 1982.

54. Bremer D, Merker HJ, Gossrau R: Ultrastructure and hydrolase cytochemistry of the developing marmoset yolk sac. *Anat Embryol* 172:101–113, 1985.
55. Enders AC, Schafke S, Hendrickx AG: Differentiation of the embryonic disc, amnion, and yolk sac in the rhesus monkey. *Am J Anat* 1977:161–185, 1986.
56. Ukeshima A, Hayashi Y, Fujimoto T: Surface morphology of the human yolk sac: endoderm and mesothelium. *Arch Histol Jap* 49:483–494, 1986.
57. Jollie WP: Review article: Ultrastructural studies of protein transfer across rodent yolk sac. *Placenta* 7:263–281, 1986.
58. Fukuda T: Fetal hemopoiesis. I. Electron microscopic studies on human yolk sac hemopoiesis. *Virchows Abt B Zellpathol* 14:197–213, 1973.
59. Hesseldahl H, Larsen JF: Ultrastructure of human yolk sac: endoderm, mesenchyme, tubules, and mesothelium. *Am J Anat* 126:315–336, 1969.
60. Gitlin D, Pericelli A: Synthesis of serum albumin, prealbumin, foctoprotein, α_1-antitrypsin, and transferrin by human yolk sac. *Nature* 228:995–997, 1970.
61. Shi WK, Hopkins B, Thompson S, Heath JK, Luke BM, Graham CF: Synthesis of apolipoproteins, alphafoetoprotein, albumin, and transferrin by the human foctal yolk sac and other foetal organs. *J Embryol Exp Morph* 85:191–206, 1985.
62. Mantoni M, Pederson JF: Ultrasound visualization of the human yolk sac. *J Clin Ultrasound* 7:459–460, 1979.
63. Sauerbrei E, Coopersberg PL, Poland BT: Ultrasound demonstration of the normal fetal yolk sac. *J Clin Ultrasound* 8:217–220, 1980.
64. Anderson DJ, Johnson PM, Alexander NJ, Jones WR, Griffin PD: Monoclonal antibodies to human trophoblast and sperm antigen: Report of two WHO-sponsored workshops, June 30, 1986–Toronto, Canada. *J Reprod Immunol* 10:231–257, 1987.
65. Zola H, Brooks D: Techniques for the production and characterization of monoclonal hybridoma antibodies. In Hurrell JG (ed): *Monoclonal Hybridoma Antibodies: Technique and Applications*. Baton Raton, FL: CRC Press, 1982, pp 1–57.
66. Oi VT, Herzenberg LA: Immunoglobulin-producing hybrid cell lines. In Misnell BB, Shiggi SM (eds): *Selected Methods in Cellular Immunology*. San Francisco: Freeman, 1980, p 351.
67. Jensen M, Damjanov I, Tichy D, Brent RL: Monoclonal antibodies to the visceral yolk sac antigens. *Teratology* 31:60A, 1985.
68. Jensen M, Lloyd JB, Beckman DA, Koszalka TR, Brent RL: Monoclonal gamma globulins prepared against rat visceral yolk sac proteins. *Ped Res* 20:338A, 1986.
69. Jensen M, Damjanov I, Koszalka TR, Brent RL: Congenital malformations induced by monoclonal antibodies against rat visceral yolk sac antigens. *Teratology* 35:71A, 1987.

15
From Megaloblastosis to Molecular Definition in Methylmalonic Acidemia

GRANT MORROW III

In 1965 I joined Dr. Barness at the Hospital of the University of Pennsylvania. A year earlier Elizabeth Jamison Hodges had published a children's book[1] that described a story with amazing similarities to many of the adventures that the three of us – ie, Bill Mellman, Frank Oski, and I – had with the "Chief." Let me quote from the introduction of that book.

"Long, long ago in a land far off at the end of the Earth, there lived three princes: Balakrama, Vijayo and Rajahsingha, all three full of wisdom and great learning. When they came to maturity, the King sent them forth to other lands to complete their education and to find the secret formula, death to dragons, that would rid the seas around their homeland of great beasts that hindered travel. The three princes journeyed far seeking the formula, but happening always instead upon adventure and rare treasures."

Serendip is the ancient name for Ceylon, and our word, serendipity, comes from the unexpected rewards the princes received for their kindness and knowledge as well as from the intellectual wonders of the time spent in their kingdom. For me, one of the most exciting and rewarding adventures in my career dealt with the story of methylmalonic acid (MMA). It's really Lew's story, but I was privileged to have the opportunity to participate in it.

What I would like to do at this point is to return to the year 1965 to a kingdom on the 8th floor of the Maloney Building at the Hospital of the University of Pennsylvania, which was ruled by the Chief.

Dr Barness had the idea that adult patients with pernicious anemia should not be able to metabolize Methylmalonyl CoA (MMCoA) to succinylCoA because the B_{12} cofactor required at that particular biochemical step would be deficient, with the result that there would be decreased enzyme activity. Therefore, the appearance of MMA in the urine would become a sensitive, diagnostic biochemical marker. It worked, and the result was reported in his landmark paper in the

From the Department of Pediatrics, Ohio State University College of Medicine, Columbus, Ohio.
Presented in honor of Lewis A. Barness, MD, November 12, 1988.

TABLE 15.1. Metabolism of propionate-1-^{14}C by liver homogenates.

	^{14}C-methylmalonate cpm/3 mg liver protein		^{14}C-succinate cpm/3 mg liver protein	
Patient	No DBCC	DBCC added	No DBCC	DBCC added
LA	3,820	3,690	72	89
DW	2,140	3,420	32	142
CD	2,820	3,400	26	40
RH	2,600	689	190	6,200
Control 1	617	300	3,480	5,140
Control 2	1,400	570	2,740	5,300
Control 3	612	166	2,910	5,200

The incubation mixtures contained (in μmole): propionate-1-^{14}C, 0.43 (2.18 μc); Mg^{++}, 2.5; ATP, 1.2; CoA, 0.52; glutathione (reduced form), 2.5; $KHCO_3$, 5.0; and TRIS-HCl, 25.6 (pH 7.3). Twelve micrograms of DBCC was added as indicated. From 2.2 to 4.6 mg liver protein was added to initiate the reaction in a total volume of 375 μl.
Data from Morrow et al.[4]

New England Journal of Medicine.[2] When the tests were positive, the two-way chromatograms would demonstrate a small but distinct, yellow spot. One day, I saw the Chief as excited as I have ever seen him because a urine specimen from a child referred from Drs Bob Kaye and Lester Baker had a spot that almost filled the entire chromatogram. Instead of the milligram amounts of MMA expected in B_{12} deficiency, there appeared to be gram quantities. Dr Barness confirmed that it was MMA, that it was indeed massive, that the child did not have any evidence of B_{12} deficiency, and, in fact, had a new metabolic disorder. This serendipitous observation launched us on a fascinating foray into a field which permitted direct application of biochemical dicta to our patients.

Lew told me to start "working up" Lee so that we could find out what mechanisms had gone awry in this 9-month-old boy. Although severely acidotic, Lee did not display any of the stigmata of vitamin B_{12} deficiency. During the course of our investigations, among the many observations that were made in this particular patient, it was apparent that large parenteral doses of cyanocobalamin did not lower his methylmalonic acid levels. One perplexing finding that we could not explain was his consistently elevated plasma glycine levels. As a result of this glycine association, the Chief sent me on the first of a series of voyages of which this one ultimately ended up in the bottom of a freezer in North Philadelphia. Dr Barness remembered that Drs Angelo DiGeorge and Victor Auerbach, at St. Christopher's Hospital for Children, had taken care of the first child with "ketotic hyperglycinemia," and he assumed that there might be some urine stored somewhere from earlier studies. Although there was no frozen urine from the original patient, there was a postmortem liver specimen from a child who had died with hyperglycinemia 3½ years earlier. We assumed, incorrectly, that this specimen could be used as a control.

During the next 2 years Dr Barness was able to detect four additional acidotic children who excreted massive amounts of MMA in their urines.[3] As a result of

TABLE 15.2. Metabolism of ^3H-methylmalonylCoA by liver homogenates.

Patient	^3H-succinate cpm/mg liver protein	
	No DBCC	DBCC added
LA	6	17
DW	44	189
CD	16	41
RH	452	7,770
Control 1	4,920	6,010
Control 2	3,040	4.540
Control 3	3,710	5,000

The incubation mixtures contained ^3H-methylmalonylCoA, 0.11 μmole (62,500 cpm); TRIS-sulfate pH 7.3, 20 μmole; and DBCC, 12 μg. From 1.3 to 2.8 mg liver protein was added to initiate the incubations in a total volume of 200 μl.
Data from Morrow et al.[4]

studying these five families as well as from looking at five patients from the literature, we were able to determine that the genetic transmission of this disease was most likely via an autosomal-recessive mode.

I was then sent on my next voyage, to the Biochemistry Department at the University of Pennsylvania, to work with Joel Flaks and to develop the enzyme assay for MMCoA mutase. The results of our first series of assays in liver homogenates were dramatic.[4] In our first series of experiments, when no coenzyme was added to the homogenates, all four patients accumulated radioactive label from propionate into methylmalonic acid, as noted in Table 15.1, but not the next compound in the pathway—ie, succinate. (The terminology we used at that time for the coenzyme adenosylcobalamin was its chemical name, DBCC or 5,6-dimethylbenzimidazolylcobamide 5′-deoxyadenosine.) Our "control" patient (R.H., from St. Christopher's Hospital) was quite different. He had abnormal activity without added coenzyme but was similar to controls when coenzyme was added. Since, at that point, we could not be absolutely certain whether the racemase or the mutase was affected, our next challenge was to reassay those same liver homogenates with the proper substrate—ie, methylmalonylCoA. The results in Table 15.2 again strongly pointed to the mutase as the point responsible for the metabolic block. However, as can be noted, R.H. had significant activity without added coenzyme.

Dr Barness geared up again and told me that I had to take another trip, this time to Brandeis University to work with Bob Abeles and George Cardinale in order to determine what the actual coenzyme content (DBCC) of the liver homogenates was. To our great excitement, as noted in Table 15.3, all were normal as predicted, except for R.H., who had low levels of coenzyme despite normal apoenzyme activity when supplemented with adenosylcobalamin. We felt that the differences noted in R.H. were not simply due to prolonged storage, since he

TABLE 15.3. Source of liver samples and DBCC content.

Patient	Age at death	Cause of death	Time frozen before assay	Liver content of DBCC[a]
LA	22 mo	Methylmalonic acidemia	1½ mo	0.10
DW	4 mo	Methylmalonic acidemia	10 mo	0.09
CD	36 mo	Methylmalonic acidemia	13 mo	0.14
RH	21 mo	Methylmalonic acidemia	40 mo	<0.01
Control 1	70 yr	Lymphoma	1 day	5.8
Control 2	5 mo	Meningococcemia	1 mo	0.15
Control 3	48 mo	Acute lymphocytic leukemia	13 mo	0.29
Control range				0.08–0.25[b]

[a] DBCC values are expressed in μg/g wet liver.
[b] The range consists of seven additional controls in whom only DBCC was assayed.
Data from Morrow et al.[4]

had normal activity when supplemented with coenzyme. This was the first time that the existence of two variants had been proved–one that might respond to coenzyme, and the other that would not. Now, we were off to the races.

During this same period of time Lee Rosenberg at Yale University was studying a vitamin B_{12}-responsive patient, and he demonstrated[5] that the theoretical treatment implied from our in vitro liver studies could, in fact, be very effective in a responsive patient.

The next, extremely important milestone was passed when we were able to demonstrate that the biochemical pathway involved in this genetic defect was operative in normal fibroblasts. Fortunately, Bill Mellman and Ted Tedesco were in situ, so we didn't have to set sail on another voyage. The rest of the story is possible from the in vitro studies that were subsequently accomplished utilizing fibroblasts cultured from patients. Let me quickly touch on these exciting areas.

Prenatal diagnoses became possible through the vehicle of amniocentesis[6] and analysis of cultured amniocytes as well as amniotic fluid itself. In the vitamin B_{12}- responsive forms of MM-emia, successful prenatal therapy has been accomplished with intramuscular injections of hydroxocobalamin in the fetus.[7]

Measuring enzyme kinetics in fibroblasts became possible, and early in the story we were able to demonstrate that one of our responsive patients had defective binding of his B_{12} coenzyme.[8]

Distinct genetic variants could now be defined and used as valuable adjuncts to counseling. Lee Rosenberg's group was able to further define these defects through a series of elegant studies using the tool of complementation with hybridized cell lines in vitro.[9] Initially, they found two defects in apoenzyme synthesis and three defective variants of cobalamin metabolism. Other mutant cell lines have been described, so at the present time there are seven genetically distinct variants of cobalamin metabolism alone.

Figure 15.1 depicts the metabolism of vitamin B_{12} in the human. B_{12} is carried in the plasma by transcobalamin II (TC II), taken up by the process of endocytosis, processed, and released from the lysosome by protease activity. It

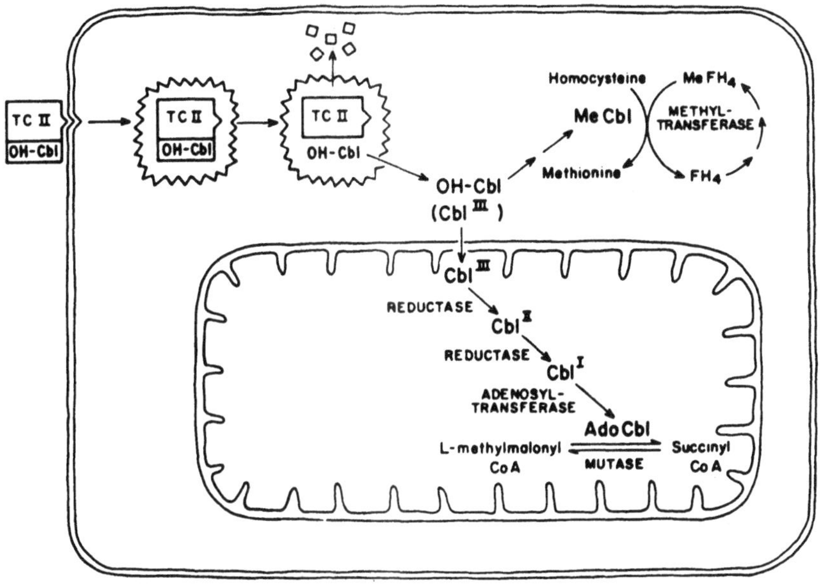

FIGURE 15.1. General pathway of the cellular uptake and subcellular compartmentation of cobalamins, and of the intracellular distribution and enzymatic synthesis of cobalamin coenzymes. Abbreviations: TC II, transcobalamin II; OH-Cbl, hydroxocobalamin; MeCbl, methylcobalamin; AdoCbl, adenosylcobalamin; Cbl^{III}, CBl^{II}, Cbl^{I}, cobalamins with cobalt valence of 3^+, 2^+, and 1^+, respectively. Reprinted with permission from JB Stanbury et al., *The Metabolic Basis of Inherited Disease*, 5th Edition, McGraw-Hill, New York, 1983.

can then be metabolized to the methyl form of the coenzyme (MeCbl) in the cytosol and be reduced in the mitochondrion to adenosylcobalamin form of the coenzyme (AcoCbl). We now know of variants that cannot process and release B_{12} from the lysosomes so that neither form of B_{12} coenzyme is synthesized. There are also mitochondrial defects in the reductases as well as in adenosyltransferase. This series of observations points out an important principle that Dr Barness emphasized—ie, that if we look hard enough, we will discover clinical expressions of defects in every enzyme step in any particular metabolic pathway.

At point after point, I used to think that the story of MM-emia must be complete. However, even in 1988, there continue to be new, important observations being made in this group of diseases. Looking at the mechanisms of brain damage in this disorder,[10] detecting new variants of defects in metabolism of vitamin B_{12},[11] describing techniques for detecting affected fetuses,[12] and, finally, mapping the locus for the gene,[13] all subjects of manuscripts published in 1988. The gene locus has been located on chromosome 6 with the long-term implication that gene therapy may be possible at some time in the future.

In December 1971 I left the University of Pennsylvania and joined the University of Arizona. On New Year's Day, 1972, I was asked to consult on an 11-month-old boy who had been admitted to the hospital for a second time with severe dehydration and metabolic acidosis. Because of his profound ketoacidosis with a large anion gap, we were quickly able to diagnose methylmalonic acidemia and to begin vitamin B_{12} therapy. In the intervening 16.5 years, this lad has done well on weekly injections of hydroxocobalamin and a low-protein diet. Matt has never met you, Lew, but he knows that you were the one who had first described his genetic problem, which, by the way, is a reductase defect of the group A complementation.

This wonderful medical story about a potentially lethal disease has brought us full circle. It was a quarter of a century ago that the Chief made his observations about urinary methylmalonic acid. These ideas were spawned from dealing with patients. We turned to the laboratory and finally successfully applied those data to the therapy of children. It was Lew's tenacity about asking questions and making certain that there were answers, and some serendipity, that have resulted in the blossoming of an extremely complex biochemical awareness with a very happy ending; ie, what initially could have been viewed as a hopeless genetic anomaly is not, and many of these patients now live active, healthy lives. Truly, Dr Barness has rid the seas around this group of medical perturbations from the great beasts and dragons so that our medical travels in those seas are much safer for our patients. Also, we are now much more focused on our ultimate destination.

References

1. Hodges EJ: *The Three Princes of Serendip.* New York: Antheneum, 1964.
2. Barness LA, Young D, Mellman WJ, Kahn SB, Williams WJ: Methylmalonate excretion in a patient with pernicious anemia. *N Engl J Med* 268:144–146, 1963.
3. Morrow G, Barness LA, Auerbach VH, DiGeorge AM, Ando T, Nyhan WL: Observations on the coexistence of methylmalonic acidemia and glycinemia. *J Pediatr* 74: 680-690, 1969.
4. Morrow G, Barness LA, Cardinale GJ, Abeles RH, Flaks JG: Congenital methylmalonic acidemia: Enzymatic evidence for two forms of the disease. *Proc Natl Acad Sci USA* 63:191–197, 1969.
5. Rosenberg LE, Lilljeqvist A, Hsia YE: Methylmalonic aciduria: An inborn error leading to metabolic acidosis, long-chain ketonuria and intermittent hyperglycinemia. *N Engl J Med* 278:1319–1322, 1968.
6. Morrow G, Schwartz RH, Hallock JA, Barness LA: Prenatal detection of methylmalonic acidemia. *J Pediatr* 77:120–123, 1970.
7. Ampola MG, Mahoney MJ, Nakamura E, Tanaka K: Prenatal therapy of a patient with vitamin-B_{12}- responsive methylmalonic acidemia. *N Engl J Med* 293:313–317, 1975.
8. Morrow G, Lebowitz J: Studies of methylmalonyl- coenzyme A carbonylmutase activity in methylmalonic acidemia. II. In vitro binding kinetics with adenosylcobalamin. *Biochem Med* 15:241–245, 1976.
9. Gravel RA, Mahoney MJ, Ruddle FH, Rosenberg LE: Genetic complementation in heterokaryons of human fibroblasts defective in cobalamin metabolism. *Proc Natl Acad Sci USA* 72:3181–3185, 1975.

10. Wajner M, Eneida CB, Dutra JC, et al: Diminished concentrations of ganglioside N-acetylneuraminic acid (G-NeuAc) in cerebellum of young rats receiving chronic administration of methylmalonic acid. *J Neurol Sci* 85:233–238, 1988.
11. Carmel R, Watkins D, Goodman SI, Rosenblatt DS: Hereditary defect of cobalamin metabolism (cblG mutation) presenting as a neurologic disorder in adulthood. *N Engl J Med* 318:1738–1741, 1988.
12. Fowler B, Giles L, Sardharwalla IB, Donnai P, Clayton JK: First trimester diagnosis of methylmalonic aciduria. *Prenat Diagn* 8:207–213, 1988.
13. Ledley FD, Lumetta R, Zoghbi HY, Vantuinen P, Ledbetter SA, Ledbetter DH: Mapping of human methylmalonyl CoA mutase (MUT) locus on chromosome 6. *Am J Hum Genet* 42:839–846, 1988.

16
Cerebral Phosphorus Magnetic Resonance Spectroscopy in Perinatal Distress

MARIA DELIVORIA-PAPADOPOULOS

Perinatal asphyxia occurs in 1% to 5% of all births and frequently results in a permanent neurological handicap.[1] The extent of brain damage is probably related to the duration and degree of fetal hypoxia and ischemia and to resultant changes in cerebral metabolism. Following hypoxic-ischemic insults, cortical metabolism changes from aerobic to anaerobic glycolysis and has secondary changes in phosphorus-containing metabolites, lactate accumulation, and acidosis.[2] These changes may represent the final common pathway of hypoxic cerebral damage that occurs after hypoxia or ischemia.[3]

Theory

The control system of body processes follows the well-known Michaelis-Menten hyperbola where the abcissa is the concentration of the control chemical, and the ordinate is the velocity of the process[4] (Fig. 16.1). The abscissa is the adenosine diphosphate (ADP) concentration (or Pi/PCr value) which control adenosine triphosphate (ATP) systems. It is useful to apply this diagram to the production of ATP by oxidative metabolism of the mitochondria.

If we recognize that the maintenance of the living state requires that the rate of ATP synthesis equals the rate of ATP breakdown (ie, cellular work), we can see from Fig 16.1 where stable and unstable states of metabolism exist. The required metabolic velocity, V, allows the organ to operate in the lower portion of the hyperbola (a small perturbation of metabolism is corrected by a small change of ADP, and the V/V_{max} is small). If, however, the stress of metabolism requires V to approach V_{max}, much higher concentrations of the control chemical ADP are required, and cellular metabolism operates near the asymptote of the hyperbola. Here, a small further change of metabolic stress will lead to lack of control, and

From the Departments of Pediatrics and Physiology, University of Pennsylvania School of Medicine, Philadelphia.
Presented in honor of Lewis A. Barness, MD, November 11, 1988.

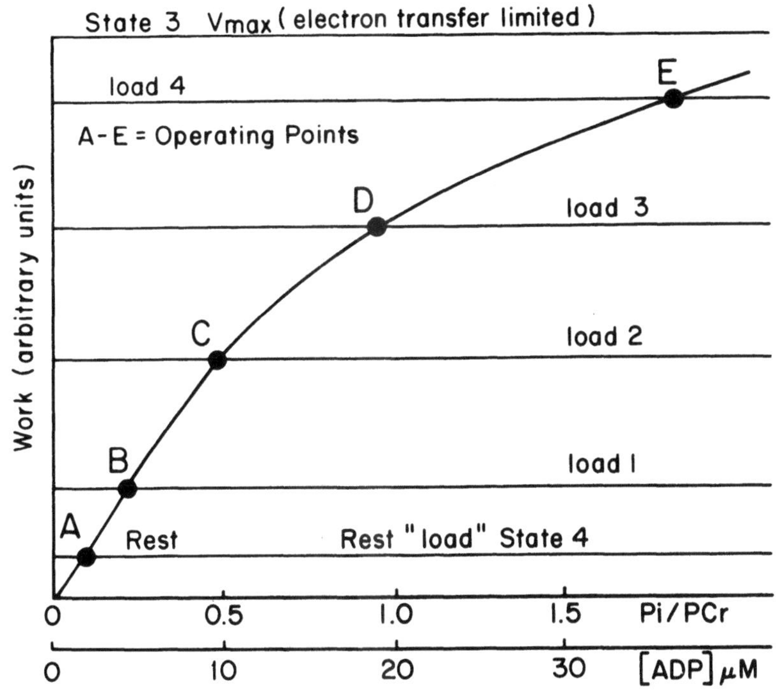

FIGURE 16.1. Relationships between steady-state work (V) of the cell (ordinate) and the increase of ADP concentration necessary to activate metabolism to the appropriate value of V. The analysis shows that Pi/PCr is proportional to ADP and the proportionality constant is evaluated.

in fact, negative feedback control is no longer possible. The metabolic needs of the brain are no longer satisfied by its metabolic machinery.[5] In biochemical terms, the rise of ADP and inorganic phosphate (Pi) stimulates glycolosis, lactate acidosis rises, ATP is depleted and ADP is lost through its conversion to adenosine monophosphate (AMP), inosine monophosphate (IMP), adenine, and finally, hypoxanthine and uric acid (see Fig. 16.2).

Insufficient ADP remains to allow resynthesis of ATP. Furthermore, if therapeutic intervention allows reflow of oxygen into previously ischemic regions, free-radical damage may further impair the capacity for recovery. In short, when V and V_{max} become equal, control is lost and life may be lost. This is a very simple concept and one that applies particularly to the brain of the preterm neonate where oxygen delivery to tissues is jeopardized by the many complications in the birth process and the preterm neonate.[6] If the hypothesis is correct, its applicability to the neonatal brain is of importance since brain-damaged neonates may incur severe functional disabilities which will cause handicaps in their later life.

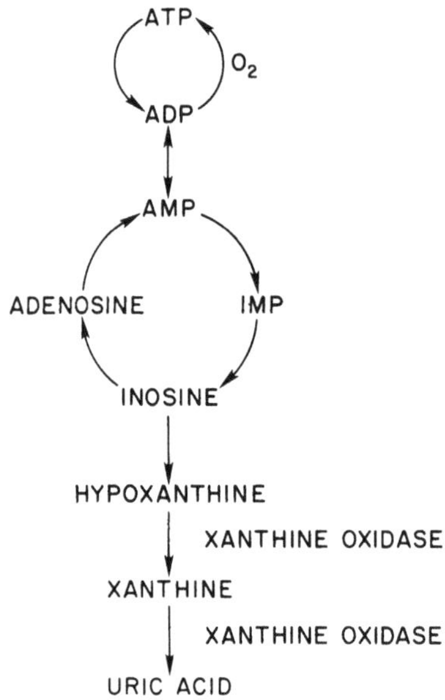

FIGURE 16.2. Pathway for a breakdown of ADP finally to uric acid which may occur in ischemic hypoxic tissue.

In order to determine the V/V_{max} for the newborn brain in a noninvasive, nondestructive, safe, and quantitative procedure, we applied phosphorus magnetic resonance spectroscopy (P MRS). This device measures ATP directly in living tissues together with its "backup" system—phosphocreatine (PCr) and creatine kinase (Cr). In the cortical neuron there are mitochondria in the cytoplasm of the cell and thus there are many places where ATP can be used at synaptic junctions, axons, etc, as well as in the cell body itself.[7] Loss of ATP immobilizes the ion pumps and allows effusion of potassium and entry of sodium and water. At the same time, Rothman emphasizes the release of large amounts of neurotransmitters particularly glutamate, resulting in severe osmotic stress of the neuronal membrane.[8] This results in osmotic forces that rupture the membrane. Irreversible structural damage follows the biochemical catastrophe mentioned above.

The interplay of cell ATPases and mitochondrial ATP synthesis in a steady-state system (V/V_{max}) is reviewed in Figure 16.3. ATP utilization in the cytosol is immediately reversed by the creatine kinase equilibrium, resulting in the production of Cr and Pi, which diffuse to the mitochondria. Phosphate directly activates oxidative phosphorylation, and creatine is reconverted to ADP, which enters the mitochondria for rephosphorylation. This cycle is rapid, near equilibrium, and the key to the maintenance of metabolic stability in the brain.[9,10]

NMR Function

Nuclear magnetic resonance (NMR) is an energy absorption method similar to optical absorption, but instead of involving electronic transitions, it involves nuclear spin transitions. One of the difficulties of measuring phosphorus com-

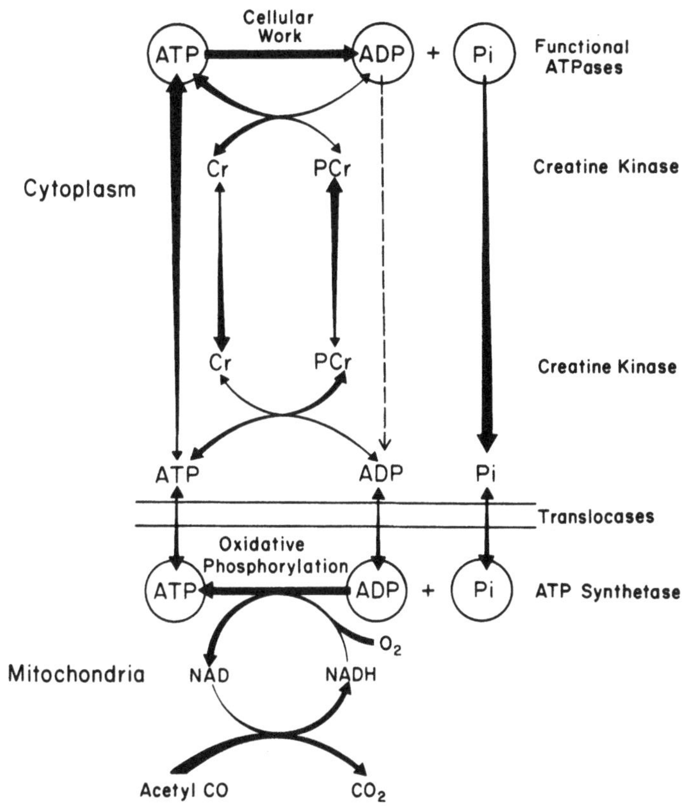

FIGURE 16.3. Kinetic couplings of the mitochondria and the cell ATPase(s) via shuttles and translocases. The bold arrows represent the main pathways of transfer of phosphate and adenine nucleotides via the creatine kinase shuttle.

pounds in vivo is the low sensitivity of the NMR method and the small amounts of phosphate present in the cell where sensitivities appropriate for concentration as low as 0.5 mM are required. Times of data acquisition should be 5 min or less. Figure 16.4 displays representative data of the absorption of radiofrequency energy at specific frequencies appropriate to the three phosphates of ATP and the single phosphates of Pi and PCr. This spectrum is from an extract of a rat brain and, although sacrifice was made as rapidly as possible, the model is incorrect in many respects when compared with in vivo data because of the rapidity with which cell metabolism deteriorates even during the short time it takes to freeze the brain. A variety of NMR spectrometers have been developed for studying organic chemical molecules, but a much greater sensitivity is required for in vivo spectroscopy, and most of the worldwide data on neonates and human limbs have been recorded using systems manufactured by Phospho-Energetics (P-E) or Oxford Research Systems; the former has made special modifications to ensure the safety of the neonate.

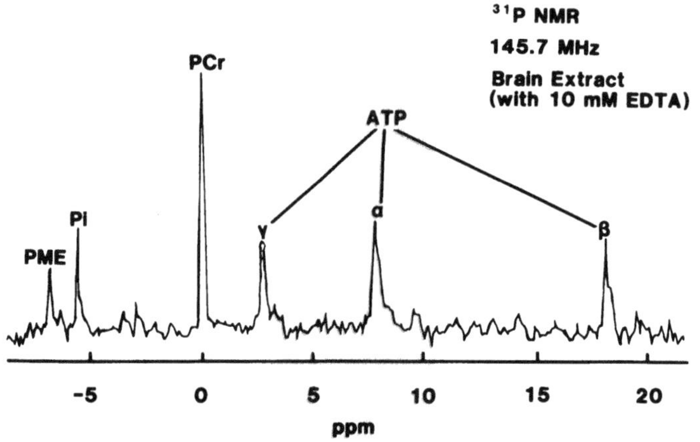

FIGURE 16.4. NMR spectrum of a rat brain extract, illustrating the ^{31}P NMR spectrum of phosphorus metabolites in vitro and deionized medium. There is excellent resolution of the peaks because the cells are destroyed, and peak broadening interactions do not exist.

Safety of the Neonate

In Figure 16.5 are listed the devices necessary for neonate brain study to be done safely. All health care monitoring devices must be available and employed in such a way that the use of one does not defeat the use of another. Thus, EKG, transcutaneous oxygen, and CO_2, together with various leads for blood sampling, may be required. In addition, an endotracheal tube or an appropriate oxygenated atmosphere must be available.

It is most important to maintain appropriate temperature and to ensure that no abrasion of the head occurs by contact with the probe. For this reason, the baby is placed on an airbag and gently raised to contact the NMR coil. Since 25- to 30-week-old neonates may weigh less than a kilogram, they are placed within the isolette with all monitoring devices in operation and with a special shielding system developed by our laboratory.

Safety of NMR Spectroscopy

Magnetic Field

A large number of mice have been conceived, reproduced, and grown to maturity in the 1.5-Tesla magnet used here. They have been subjected to a battery of psychological tests to determine whether they were inferior to control animals![11] The experiments lasted several months, and two batches of mice were observed over several generations. No significant differences were observed in the two groups of mice, suggesting that the static magnetic field is safe. However, rapidly varying magnetic fields can generate voltages across blood flowing in major

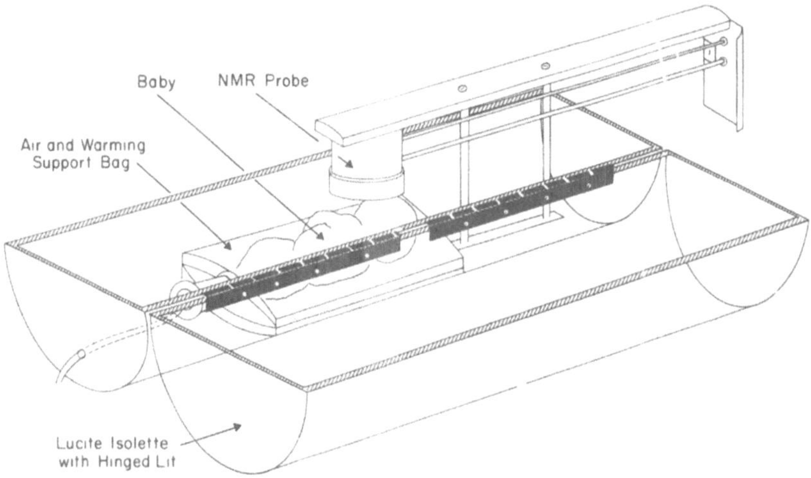

FIGURE 16.5. Drawing of the safety isolette for MRS examination of full-term and preterm neonates in 7-in. bore MRS in the intensive care nursery at the Hospital of the University of Pennsylvania and a listing of life support devices that can be used in the NMR or are readily available in the case of emergency. Endotracheal tubes can also be used in the NMR. Monitoring equipment includes (1) EKG, temperature, and pressure readings; (2) % O_2 inspired, % CO_2 inspired/expired, and respiratory rate; (3) pulse oximeter for % SaO_2 and pulse rate; (4) suction regulator; and (5) aquamatic module and warming blanket.

vessels and may also affect some neurological processes in the retina. At present, rapidly varying magnetic fields are not acceptable for neonatal studies, and the P-E spectrometer thus does not include imaging of the neonate.

RF Power Deposition

Radio-frequency (RF) power deposition may also be a serious problem with proton imagers (some transmitters have 10 and 20 of kW available for rapid imaging). A device that provides spectrometry only has power depositions by electrostatic fields that are 10^{-4} of the permissible (10 mW/cm^2) limit. A most important factor is that the acceptable power levels are based on the effect of electrostatic fields. Our shielded surface coil[12] allows no electrostatic fields to penetrate body organs, as magnetic fields would, and they have no detectable effect on the neonate.

Duration of NMR Examination

It is a significant disturbance simply to move a neonate from its isolette into the MRS isolette, and examinations must be carried out expeditiously. Five to seven minutes is usually adequate for the shim process, and adequate signal-to-noise ratio is available to obtain NMR values of PCr/Pi with an accuracy of $\pm$ 10% in 5 min. Usually both hemispheres of the brain are studied; however, the very nature of the undifferentiated neonate brain makes NMR examination of the total volume adequate. Because of the brief time available, imaging methods have not been applied to neonates, and benefit/risk advantage has not been assessed. Furthermore, the complex structure of the adult brain is not expected in the undifferentiated preterm neonatal brain. Thus, the surface coil evaluation of metabolism in one portion of the brain may be representative of metabolism elsewhere. However, as mentioned above, when time permits, several regions of the brain are studied.[6,13] Depth selection in the neonatal brain has not been employed, again, because the skull is thin, muscles are undeveloped, and a surface coil placed on the side of the head appears to give signals attributed wholely to brain tissues as demonstrated by spectra of "dead brain" (see below). The studies of other organs are also simplified.[14] The sternum is thin, and in heart disease the hypertrophic tissue gives large and clear signals attributed almost completely to cardiac tissue, a case distinctly different from that of the adult human, where significant difficulties have been reported.[15] In the case of neonatal liver carcinoma, signals identified with the tumor are obtained,[16] and studies of the arms and legs are obviously possible.[17,18] To date, little has been done with the neonatal kidney, but indications are that the signals may be clearer in the neonate than in the adult. In summary, P MRS studies are rapid and accurate. Both research and clinically useful information in the preterm and full-term population can be obtained.

Location of the Spectrometer

P MRS is used for detecting the early phases of diseases that may lead to loss of the steady state of metabolism and eventual death of the tissue. For example, studies of neonates shortly after birth trauma make possible an early diagnosis of possible potential brain damage. Examinations of older neonates in acute phases of disease are highly desirable. These examinations of endangered, unstable neonates cannot involve extensive and complicated transportation procedures to a distant P MRS center. For this reason, we have found it essential to keep the spectrometer in the intensive care nursery 10 to 20 feet away from the population of neonates in their appropriate isolettes. P MRS is useful because (1) it is available at any time for study of the neonate; (2) transportation of the neonate is not a problem; (3) all emergency devices are readily available; and (4) it occupies a minimum of space.

For these reasons, we have designed a special neonatal spectrometer with a restricted fringe field yet an adequate bore to take care of all preterm neonates. This magnet allows the isolette containing the neonate to be conveniently slid into the 7-in. bore of the spectrometer. We do not predict that a high field adult spectrometer (1-M bore) can possibly be located within intensive care nurseries.

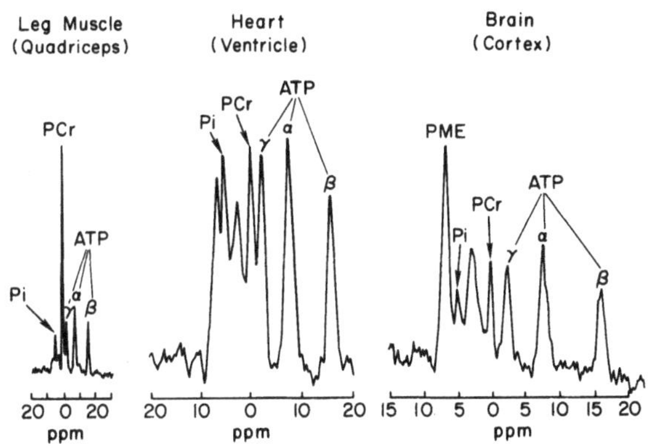

FIGURE 16.6. MRS of human body showing ATP signals in functioning organs of neonate (4-min scans). A comparison of the spectra of skeletal tissue (leg muscle from a healthy adolescent), heart (of a young child 1.5 to 2 years), and brain (of normal term infants, average weight and size, uncomplicated pregnancy/delivery). Data were acquired under the conditions described in the text. Note the different Pi/PCr values of the resting muscle and the active heart and brain. Also, PME appears as a highly significant peak in the neonate brain.

Types of Tissues Surveyed by P MRS in the Neonate

Skeletal Tissue

As mentioned above, the favorable conditions for observation of the neonatal heart and brain make studies of these organs uniquely precise in the neonate.[14,15,19] Figure 16.6 compares the P MRS spectra of skeletal tissue, heart, and brain acquired in relatively short intervals. First, the quality of the spectra is good, and the baseline noise is of little significance in interpreting the data. Secondly, arms and limbs show characteristic five-peak spectra with three of them due to ATP, one to PCr, and one to Pi. The lack of need for background corrections makes these spectra sufficiently accurate that quantification by peak heights prior to computer fitting is acceptable.

Heart

The cardiac region of the neonate shows, in addition to the three peaks of ATP, a *smaller PCr* peak and a *higher Pi* peak than in the skeletal muscle. The heart is working ($V/V_{max} \sim 0.5$) while the muscle is at rest ($V/V_{max} \sim 0.1$), so the ATP is higher in the heart, and this is related to the Pi/PCr value. In addition to these peaks, two additional peaks appear; one between Pi and PCr, phosphodiester (PDE) peak, usually phosphorylglycerolcholine, and beside the phosphate peak is a phosphomonoester (PME) peak which contains phosphoethanolamine and

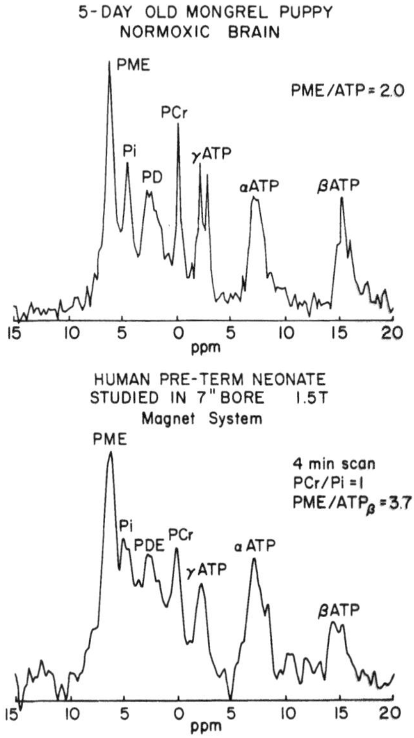

FIGURE 16.7. P MRS signals of the neonate dog and neonate human are similar. The PME peak is distinctive, and in the full-term puppy, the Pi/PCr is lower than in the human neonate. The neonatal spectrum is typical of a preterm infant, 32 weeks' gestation, 1,840 g at birth, average weight and size for birth age (postconceptional age, 33 weeks, body weight, 1,730 g).

phosphocholine. The thin sternum adds very little due to its muscle content, and the low Pi/PCr of resting tissue is thus not observed. In the neonate, then, the thin overlying muscle does not interfere with the observation of the much lower values of the cardiac tissue. Some contribution from 2,3-diphosphoglycerate acid in the red blood cells within the ventricles may be observed as a peak at ~ 6 ppm.

Brain

Finally, and most important, is the P NMR spectrum of the neonatal brain. As before, the three ATP peaks, PCr, and Pi are distinct. The Pi/PCr value is high as in the heart because this is a working tissue ($V/V_{max} \sim 0.5$). ATP and Pi/MCr must rise in order to sustain a metabolic rate equal that of the ATPase. A striking feature of the spectrum is the PME peak. Biochemical analysis of puppy brains shows this peak to be largely attributed to phosphorylethanolamine. The phosphoglycerolcholine peak lies between that of PCr and Pi.[20]

Species Differences

The puppy and the human preterm neonate have very nearly identical P MRS signatures, as indicated in Figure 16.7. The high PME/ATP value if presumably

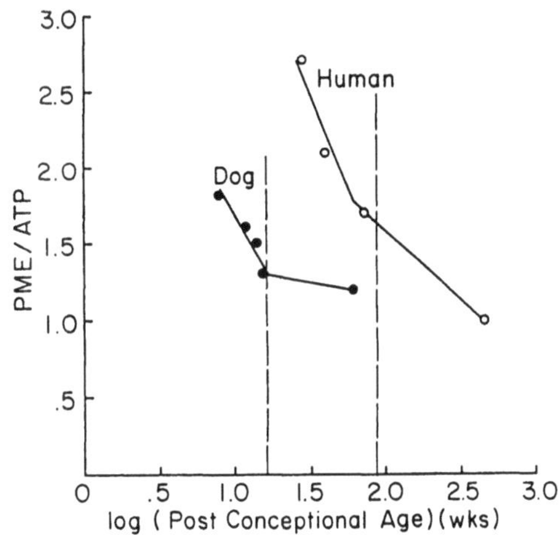

FIGURE 16.8. Developmental progression of PME illustrating the "maturation" of brain biochemistry in the neonatal dog and human as measured by P MRS. The dashed vertical lines indicate structural maturation.

characteristic of the rapid growth phase of the neuronal tissues. The Pi/PCr value of the puppy brain is slightly lower than that of the preterm neonates, who are generally stressed in order to obtain adequate oxygen for their body tissues. We conclude that the puppy provides an acceptable model for the P MRS study of the human neonate and have found similar biochemical patterns in the piglet and lamb.

Age Dependence of PME/ATP

Figure 16.8 plots the logarithm of the PME/ATP value as a function of log time and indicates that the PME falls toward the adult values upon maturation of the neuronal connections.[21] Thus, the PME peak is a marker of the rapidly maturing neuronal tissue. In other studies of tumor tissue PME/ATP is ~ 2.0.

Brain Death

Two examples of P MRS spectra of the neonatal brain show global and local cell death.[22] The biochemical changes that occur immediately upon death of the neonate show that ATP and PCr are no longer detectable. The Pi accumulation appears as a single peak in Figure 16.9, with PME remaining as a metabolically inactive component. The absence of PCr and of ATP in a tissue signifies that the steady state is no longer maintained, $V > V_{max}$, and that cell death ensues.

Localized Brain Damage

The infant whose spectra are shown in Figure 16.10 had a localized infarct in the left hemisphere, which has a distinctive NMR signature different from that of three other places tested with the surface coil which gave approximately equal

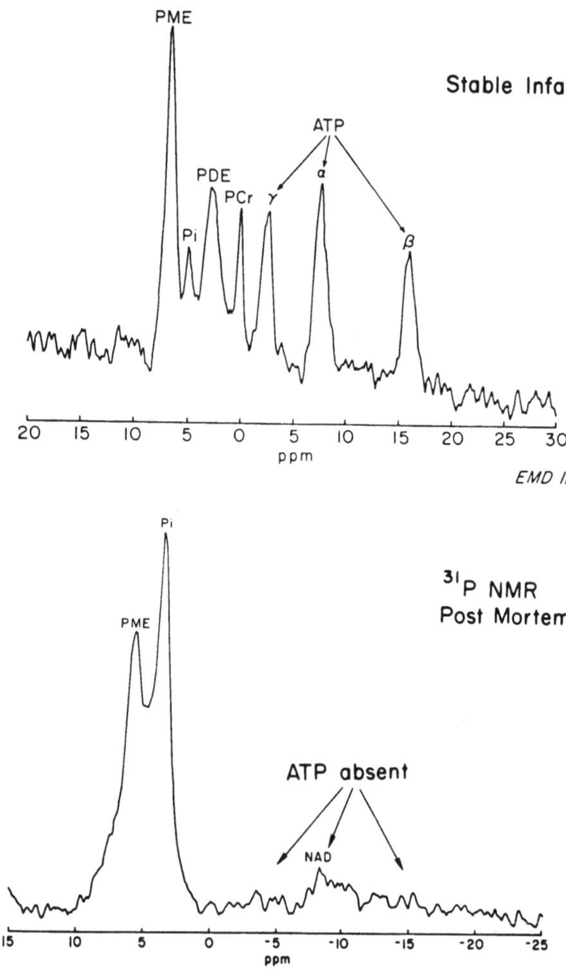

FIGURE 16.9. MRS study of living and dead brain tissue in the preterm neonate. Comparison P MRS of stable and unstable states of brain metabolism. ATP and PCr are not seen, and Pi is very high in the dead brain; PME remains.

and normal values of ATP and of Pi/PCr. The infarct is characterized by the lack of any phosphate compound, and, presumably, it has been filled with cerebral spinal fluid. The region of the infarct identified by P MRS is identical with the region identified in the CT scan.

Prognosis of Infarct

Since P MRS permits safe and repetitive monitoring of the neonatal brain, many of the studies presented here have been followed longitudinally in time. An example similar to that of the previous one (Fig. 16.11) shows that the region deficient

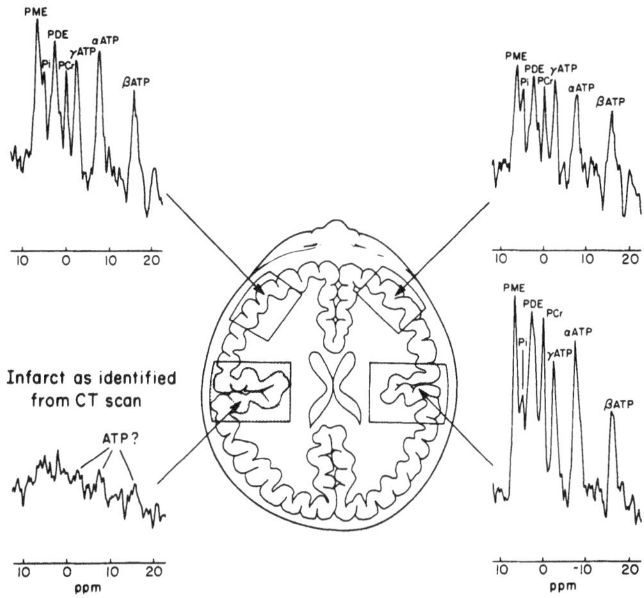

FIGURE 16.10. MRS localization of neonate infarct showing lack of ATP in the infarct. An illustration of the use of the surface coil to compare the P MRS signal in different quadrants of the brain, one of which includes a CT-identified infarct and which showed presence of no recognizable biochemicals. Baby M.P. was a full-term infant of average weight and size, the product of an uncomplicated pregnancy; at birth, the baby had a cyanotic right arm. Arteriography showed occlusion of artery to arm and also occlusion of carotid artery, causing chronic ischemia of left frontal lobe. CT scan showed left hemisphere infarct.

in ATP and PCr will show no recovery, whereas the contralateral hemisphere showed increasing Pi/PCr, characteristic of the normal developing brain. If there was a diacrisis present initially, it disappeared with growth and development of the neonate.

Partial Loss of Neuronal Population

The most frequently encountered state of a population of neurons that are threatened with hypoxia is a heterogeneous state, in which those neurons capable of the steady state ($V/V_{max} \sim 0.5$) exhibit normal values of PCr and ATP, while those that are incapable of maintaining a steady state ($V > V_{max}$) show rapid deterioration of concentrations of PCr and ATP.[22] Since steep oxygen gradients may be involved in rapidly respiring tissues such as the neonatal brain, neurons that are in steady state and in an unsteady state may be a few hundred microns from one another, leading to diffuse brain damage on a scale that is impossible to image by available NMR and CT techniques. However, this region is identified

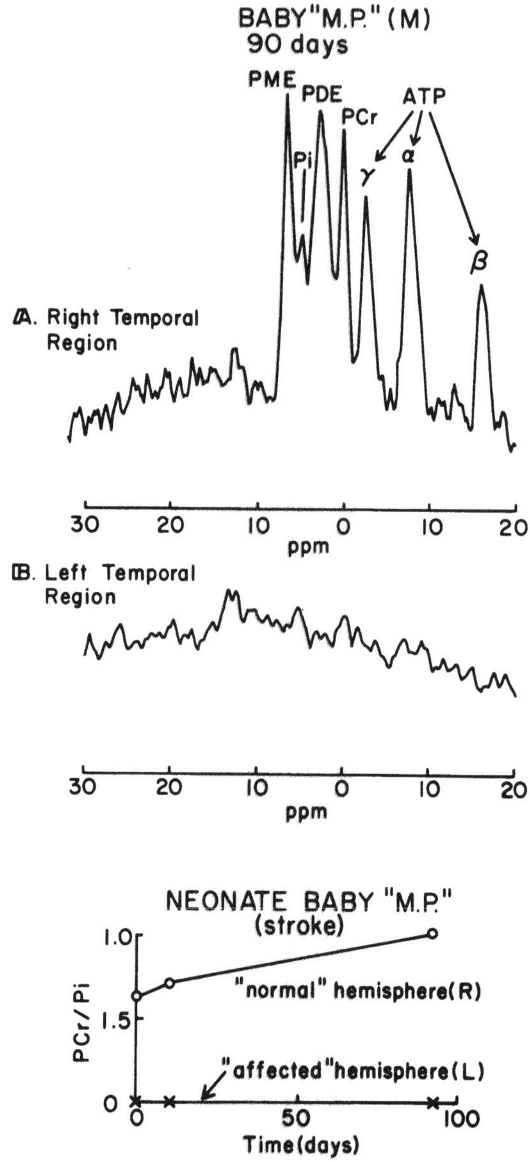

FIGURE 16.11. Time course of P MRS signals in a brain-damaged hemisphere (lower trace) and the contralateral hemisphere in baby M.P. (male, 90 days). The longitudinal study shows no improvement of the damaged hemisphere.

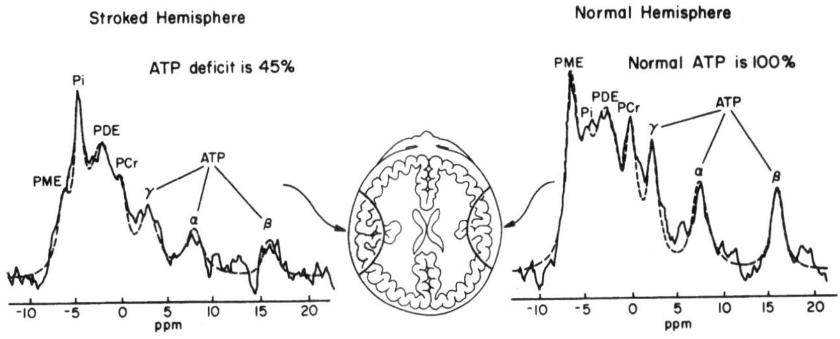

FIGURE 16.12. An illustration of NMR signals from two hemispheres of the neonatal brain in which hypoxia and ischemia selectively affected the left hemisphere; the right hemisphere appears to be normal as compared with age-matched neonates. The significant feature of the spectrum is that the ratio of the ATP has occurred in one hemisphere. Two types of traces are presented, the original data and the computer fits to the original data. Baby H.______, full-term infant, average weight and size, uncomplicated pregnancy. Fetal distress; on day 1, seizure activity present, EEG showed focal status left hemisphere, CT scan showed infarct in left hemisphere.

by P MRS as having a global loss of ATP, which we propose to be proportional to the fraction of the now endangered steady-state neurons.

An example of this is afforded in Figure 16.12, which shows, on the right-hand side, a near normal hemisphere, and on the contralateral side, an afflicted hemisphere in which half of the ATP has been hydrolyzed.[23] This results in a very high phosphate peak due to the contribution to phosphate from ATP breakdown and from PCr breakdown. An analysis of these results indicates that the Pi/PCr value of the surviving cells (50% of the total in that hemisphere) is less than 1.0. Animal experiments simulating this phenomenon suggest that in a brain endangered by hypoxia and ischemia, as much as 10% per hour of the neuronal population may make a transition from a viable steady state to a nonviable, nonsteady state. Thus, time is of the essence in detecting such a state and countering it with aggressive therapeutic measures.

Distribution of Patients

The population of all preterm neonates of our studies (over 500), together with the distribution of those of greater age, ranged in gestational age from 23 to 41 weeks and had birth weights from 550 to 4,540 g. In this study postconceptional ages ranged from 25 to 62 weeks, and the study weights ranged from 590 to 4,450 g. From observations in a variety of models and, indeed, based upon studies in both Philadelphia[6] and London,[24] no infants have survived with PCr/Pi values of less than 0.6, and several of those noted in that portion of distribution have died.[6,24] When the ADP value rises and V approaches V_{max}, the steady state may be lost and the cells may die.

Intraventricular hemorrhage (all bilateral grade III–IV bleeds) with associated increases in ICP (intracranial pressure) and possible ischemia was associated with prematurity and occurred in the 29-to-32-week gestational age group with birth weights ranging from 900 to 1,300 g. The postconceptional age range was 30 to 38 weeks, and the weight range was 900 to 2,000 g.

Relation to Adult Infarcts

As indicated by Figure 16.10, infarcted regions may show no detectable biochemicals and presumably are filled with cerebrospinal fluid. This contrasts significantly with the adult stroke where, so far, studies of brains after stroke[15] indicate the presence of survivor cells, presumably glia.

Relation to Functional Deficits

It is expected that many of the infarcted regions observed early in preterm neonates will mature to functional deficits of the brain. The correlation between these two may not be easy because of the plasticity of the neonatal brain and because of the variety of regions that can be affected. However, matured infarcts detectable by magnetic resonance imaging, computerized tomography, and ultrasound may exist in the brains of neonates with functional deficits.

^{31}P NMR spectroscopy adds a new tool to the investigation of neurological problems in human newborn infants and raises a number of important but unanswered questions concerning brain metabolism. The results of our neonatal studies suggest that newborn cortical metabolism may be unique and is considerably different from that in mature animals and previous neonatal animal models.

References

1. Nelson KB, Ellenberg JH: Neonatal signs as predictors of cerebral palsy. *Pediatrics* 64:225–232, 1979.
2. Holowach-Thurston J, Hauhart RE, Jones EM, et al: Decrease in brain glucose in anoxia in spite of elevated plasma glucose levels. *Pediatr Res* 7:691–695, 1973.
3. Thulborn KR, Du Boulay GH, Duchen LW, Radda G: A ^{31}P nuclear magnetic resonance in vivo study of cerebral ischemia in the gerbil. *J Cereb Blood Flow Metab* 2:299–306, 1982.
4. Michaelis L, Menten M: Die Kinetic der Intervertasewirkung. *Biochem Z* 49:333, 1913.
5. Chance B, Leigh JS Jr, Nioka S: P MRS as a sensor of oxygen in the heart of brain tissue. *Society for Magnetic Research in Medicine, Fifth Annual Meeting*, 1986, Vol 4, p 1368.
6. Younkin DP, Delivoria-Papadopoulos M, Maris J, Donlon E, Clancy R, Chance B: Cerebral metabolic effects of neonatal seizures measured with in-vivo ^{31}P NMR spectroscopy. *Ann Neurol* 20:513, 1986.

7. Lentz TL: *Cell Fine Structure: An Atlas of Drawings of Whole Cell Structure*. Philadelphia: W.B. Saunders, 1971, p 357.
8. Rothman S: Synaptic release of excitatory amino acid neurotransmitter mediates anoxic neuronal depth. *J Neurosci* 4:1884, 1984.
9. Chance B, Leigh JS Jr, Clark BJ, et al: Control of oxidative metabolism and oxygen delivery in human skeletal muscle: A steady-state analysis of the work/energy cost transfer function. *Proc Natl Acad Sci USA* 82:8384, 1985.
10. Chance B, Leigh JS, Kent K, et al: Multiple controls of oxidative metabolism of living tissues as studied by ^{31}P MRS. *Proc Natl Acad Sci USA* 83:9458–9462, 1987.
11. Maris J, Argov Z, DaMico L, Leigh JS Jr, Chance B: ^{31}P NMR in hamster dystrophy: Skeletal muscle bioenergetics in an animal model of inherited myopathy. *Society for Magnetic Research in Medicine, Fifth Annual Meeting*, 1986, Vol 2, p 442.
12. Chance B, Eleff S, Leigh JS Jr: Noninvasive, nondestructive approaches to cell bioenergetics. *Proc Natl Acad Sci USA*, 77:7430, 1980.
13. Lawson B, Guillet R, Sinnwell T, Gradwell L, Chance B, Delivoria-Papadopoulos M: Nuclear magnetic resonance (NMR) spectroscopy as a predictor of survival in the severely ill neonate. *Pediatr Res* 20:352, 1986.
14. Chance B, Clark BJ, Nioka S, Harihara Subramanian V, Maris JM, Bode H: Phosphorus NMR spectroscopy in-vivo. *Circulation* 72(Suppl IV):103, 1985.
15. Bottomley PA, Smith LS, Brazzamano S, Hedlund L, Redington RW, Herfkens RJ: The fate of Pi and pH in regional myocardial infarction: A noninvasive ^{31}P NMR study. *Society for Magnetic Research in Medicine, Fifth Annual Meeting*, 1986, Vol 3, p 608.
16. Maris JM, Evans AE, McLaughlin AC, et al: ^{31}P Nuclear magnetic resonance spectroscopic investigation of human neuroblastoma in situ. *N Engl J Med* 312:1500, 1985.
17. Chance B, Eleff S, Leigh JS Jr, Sokolow D, Sapega A: Mitochondrial regulation of phosphocreatine/inorganic phosphate ratios in exercising human muscle: A gated ^{31}P NMR study. *Proc Natl Acad Sci USA* 78:6714, 1981.
18. Arnold DL, Matthews PM, Radda GK: Metabolic recovery after exercise and the assessment of mitochondrial function in-vivo in human skeletal muscle by means of ^{31}P NMR. *Mag Res Med* 1:307, 1984.
19. Whitman GJ, Chance B, Bode H, et al: Diagnosis and therapeutic evaluation of a pediatric cardiomyopathy using ^{31}P NMR. *J Am Coll Cardiol* 5:745, 1985.
20. Gyulai L, Bolinger L, Leigh JS Jr, Barlow C, Chance B: Phosphorylethanolamine—the major constituent of the phosphomonoester peak observed by ^{31}P NMR on developing dog brain. *FEBS Lett* 178:137, 1984.
21. Nioka S, Mayevsky A, Chance B, et al: Age dependent metabolic control parameters in the neonate puppy brain from birth to 21 days age. *Society for Magnetic Research in Medicine, Fifth Annual Meeting*, 1986, Vol 3, p 674.
22. Chance B, Nioka S, Smith D, Leigh JS Jr: Biochemical heterogeneity in brain ischemia. *Society for Magnetic Research in Medicine, Fifth Annual Meeting,* 1986, Vol 4, p 1372.
23. Lien RI, Sinnwell T, Chance B, Delivoria-Papadopoulos M: Analysis of cerebral metabolism in a neonatal population. *Society for Magnetic Research in Medicine, Fifth Annual Meeting*, 1986, Vol 2, p 293.
24. Hope PL, Cady EB, Tofts PS, et al: Cerebral energy metabolism studied with phosphorus NMR spectroscopy in normal and birth-asphyxiated infants. *Lancet* 2:366, 1984.

17
Retinopathy of Prematurity: Overview and Findings in the Anterior Segment of Affected Eyes

MARY M. GILBERT, M. ELIZABETH HARTNETT,
THOMAS M. RICHARDSON, JOSEPH H. KRUG, TATSUO HIROSE

Background and Risk Factors

Our understanding of the disease known as retrolental fibroplasia (RLF) has changed enormously since the 1950s. Even its name has been changed to the more appropriate "retinopathy of prematurity" (ROP), which emphasizes the current thinking that the disease is due mainly to the immaturity of the infant's retina. The fibrotic changes characteristically seen behind the lens in the advanced stages of this disease, and for which the term retrolental fibroplasia (RLF) was given, are now thought to be a common end-stage manifestation of many diseases of the retina.

Opinions as to causes and risk factors in this disease have also undergone significant changes in the past 30 years. Supplemental oxygen was initially felt to be solely responsible for irreversible retinal damage seen in prematurely born babies.[1] The incrimination of oxygen in the 1950s led to drastic reduction in its use in the management of premature infants and brought about a concomitant decrease in the incidence of ROP. However, in the 1960s and early 1970s, neonatologists began recognizing increasing morbidity[2] and mortality[3] associated with the rigid restriction of oxygen. Additionally, many causes and risk factors other than oxygen began to appear in the literature during the ensuing years. Repeated occurrences of typical retinopathy in premature infants who had never been exposed to supplemental oxygen were recorded. Consequently, there was a trend toward the liberalization of oxygen use in nurseries, with the hope of reducing the risks of brain damage and death while only minimally increasing the risk of eye damage.[4]

From the Eye Research Institute, Retina Associates, Massachusetts Eye and Ear Infirmary, and the Department of Ophthalmology, Harvard Medical School, Boston, Massachusetts.
Portions of this material were presented at the Annual Meeting of the Academy of Ophthalmology, October 1988.
Supported in part by a grant from the Charles de Gunzberg Fund.
Presented in honor of Lewis A. Barness, MD, November 12, 1988.

The ophthalmic literature has been replete with reports of causative agents and risk factors for ROP. Most of the reported determinants of ROP, however, were analyzed in such small trials that it was difficult to assess their importance.[4] In the more recent and larger studies, however, low birth weight has been found to be the most significant and reproducible risk factor in ROP. Numerous investigators have shown an inverse relationship between the birth weight and the incidence and severity of ROP.[5-8]

Other risk factors with some current popularity include gestational age, episodes of hypoxemia, apnea treated by mask-and-bag ventilation, ventilator hours, prolonged parenteral nutrition, repeated blood transfusions, hypercarbia, hypocarbia, xanthine administration, maternal bleeding, and bright ambient light in the neonatal unit.[5-9] Current thinking is that ROP is a multifactoral disease, the most significant risk factor being low birth weight.

Incidence

With increased survival rates of low-birth-weight premature infants due to advances in neonatal intensive care, we have seen a recent resurgence in the incidence of ROP.[5-7] For infants weighing less than 1,250 g, investigators have reported incidences in the range of 38%[10] to 52%.[6] Phelps[11] reports that, of infants weighing 1,000 g or less at birth, 30% will develop the severe stages of ROP and 8% will go on to blindness. Infants of birth weights between 1,001 and 1,500 g have much better prognosis—only 2.2% will develop the late stages of ROP, and only 0.5% will be blind. ROP is currently a major cause of blindness among children.[11]

Classification

The advent of newer methods of evaluating and treating ROP brought the need for an international standard of classification, so that results could be compared. The international classification was published in *Pediatrics* in July 1984[12] and in the *Archives of Ophthalmology* in August 1984.[13] Refinements of the classification were published by the international committee in 1987.[14]

The international classification of ROP is determined by three parameters: location, extent, and staging.

Location

The retina is divided into three circular zones (I, II, III) centered on the optic disc. Zone I is the innermost portion of the retina which centers on the optic disc and has a radius of twice the distance from the optic nerve to the fovea. Zone II includes the circumferential area from the edge of zone I and extends nasally to the anterior edge of the retina (the ora serrata). It extends the same radial distance from the edge of zone I 360°, so the temporal edge of zone II is approximately at the equator of the globe. Zone III is the remainder of the retina and forms a crescent temporally. This is the area that is vascularized last in the developing eye and is therefore the most frequently involved in ROP.

Extent

The extent of the disease is described by the clock hours of involvement.

Staging

There are five stages which represent a gradual continuum of the peripheral vascular response observed in these eyes. Two additional descriptors are used to help classify the staging: *plus disease*, which describes the vascular response seen posteriorly, and *regressed disease*, which recognizes the multiple vascular and retinal changes that are seen as the disease regresses.

Stage 1 – Demarcation Line

Stage 1 is manifested by a thin, white line separating the vascular retina posteriorly from the avascular retina anteriorly. It is flat, lying in the plane of the retina. The retinal vessels leading up to the line may appear slightly abnormal.

Stage 2 – Ridge

In stage 2 the line is enlarged, so that it has height and width and extends out of the plane of the retina. The ridge may have a pink color, and tufts of vessels may be seen on the posterior edge of the ridge.

Stage 3 – Ridge with Extraretinal Fibrovascular Proliferation

The next stage of ROP is characterized by the ridge described in stage 2, with the presence of fibrovascular proliferative tissue. The proliferative tissue may be seen on the ridge, just posterior to it, or extending into the vitreous.

Stage 4 – Partial Retinal Detachment

The description of stage 4 includes the findings of stage 3 with the presence of a partial retinal detachment. This may be caused by an exudative effusion, or traction, or both. The detachment may be located in the area of the fovea, where the visual prognosis is poor, or in the extrafoveal area, where the visual prognosis is relatively good.

Stage 5 – Total Retinal Detachment

The total retinal detachment seen in ROP is funnel-shaped. The configuration of the funnel appears to be an important factor in predicting the success of the various vitreoretinal surgery techniques. Ultrasonography is often used to evaluate this stage.

Plus Disease

The previously outlined stages concentrate on the vascular changes that occur at the leading peripheral edge of the retinal vasculature. Vascular changes may also be seen posteriorly in ROP, and include engorgement of the veins and increased tortuosity of the arterioles. When plus disease is present, there may be very rapid progression of the vascular abnormalities. Other findings typical of plus disease include iris vascular engorgement, pupillary rigidity, and vitreous haze and/or hemorrhage.

Regressed ROP

This category details the multiple vascular and retinal changes that are seen as the disease regresses. Findings consistent with these changes represent the most common outcome of ROP.

Prevention and Treatment

As we gain greater understanding of this disease, it becomes clear that the prevention of ROP is probably impossible. In the 1950s oxygen was felt to be the sole culprit, and it was the popular opinion that strict oxygen restriction would be preventive. Another modality of preventive management that has been given considerable attention is vitamin E. It has waxed and waned in popularity since it was first reported to decrease the severity of the disease in 1949 by Owens and Owens.[15] The data from prospective studies are conflicting, and there does not seem to be a consensus regarding the effect of vitamin E on the prevention of ROP.

Ophthalmic instrumentation and techniques have shown great advances over the past two decades. We are now able to intervene with treatment modalities which, although far from perfect, help to reduce the incidence of blindness in these children. The two mainstays of treatment are cryotherapy (or laser photocoagulation) and vitreoretinal surgery.

Cryotherapy has been shown to prevent in part the more severe complications of active angiopathy. Most authorities recommend that treatment be given at stage 3 of the international classification. A multicenter national study to evaluate the effects of cryotherapy published its preliminary results in 1988.[16] These researchers found that cryotherapy conferred a clear benefit 3 months after treatment and that there was a 50% reduction in unfavorable outcomes.

Modern vitreoretinal surgery techniques have been developed for the treatment of the severe stages of ROP (stages 4 and 5) and have achieved some anatomic success in reattaching these retinas, as well as achieving some degree of functional visual success. In 1986, Trese[17] reported anatomic success in reattachment of the retina in 48% and functional success in 31% of 85 eyes undergoing surgery. Another large retrospective vitrectomy study was published by Chong et al[18] in 1986. Of the 58 eyes undergoing vitrectomy, anatomic success was achieved in 43%, but the recovery of postoperative useful vision was only 19%. Hirose and Schepens[19] reported that of 184 consecutive cases of vitrectomy, 38% had anatomic reattachment of the retina and that 46% of the cases that were anatomically successful obtained ambulatory vision. Despite the seemingly low rate of visual recovery seen in these series, they do represent advancements: Only 15 years ago, we could only watch passively as the disease took its course, leading to the blindness of these children.

Late-Onset Blindness – Glaucoma

Despite the accomplishments of the newer treatment modalities in preventing and reattaching retinal detachments in the posterior segment, glaucoma (and possibly other problems of the anterior segment) may continue to be a significant late manifestation of advanced ROP. Glaucoma has been reported to occur in 25% to 35% of cases with untreated stage 5 ROP.[20-23]

Proposed mechanisms of glaucoma in patients with severe ROP have included angle closure,[24] ciliary block,[25] and inflammation.[26] Methods of treatment have been designed to correct the presumed abnormality. Iridectomy,[22] which is the treatment for angle closure glaucoma; lensectomy,[27] which is the treatment for ciliary block glaucoma; and corticosteroid administration,[26] which quiets the inflammatory response, have been tried. Unfortunately, these treatments have, at best, met with only limited success, leading us to believe that there may be other mechanisms that are contributing to the development of glaucoma in these eyes.

To study this, we performed detailed clinical examinations of the eyes of infants with untreated stages 4 and 5 ROP who were undergoing examination under anesthesia for possible vitreoretinal surgery. We are following these children prospectively for the development of glaucoma. At the time of examination, intraocular pressure (IOP) measurements are taken, and detailed examinations of the anterior segment are performed including microscopic evaluation and gonioscopy (a technique using a contact lens that allows viewing of the angle structures). The posterior segments are evaluated using binocular indirect ophthalmoscopy and B-scan ultrasound when indicated. We have documented and classified some of the structural characteristics of these eyes, and we hope to identify the findings that may predispose the premature infant with ROP to glaucoma. Ultimately, data collected in sequential examinations of these children could lead to better understanding of the mechanisms of glaucoma in ROP.

Posterior segment findings in these eyes included total retinal detachment (stage 5 ROP) in 77% and partial retinal detachment (stage 4 ROP) in 23%.

The anterior segment and gonioscopic findings of the 26 previously untreated eyes were recorded. Of the eyes studied, 35% had 90° or more of angle closure. Buphthalmos (corneal diameter greater than 12 mm) occurred in both eyes of one patient. Endothelial dystrophy occurred in 22%, and a prominent Schwalbe's line was seen in 15%. A high degree of iris convexity was noted in 58% of the eyes.

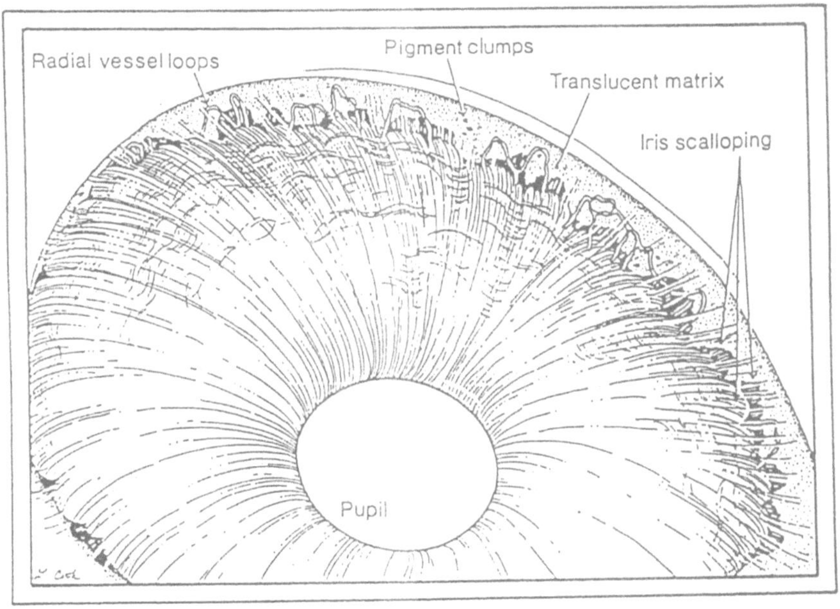

FIGURE 17.1. Drawing traced from a photograph taken during an examination of an infant with stage 5 ROP. It shows the condensed translucent "Barkan's-like" matrix which enmeshes radial blood vessel loops. Small pigment clumps suspended in the matrix are noted in the angle.

Of interest is that 69% of the eyes examined had a translucent "Barkan's-like" matrix in the angle. Peripheral anterior synechiae were seen in 26%, and posterior synechiae were seen in 62%. Synechiae suggested that an inflammatory process might be contributory. A very high percentage (70%) of the eyes exhibited abnormal iris or angle vessels. Pigment clumping in the angle recess was seen in 46%, and white tissue posterior to the ciliary body band (scleral show) was seen in 12% of the eyes. Figures 17.1 and 17.2 are drawings traced from photographs taken during the examinations and are representative of many of the structures that have been described.

Some of the findings in these immature eyes may represent normal ocular development. Unfortunately there are few reports in the literature of the clinical microscopic and gonioscopic appearance of the anterior segment of normal newborns, or of premature babies without ROP.

Other characteristics we have described may indeed be abnormalities. They may be a direct consequence of the ROP, or they may be a result of other influences concomitant with prematurity. Although there are probably multiple mechanisms contributing to the development of glaucoma, which of these findings are significant? Studies in the future should help to answer this question. Sequential examinations of the anterior segment including the angle are essential for understanding the

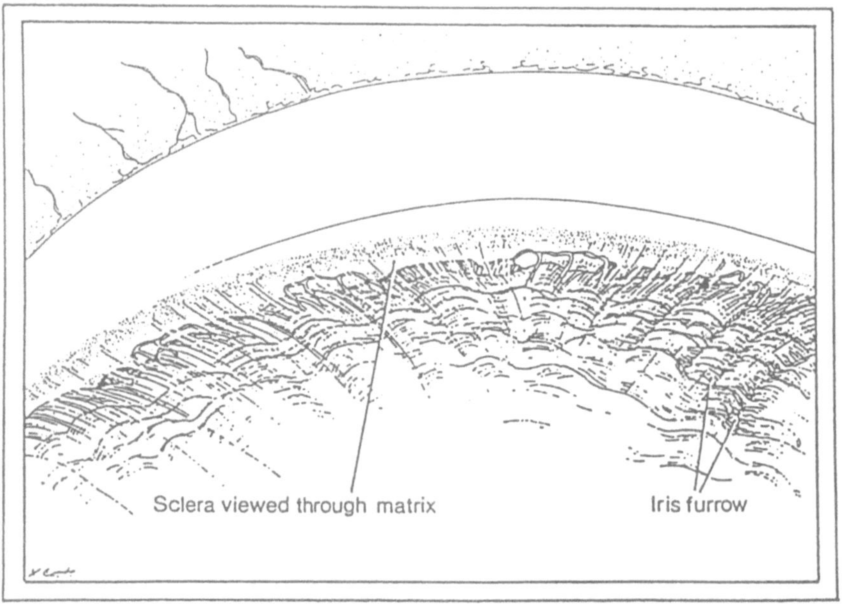

FIGURE 17.2. Drawing traced from a photograph showing the white tissue believed to be sclera (scleral show) that is seen posterior to the broad gray ciliary body band/trabecular meshwork area. Vascular loops are also depicted within a translucent matrix.

mechanisms of glaucoma in ROP. Ultimately, data collected in this and subsequent studies could lead to a better understanding of ROP and perhaps suggest better methods for its treatment and prevention.

Conclusion

Major advances in instrumentation and patient management in the neonatal intensive care units are increasing the survival rates of very low-birth-weight infants. With the increased survival has come resurgence of the disease now known as retinopathy of prematurity (ROP). We have a much greater understanding of ROP now than when it was first described over 40 years ago, and we are beginning to make inroads into the successful treatment of the disease. With new ablative and surgical treatment modalities, useful vision is sometimes able to be restored even in eyes with very advanced disease.

We must not forget that late-onset manifestations, especially glaucoma, may occur in our patients with ROP. Awareness of, and prompt attention to, these potentially blinding sequelae may make the difference of a sighted or a nonsighted child or adult. It is hoped that the future will see a reduction in the incidence of blindness due to ROP, and that these low-birth-weight premature babies will be able to lead full, productive, "sighted" lives.

References

1. Guy LP, Lanman JT, Dancis J: The possibility of total elimination of retrolental fibroplasia by oxygen restriction. *Pediatrics* 17:247–249, 1956.
2. McDonald AD: Neurologic and ophthalmic disorders in children of very low birth weight. *Br Med J* 1:895–900, 1962.
3. Cross KW: Cost of preventing retrolental fibroplasia? *Lancet* 2:954–956, 1973.
4. Silverman WA, Flynn JT: Overview: A "developmental" retinopathy reconsidered. In Silverman WA, Flynn JT (eds): *Contemporary Issues in Fetal and Neonatal Medicine 2: Retinopathy of Prematurity.* Boston: Blackwell Scientific Publications, 1985, pp ix–xxiii.
5. Gunn TR, Easdown J, Outerbridge EW, Aranda VJ: Risk factors in retrolental fibroplasia. *Pediatrics* 65:1096–1100, 1980.
6. Shohat M, Reisner SH, Krikler R, et al: Retinopathy of prematurity: Incidence and risk factors. *Pediatrics* 72:159–163, 1983.
7. Bossi E, Koenher F, Flury B, Zulali FM: Retinopathy of prematurity: A risk factor analysis with univariate and multivariate statistics. *Helv Paediatr Acta* 39:307–317, 1984.
8. Hammer ME, Mullen PW, Ferguson JG, et al: Logistic analysis of risk factors in acute retinopathy of prematurity. *Am J Ophthalmol* 102:1–6, 1986.
9. Glass P, Avery GB, Subramanian KN, et al: Effect of bright light in the hospital nursery on the incidence of retinopathy of prematurity. *N Engl J Med* 313:401–404, 1985.
10. Kinsey VE, Arnold HJ, Kalina RE, et al: PaO_2 levels and retrolental fibroplasia: A report of the cooperative study. *Pediatrics* 60:655–668, 1977.
11. Phelps DL: Vision loss due to retinopathy of prematurity. *Lancet* 1:606, 1981.
12. Committee for the Classification of ROP: An international classification of retinopathy of prematurity. *Pediatrics* 74:127–133, 1984.
13. Committee for the Classification of ROP: An international classification of retinopathy of prematurity. *Arch Ophthalmol* 102:1130–1135, 1984.
14. Committee for the Classification of ROP: An international classification of retinopathy of prematurity. II. The classification of retinal detachment. *Arch Ophthalmol* 105:906–912, 1987.
15. Owens WC, Owens EU: Retrolental fibroplasia in premature infants. II. Studies on the prophylaxis of the disease: The use of alpha tocopherol acetate. *Am J Ophthalmol* 32:1611, 1949.
16. Cryotherapy for ROP Cooperative Group: Multicenter trial of cryotherapy for retinopathy of prematurity (preliminary results). *Arch Ophthalmol* 106:471–479, 1988.
17. Trese MT: Visual results and prognostic factors for vision following surgery for stage 5 retinopathy of prematurity. *Ophthalmology* 93:574–579, 1986.
18. Chong LP, Machemer R, deJuan E: Vitrectomy for advanced stages of retinopathy of prematurity. *Am J Ophthalmol* 102:710–716, 1986.
19. Hirose T, Schepens CL: Open-sky vitrectomy in retrolental fibroplasia. *American Academy of Ophthalmology Annual Meeting,* Nov 12, 1984.
20. Kwitko ML: Secondary glaucoma in infancy and childhood. In Kwitko ML (ed): *Glaucoma in Infants and Children*. New York: Appleton-Century-Crofts, 1973, p 468.
21. Blodi FC: Symposium: Retrolental fibroplasia. *Trans Am Acad Ophthalmol Otolaryngol* 59:35–38, 1955.
22. Smith J, Shivitz I: Angle closure glaucoma in adults with cicatricial retinopathy of prematurity. *Arch Ophthalmol* 102:371–372, 1984.

23. Johnson DR, Swan KC: Retrolental fibroplasia—a continuing problem. *Trans Pacif Coast Oto-ophthalmol Soc* 47:129–133, 1966.
24. Pollard ZF: Secondary angle closure glaucoma in cicatricial retrolental fibroplasia. *Am J Ophthalmol* 89:651–653, 1980.
25. Kushner BJ: Ciliary block glaucoma in retinopathy of prematurity. *Arch Ophthalmol* 100:1078–1079, 1982.
26. Kushner BJ, Sondheimer S: Medical treatment of glaucoma associated with cicatricial retinopathy of prematurity. *Am J Ophthalmol* 94:313–317, 1982.
27. Pollard ZF: Lensectomy for secondary angle closure glaucoma in advanced cicatricial retrolental fibroplasia. *Ophthalmology* 91:395–398, 1984.

18

Current Concepts in the Surgical Treatment of the Infant with Facial Deformities: The Center Concept

MUTAZ B. HABAL

Introduction

Facial-cleft deformities are among the most common birth defects in newborns occurring in pediatric practice. One newborn in every 700 live births is born with a cleft: cleft lip in 25%, cleft palate in 25%, or cleft lip and cleft palate in 50%. This incidence refers to clefts reported in an isolated manner, as opposed to syndromes in which a cleft is a manifestation. Excluded from the incidence data also are the trisomy syndromes. In a given community, the number of patients born with clefts can be roughly determined from the number of live births. For example, at a referral center in the Tampa Bay area with 14,000 live births per year, about 20 newborns with clefts are treated yearly. Spina bifida (one in every 950 live births) is the second most common congenital malformation. The majority of handicapped children with treatable conditions fall into one or both of these categories of defects.

The third most common birth defect is congenital heart disease, which occurs in 1 of every 1,000 live births. Thirty percent of newborns with facial deformities have associated congenital cardiac anomalies.

Facial cleft and spina bifida occurring together demands a long, ongoing treatment plan. In turn, tight coordination of the practitioners is necessary to treat such affected children appropriately. Treatment and rehabilitation must start at birth and must be continued into their 20s in most patients. All patients born with facial clefts should be treated by a coordinated team. Solo approaches should be discouraged, since these approaches are not in the best interest of the patient. The team should initially counsel carefully the parents of a child with a birth defect. Good counseling begins with the pediatrician, who describes the possibilities for treatment and who works to reduce any guilt that such parents may feel. The pediatrician also institutes well-baby care and becomes the patient's advocate.

From the Tampa Bay Craniofacial Center, Tampa, Florida.
Submitted in honor of Lewis A. Barness, MD, November 1988.

The Team Concept

Historically, the team concept originated simultaneously in Europe and the United States (Pennsylvania). The ideal treatment team is a group of specialized professionals who work together to coordinate the patient care. Agreement on patient management should be the paramount goal of all concerned. However, honest medical disagreements may exist, and in such cases the patient's welfare should always be considered academically and not distorted by personality differences. Disruptive factors within the team result in less than ideal rehabilitation for the patient.

The team provides and executes a treatment plan designed to optimize function and development of the growing patient.

Telephonic communication between team members to plan definitive treatment for the patient is unwise. Such a plan will tend to produce an unfavorable outcome. Communication between these professionals should be in face-to-face meetings as frequently as needed.

The team members should be experts in their fields and should use their expertise on behalf of the patient's well-being. In the beginning of this team concept (the early 1950s), when the basic concern was improved patient growth and function as influenced by correction of structure, the participants typically consisted of a plastic surgeon, a speech pathologist, and an orthodontist, although a pediatrician would occasionally participate in the meetings. In recent years, the pediatrician has been assuming a far more active role on the team – as patient advocate, director of coordinated treatment-management plans, and monitor of well-baby care.

The problem of structural abnormalities should be addressed in terms of function. Coordination between appearance and function has always been the major concern. Other important considerations have included the need for speech correction and correction of occlusion.

To maintain their clinical skills, enhance their diagnostic judgment, and upgrade treatment protocols, members of a cleft lip/palate and craniofacial team should concurrently treat a minimum of 10 newborns with clefts and 10 with complex facial deformities. To have teams working on relatively few patients is not feasible, economical, or practical, nor does it advance clinical science and in the best interest of the patient.

A code of standards has been formulated for use by teams around the country. A directory of all the team professionals in the United States is published once a year by the American Cleft Palate Association. Many states are in the process of legislating guidelines and standards for the treatment of patients born with clefts to minimize duplication of care, prevent unnecessary treatments, and promote general safety for patients through quality treatment protocols.[1]

An appropriate team should meet weekly to examine, evaluate, and organize treatment plans. There are approximately 200 functioning teams at any one time in the United States available without delay to every cleft patient or family in need. Within each team, there are qualified experts to handle special or complicated problems. It is often suggested that the family may seek a second and third opinion from adjacent teams. With such coordinated efforts, parents of patients born with cleft lip and/or cleft palate can be referred to an appropriate team immediately after the child's birth.

When a child is born with cleft lip, cleft palate, or other craniofacial abnormality, a member of the team promptly visits the family in the hospital and explains the child's condition to them. This individual customarily advises the parents of the treatment methodology available before the family is influenced by friends, neighbors, or relatives to seek unconventional treatments such as ointments, massage, or herbs. A parent support group is available within every team to help to inform parents of the special care that will be required and to stress proper care and a satisfactory feeding program for the child.

As a team becomes more sophisticated, new professionals capable of working on clinical problems join the effort. In the process, they enhance their own knowledge of problems in patients with clefts. By attending comprehensive seminars while on the team, members keep their clinical skills current. A second pediatrician and a pediatric otologist, an otolaryngologist, an audiologist, a psychologist, and other health professionals are frequently necessary to complement the team effort, allowing fully comprehensive treatment to be instituted. Finally, parents should be present during any of the discussions and should be active participants on the team, for they are also the patient's advocates.

The Traditional Treatment

It is now accepted that treatment of the patient with cleft lip, cleft palate, and craniofacial abnormality must follow a carefully planned sequence of staged surgical procedures. The order of the stages is dictated by the importance of preservation of function. The cleft lip is closed first, the cleft palate second, the pharyngeal flap third. If there are other cranial constricting anomalies, further problems are addressed early. Bone grafting in the open bony cleft is next done, when necessary, and lastly, during the teen years, total nasal reconstruction is accomplished.

In the past, cleft lip was closed by the time a child weighed 10 lb and if the hemoglobin was over 10 g. This was designed to avoid serious and statistically high anesthetic complications, particularly when ether was the main anesthetic agent. Similarly, the palate was closed at 18 to 24 months to avoid interference with maxillary growth. These archaic concepts have been successfully challenged over the years. Improvements in medical care are made as different team members compare their data for peer review. These new methods should not be adopted unless the team is fully knowledgeable of the physiologic reasons for them.

Patients treated with new methods have superior function as compared with previous modalities. It is evident that the new modalities are better. Early treatment, stress-maintenance of the acquired correction, monitoring of all functions that include growth and development, stimulation of skills, and support by increasing parental bonding are the basis for any successful treatment plan. The primary reason we no longer see speech or hearing loss in patients born with clefts is due to the fact that early, controlled, definitive treatment is now the standard and is followed by close monitoring of the results.

Treatment Plan

Treatment plans for children with facial deformities use functional priorities in the correction of the deformities. Obsolete methods should not be used. Since no two deformities are alike, a treatment plan should be individualized for each particular patient.

Among facial deformities, the cleft lip and cleft palate are the most common, and every pediatrician should be immediately aware of details of the newest methods of treatment. Other complex facial deformities should also be treated early and in a similar manner. This may involve therapy to improve vision, speech, and hearing. The nutritional status of the patient should not be compromised because of the surgical procedures. Therefore the patient is fed a regular diet following the surgical procedure.

Unilateral Cleft Lip

The cleft lip should be closed within the first month of life. Microsurgical instruments and technique should be used. The closure should be tension-free. There are two basic principles in closure of cleft lips: (1) closure within the first 2 weeks of birth,[2] to reduce scarring, and (2) approximation of the muscle gap (the orbicularis oris edges) with interdigitation at any early age, in order to effect total molding of the face and good facial balance, particularly in wide-open clefts. The closure is done in one stage.[3,4] Lip adhesion surgery is inadvisable because of unwarranted extra risks. The closure of the cleft lip goes beyond devising a skin flap; it is intended to produce muscle approximation and animation, mucosal closure, and bony alignment. Especially important in such early treatment plans is the presence of a pediatric intensivist to ensure that the patient receives proper anesthesia and perioperative and postoperative care.

Bilateral Cleft Lip

The bilateral cleft lip is closed in one stage, using the modified Manchester principle of advancing the orbicularis oris muscle across the premaxilla under the prolabium which is deficient in mesodermal tissue. Ideally, complete molding of the face is seen after the corrective procedure. Closure should be done during the first month of life, utilizing microsurgical instruments and optical magnification. An experienced pediatric anesthesiologist must be present at the surgery, and proper monitoring devices must be used.[5,6]

A pulse oximeter is the most valuable monitoring equipment for small babies and children undergoing general anesthesia. It can be employed in both perioperative and postoperative periods for early detection of airway compromise. It will register cardiopulmonary changes before the patient is in serious difficulty. During the early postoperative phase oximeters provide close monitoring of the patient's cardiorespiratory physiology. The infant's heart is very sensitive to oxygen deprivation. Hypoventilation and hypoxia are manifested by a sudden onset of bradycardia.

Early closure produces improved healing with less scarring since collagen formation is minimal compared to adults. Neonates heal their wounds by excessive production of mucopolysaccharide.

Cleft Palate

The cleft palate should be closed before 6 months of age. If the palatine muscles are connected together at any early age, they provide more efficient velopharyngeal function, faster reanimation, and improved speech. Speech is dependent on the child's level of intellectual comprehension, but it is helped considerably by healthy muscle function.[2] Minimal dissection of the mucoperiosteum is done; thus no damage to the growth of the maxilla occurs. Oronasal fistulas in the anterior compartment may occur; however, they are easily corrected at a later age, particularly if the child exhibits normal function of the palatine muscles in the production of speech, their primary responsibility.[8]

The palatine muscles have to be detached from the hard palate and reoriented in horizontal fashion, in order to produce good function of the velum and to regain sphincterlike action in the velopharyngeal area. This early correction may be helpful in alleviating Eustachian tube dysfunction.[9]

Nasal Structure

Nasal tip deformity, related to the lower lateral cartilage and the columella, is corrected during the first operative procedure.[5] This may be considered by some a radical operation; however, it is wise to correct the deformity when the cartilages are in a malleable state. Whether the deformity is unilateral or part of a bilateral cleft lip and cleft palate, the cleft nose deformity should still be corrected during the first operative procedure. The complete contouring effect of the nose can be seen after a badly deformed nose is corrected and after the child achieves further growth.

Nasal appearance, which was neglected in the traditional treatment plans, is therefore now being addressed as a correction of the deformed cleft-lip nose in early childhood. Stenosis of the nostril may need to be stretched at a later stage.

Clefted Alveolus

There are two approaches used to repair the clefted alveolus. The two are equally satisfactory, when carried out in adolescence.

The clefted alveolus can be closed before expansion of the upper alveolar arch is completed, sometimes as early as 3 years of age. The expansion of the upper alveolar arch orthodontically can be pursued during the bone-healing phase since new bone regenerates slowly. This newly formed bone is usually a malleable structure, particularly when placed on the maxillary segments in the patient with open clefts. Autologous grafts are also used when the upper arch is fully expanded, and necessitate bone graft to close the air gap and stabilize the movable segment. The procedure is preferably done during the interval between deciduous and permanent tooth eruption, at about six years of age, and prior to expansion of the upper arch. This approach is currently recommended by our team. Results are excellent for over 98% of the patients. The grafts can then be functionally manipulated, expanded, and molded, even after they are healed. Teeth readily erupt through the graft and can be orthodontically manipulated for proper alignment.

Bone to be used for the procedure can be harvested from any location in the body. In children, it is physically easier if the harvest is taken from the cranial area as a splint cranial bone graft–for example, from the outer table of the skull. Membranous bone grafts over membranous bone are used to fill the air gaps, producing a superior result. The length of stay in the hospital after such a bone-grafting procedure is reducible to only 48 h.

Occlusal Problems

The occlusal problems are corrected as indicated in the growing child. The process starts with expansion plates to align the arches and to correct the open and crossed bite. Reliance on an external functional appliance is as important as the surgical procedure itself. Long-term correction of the occlusal problem is a major task, requiring the use of orthodontic manipulation for maintenance of results. External appliances in the form of face mask, and functional appliances to shift the skeletal framework are very helpful to correct the patient's functional problems and achieve facial balance.

Midface Alignment

As functional alignment in early childhood is better achieved, there will be fewer indications to correct midface deficiencies during adolescence in patients with severe clefts. It is in fact already apparent that, in 10 years of follow-up, we do not see any midface collapse in the patients who have been fully treated at an early age and who have adhered to a proper maintenance schedule.

Maintenance of Corrective Maneuvers

The goals for long-term maintenance treatment is twofold. Both patient and parents must understand the basic requirements, and all instructions provided to them by the treating physician must be followed in a systematic way. Once all major operative procedures have been performed, the patients should be evaluated every 6 months for about 6 years and every 12 months thereafter until they have completed their growth. Speech, hearing, and occlusion are evaluated at each visit. If recognized early, most problems can be treated by simple measures. If, however, problems are neglected, more serious corrections will be needed, and some sequelae may be difficult to modify.

Middle Ear, Ventilation Tubes, and Hearing Impairment

It is well known that patients born with a cleft palate frequently present middle-ear problems from Eustachian tube dysfunction. A long-lasting ventilation tube should be installed in the child's middle ear at the first operative procedure, before the child develops serious otitis media. Whether cleft lip or cleft palate is being closed, the ventilation tubes are inserted at the time of the first operative procedure and anesthetic exposure.

The majority of patients already have fluid accumulated in the middle ears when ventilation tubes are first inserted. Obviously, hearing impairment is detrimental to the developing child, particularly during the language acquisition phase. A 20% to 30% loss will fundamentally handicap a child born with cleft palate, particularly when there are already borderline speech problems. Monitoring of the hearing and ear function is done during the patient's subsequent visits.

Pharyngeal Flaps

Pharyngeal flaps are needed when a child has a speech abnormality of excessive nasal quality. Speech can be evaluated as early as 2 years. The flap can be created as early as 3 years of age, although the mean age is about 5 years. The accepted flaps now are based superiorly, with lateral port control, or a retropositioned pharyngeal flap with a nasal resurfacing flap is used (Stanford). The need for such procedures is decreasing with early functional prospective protocols.[2]

The Fourth Dimension

The fourth dimension in any treatment plan is scrupulous observation of the correct timing for any given intervention or activity, particularly at times of rapid growth. A child grows at an extremely fast rate during the first 18 months of life. The face is also growing at a highly accelerated rate, with continuous shifts in facial proportions during adolescence until the adult status is finally reached.[10]

What is missed during that stage can never be recovered. Therefore attention should be directed toward realizing this "fourth dimension." The surgeon must work closely with the rest of the team to achieve their common objective—the welfare of the handicapped child. The timing for closure of the different components, and the timing of identifying any abnormality, are extremely critical. Procrastination by members of the team, for reasons of convenience is not acceptable.[11]

Conclusion

The treatment of patients with facial clefts and complex facial deformities is complex and requires a team effort by professionals. This principle is more important than any detail of surgical technique. A patient with congenital facial deformities must not be treated in the 1990s by a single surgical practitioner. Such a decision disregards functional derangements that may result.

The professional team should coordinate their treatment plans and efforts in face-to-face meetings. There must be a uniform code of standards of care accepted both by the team and on a statewide basis. Team members should improve their expertise by ongoing educational programs, including reading, and by participating in workshops on the subject. Finally, state-of-the-art treatment should be practiced within the team.

Prospective

Failure of fusion of early embryonic structures produces the common birth defects detailed here – some developmental and others inherited. Perhaps, in the future, treatment of the child born with facial deformities can be instituted in utero. The cleft stigma, no matter how acquired, is something children should not be forced to live with, particularly when any apparent external scar can be surgically eliminated. Our closest approach to ideal correction is treatment in the neonatal period.

References

1. *Guidelines for Care of Patients with Cleft Lip, Cleft Palate, and Craniofacial Deformities for the State of Florida*. Tallahassee: Health and Rehabilitative Services.
2. Barimo JP, Habal MB, Scheuerle J: Post natal palatoplasty. *Scand J Plast Reconstr Surg* 1:139–144, 1987.
3. Giraldes J: The rotation advancement principle. In McDowel F (ed): *The Source Book*. Baltimore: Williams and Wilkins, 1982.
4. Millard DR: A radical rotation in single harelip. *Am J Surg* 95:318, 1958.
5. McComb H: Primary repair of bilateral cleft lip nose. *Plast Reconstr Surg* 77: 701–713, 1986.
6. Manchester WM: Bilateral cleft lip closure. *Br J Surg* 95:878, 1965.
7. Habal MB, Scheuerle J: *Clefts in the Black Patient*. Cole L (ed). Rockville: American Speech and Hearing Association, 1988.
8. Trier W: Cleft palate closure. *Adv Plast Reconstr Surg* 2:193–226, 1986.
9. Habal MB: Cleft palate closure. Discussion, *Adv Plast Reconstr Surg* 2:225, 1986.
10. Jackson I: Cleft craft revisited. *Adv Plast Reconstr Surg* 1:205–237, 1987.
11. *Fourth International Congress of Cleft Lip, Cleft Palate, and Craniofacial Abnormalities*, Monte Carlo, Monaco, 1985.

19
Who Are Today's Pediatricians and What Do They Do?

ROBERT KAYE

Today, pediatric practitioners are predominantly young[1]; 59% are 44 years or younger, and only 20% are 55 and older (Table 19.1). A slight majority (53%) are certified by the American Board of Pediatrics[1] (Table 19.2). The number certified annually has increased from 339 in 1935 to 1,812 in 1986[2] (Fig. 19.1). The rapid increase in the number of certifications has leveled off since 1979, at around 1,600 per year[3] (Table 19.3). The number of pediatric practitioners has increased since 1970 at a greater rate than has the number of all physicians[1] (Table 19.4). In the period 1970 to 1983, the increase was 83% for pediatricians and 55% for all physicians. The percentage of women pediatricians has increased from 21% to 32% and is greater than that of women physicians as a whole. American Board of Pediatrics data reveal that women made up 48% of the third-year residents completing training in June 1988.[2]

The growth in numbers of certified pediatric subspecialists and training programs has been rapid (Table 19.5) since initiation of certification in cardiology in 1961. Inroads into consultative activities resulted in an increased primary-care focus. There are now 309 approved training programs that have certified 4,125 pediatric subspecialists.[2] The large number of neonatologists resulted in an increased tendency to practice in community hospitals, with further inroads into the consultative activities of pediatric practitioners.

The demographics of the population served by pediatricians raises some major problems for the future. With the decline in U.S. birth rate that has followed the baby boom of the 1960s, the number of children per pediatrician has decreased from about 3,100 in 1970 to a projected 1,300 in the year 2000 (Fig. 19.2). Including in the calculation family and general practitioners, who devote about 25% of their practice to children, the ratio is projected to decline to about 900.[4]

The actual and projected number of individuals under the age of 19 is projected to decline from about 77 million in 1970 to about 73 million in the year 2010[5] (Table 19.6). However, the age group constituting the bulk of pediatric patients,

---

From the Department of Pediatrics, Medical College of Pennsylvania, Philadelphia, Pennsylvania. Presented in honor of Lewis A. Barness, MD, November 11, 1988.

TABLE 19.1. Distribution of pediatricians by age.

Age	Number	Percent
< 35	11,809[a]	21
35–44	10,017	38
45–54	5,573	21
55–64	3,811	14
65+	1,621	6
Total	26,704	100

Source: AMA, 1984.
[a]Totals exclude 6,127 residents who were assumed to be < 35 years old.

TABLE 19.2. Board certification status of pediatricians, 1983.

Certified by corresponding board only	17,524
Certified by corresponding board and other board	289
Certified by noncorresponding board	253
Not board-certified	14,765
Total	32,831

Source: AMA, 1984.

TABLE 19.3. General certificates issued by the American Board of Pediatrics.

1975	1,197
1977	1,110
1979	1,547
1981	1,659
1983	1,301
1984	1,606
Total	8,417

Source: American Board of Medical Specialties, 1985.

TABLE 19.4. Number of all physicians and pediatricians: Total, women, and foreign medical graduates ×1,000.

	All physicians			Pediatricians		
Year	Total	Women	Foreign medical graduates	Total	Women	Foreign medical graduates
1970	334 (100%)	25 (7.7%)	57 (17.1%)	18 (100%)	3 (20.8%)	3 (20.1%)
1983	519 (100%)	69 (13.4%)	112 (21.6%)	33 (100%)	10 (32.3%)	8 (26.3%)

Source: Roback, et al.[1]

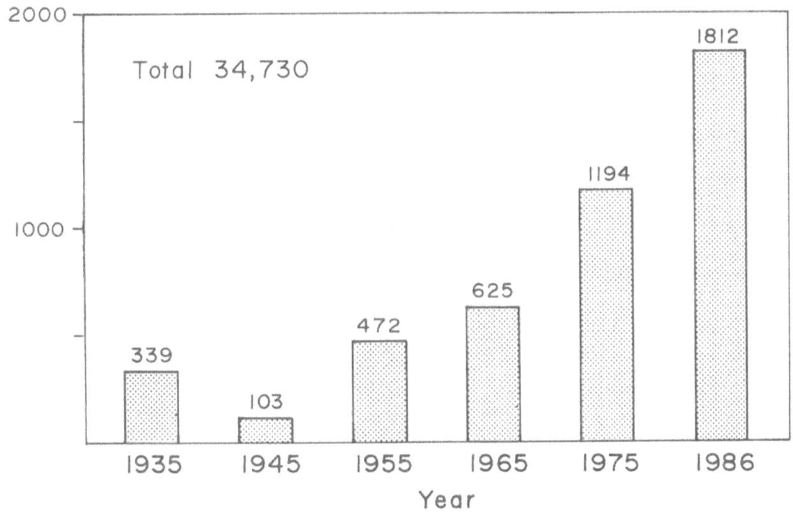

FIGURE 19.1. Numbers of pediatricians certified by ABP, by year. *Source*: ABP 1987.

0 to 4 years, will remain stable at about 18 million, or about 500 children in this age group per pediatrician. The age distribution[6] of the patients in the typical pediatric practice is shown in Figure 19.3. The large contribution of hospital service to care for infants under 1 year reflects the prominence of newborn care, the pediatrician's major inpatient activity. The figure also reveals the decreasing proportion of older children in a pediatric practice. It suggests the difficulty that pediatricians will encounter in attempting to replace the anticipated shortage of young children by acquiring more patients in the adolescent and young-adult group. Also, adolescents are the healthiest segment of the population and the least frequent users of physician services.

The source of medical care of children differs in urban and rural sites[7] (Table 19.7). Pediatricians predominate in urban areas, with 61% of office visits, but provide only one third of the child care in rural areas. This reflects the relative availability of pediatricians and family practitioners in communities of various

TABLE 19.5. Subspecialty certification.

Program	Year initiated	No. programs	No. certified
Cardiology	1961	44	775
Hematology-oncology	1974	47	730
Nephrology	1974	31	350
Neonat-perinatology	1975	102	1619
Endocrinology	1978	50	493
Pulmonology	1986	35	158
Critical care	1987	0	0

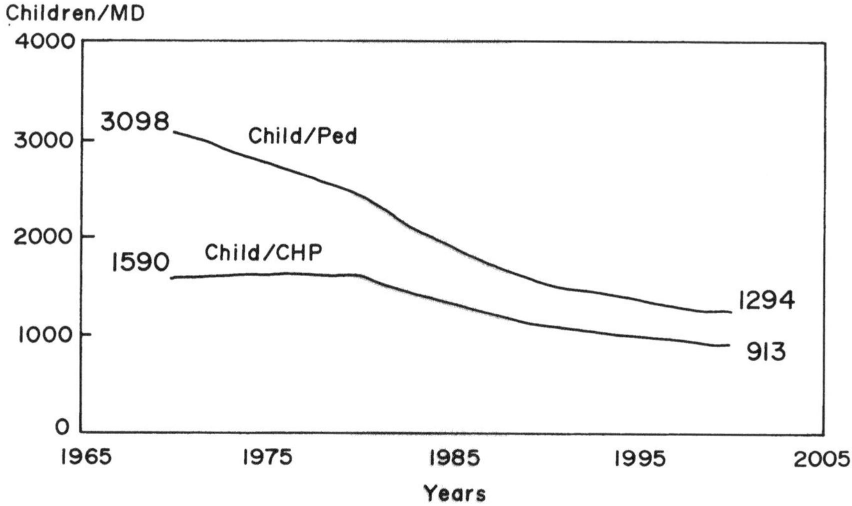

FIGURE 19.2. Physician/child ratios in U.S., by year. *Source*: AMA-AAP, 1986.

sizes[8] (Table 19.8). In 1970 and 1979, all communities with populations greater than 30,000 were staffed with general or family physicians and pediatricians. Almost all U.S. communities, even those with only 2,500 to 10,000 inhabitants, were well served by general or family practitioners. Pediatric presence was only 12% to 25% in communities of this size. Smaller towns and villages, which are relatively lacking in employment opportunities for spouses and in social, educational, and professional resources, may become more attractive to pediatricians as economically viable locations diminish in the future. A minor trend in this direction is seen in the increasing number of small communities served by pediatricians from 1970 to 1979.

In recent years there has been a tendency of physicians to leave solo practice for some form of group practice[4] (Table 19.9). Incentives fostering this change

TABLE 19.6. Actual and projected number of children 0–19 years old (in thousands) in the U.S., selected years 1970–2010.

	Years			
Age (years)	1970	1985	2000	2010
0–4	17,163	18,453	17,626	17,974
5–9	19,969	16,611	18,785	17,597
10–14	20,804	16,797	19,519	17,957
15–19	19,084	18,416	18,943	19,114
0–19	77,020	70,277	74,846	72,642

Source: U.S. Bureau of the Census, May 1984.

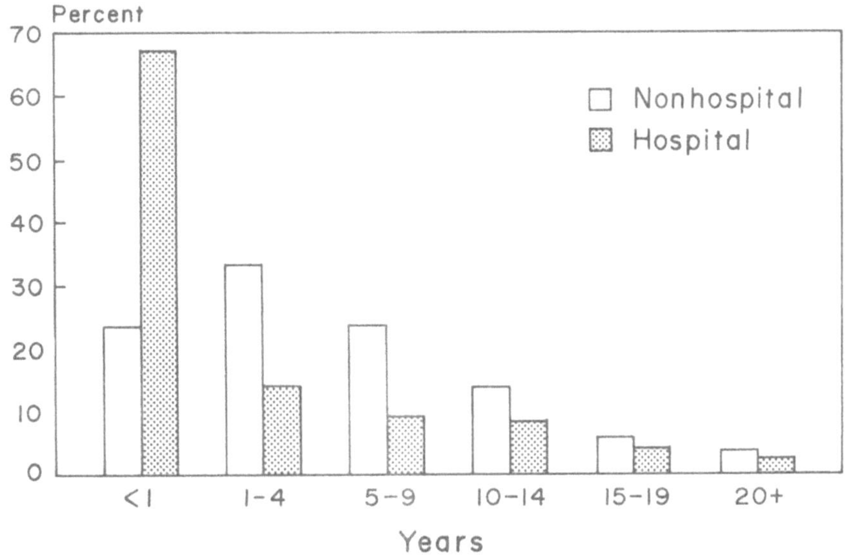

FIGURE 19.3. Hospital and nonhospital U.S. pediatric patients by age. *Source*: University of Southern California, 1978.

include economies of shared practice overhead, opportunities for scheduled time off, and the stimulation of working with professional colleagues. The percentage of pediatricians practicing in groups of two or more was 64% in 1983, an increase from about 56% in 1975. This is a marked change from the model before World War II, when solo practice was the norm.

Examination of the composition of modern pediatric practices reveals that pediatricians are engaged chiefly in primary care. Some have questioned the appropriateness of the primary-care role, advocating instead that of a consultant to other physicians and a supervisor of non-MD practitioners. The expected surplus of pediatricians suggests that economic necessity will determine that most will continue to practice in the primary-care mode. Ray Helfer has proposed that

TABLE 19.7. Percentage of office visits by patients less than 15 years of age, by physician specialty and area, 1980–81.

Specialist visited	Urban	Rural	All areas
Pediatrics	61.2%	33.8%	54.7%
General/family practice	16.8	48.9	24.5
Other	22.0	17.3	20.8
Total	100.0	100.0	100.0

Source: Reproduced from Hoekelman[7] by permission of *Pediatrics*, 74:460–477, copyright 1984.

TABLE 19.8. Percentage of communities with nonfederal pediatricians or general/family practitioners, 1970 and 1979.

	Community population				
	2,500–5,000	5,000–10,000	10,000–20,000	20,000–30,000	30,000+
Pediatrics					
1970	6%	17%	57%	92%	100%
1979	12	25	68	92	100
General/family practice					
1970	89	96	99	100	100
1979	86	96	99	100	100

Source: Reproduced from Newhouse et al,[8] *JAMA* 247:2392–2396. Copyright 1982, American Medical Association.

TABLE 19.9. Distribution of pediatricians and all physicians by size of practice, 1975 and 1983.[a]

Number of physicians in practice	All physicians		Pediatricians	
	1975	1983	1975	1983
1	54.2%	49.2%	44.3%	36.0%
2	14.1	12.5	14.2	16.4
3–4	15.0	15.9	22.7	24.4
5–7	6.3	8.5	5.4	8.9
8–25	6.0	8.8	5.4	5.3
26+	4.5	5.2	7.9	8.9
Total	100.0	100.0	100.0	100.0

Source: AMA, 1975, 1983.
[a] Excludes employee physicians.

TABLE 19.10. Major professional activities of pediatricians, 1983.

	Number	Percent
Total in patient care	28,019	91.4
Office-based	19,380	63.2
Residents	6,127	19.9
Hospital-based	2,512	8.2
Administration	857	2.8
Teaching	645	2.1
Research	1,015	3.3
Other	118	0.4
Total	30,654	100.0

Source: AMA, 1984.

TABLE 19.11. Distribution of pediatricians' patient encounters, by location and type of encounter, 1977.

Encounter location	Type of encounter				
	First	Episodic	Principal	Consultative	Specialized
Nonhospital	14.0%	3.5%	77.9%	2.2%	2.4%
Hospital	22.8	6.5	44.4	20.8	5.6
Total	15.5	4.0	72.3	5.3	3.0

Source: Pediatrics Practice Study Report.[6]

pediatricians might do well to stop apologizing for performing primary care and admit that facilitating the healthy growth and development of children and their families is "not a bad way to make a living."[9] Other professionals also spend a good part of their time in the less glamorous activities of their occupations. He further suggests that practitioners might gain considerable satisfaction from cultivating an interest in some subspecialty area of pediatrics.

Most pediatricians, about 91%, are engaged in patient care, two thirds are office-based, and 8% practice in hospitals[1] (Table 19.10). About 10% are divided about equally between administration, teaching, and research. Most office encounters are with regularly enrolled patients, and only about 2% are for consultations. The latter are a larger part of hospital activities, with many focused around care of newborns (Table 19.11). About 45% of hospital care is with regularly enrolled patients.[6]

The number and frequency of visits are greatest for children 4 years and under, about 63% (Table 19.12). Infants under 1 year are seen with an average frequency of 3.45. The relatively small contribution of children over 10 to pediatricians' practices is striking, with care of adolescents amounting to only about 4% of the total.[7]

Pediatricians see about the same number of patients per week as other physicians, but more in the office and fewer in hospitals[10] (Table 19.13). Both groups have experienced a decline in the volume of visits in the period 1975 to 1984. Pediatricians have registered a small gain in hospital visits over this time. The

TABLE 19.12. Annual number of visits to office-based pediatricians.

Patient age (years)	Average number visits/year	Percent of all visits
< 1	3.45	25.3
1–4	1.36	37.3
5–9	0.55	21.7
10–14	0.26	11.3
15–19	0.09	4.3
Total	0.60	99.9

Source: Hoekelman.[15] Copyright 1983, American Medical Association.

TABLE 19.13. Mean no. of patient visits per week, 1975 and 1984.

	All physicians			Pediatricians		
	1975	1984	Percent change	1975	1984	Percent change
Total visits	139.2	119.4	−14.2	140.2	126.5	− 9.8
Office visits	100.8	74.7	−25.9	123.9	94.9	−23.4
Hospital visits	32.6	28.1	−13.8	17.3	19.4	+12.1

Source: Reynolds and Duann.[10]

decline in physicians' activity is probably a consequence of the increase in the number of physicians.

Looking at pediatric practice time and its location from 1982 to 1984, a long work week of about 51 h and a falling off of patient volume are again apparent[10] (Table 19.14).

The variety of clinical situations dealt with by pediatricians is rather limited[5] (Table 19.15). The majority of problems seen in office practice involve young patients, are not complex, are dealt with in an average of about 11 min and include only a handful of categories. The short time spent with the individual office patient indicates that time-consuming hospital visits may not be cost-efficient, particularly for the solo practitioner. Routine examinations make up about 25% of the total; respiratory tract, pharyngeal, and ear infections, 35%; diarrhea and skin diseases, 5%; and all other problems, about 35%.

Hospital activities deal especially (about 20%), with care of the full-term or premature newborn infant[6] (Table 19.16). Management of pneumonia, meningitis, diarrhea, and diabetes mellitus together represents 11% of hospital effort. A variety of other conditions entail about 40% of hospital-based activity, suggesting a greater scope for application of medical knowledge than that required for office practice.

How does the hard-working pediatrician compare in earnings with his colleagues and those in some other activities? (Fig. 19.4). Pediatricians have increased their net income, before taxes, somewhat less than all physicians—from $34,800 in 1970 to $74,500 in 1985. Adjusting for inflation, they experi-

TABLE 19.14. Practice time and patient volume of pediatricians—mean (1982–1984).

	1982	1983	1984
Weeks practiced/year	47.1	47.3	47.4
Hours in patient care activity/week	51.3	51.0	50.7
Office hours/week	32.1	31.5	29.8
Hours on hospital rounds/week	8.5	8.4	7.4
Patient visits/week	134.9	134.7	126.5
Office visits/week	100.8	102.2	94.9
Visits on hospital rounds/week	23.6	24.0	19.4

Source: AMA, 1985.

TABLE 19.15. Leading primary problems presented to pediatricians by type of care, 1977 (nonhospital care).

Primary problem/diagnosis	Percent	Mean length of encounter (min)	Mean patient age (years)
Medical or special examination	25.5	13.0	3.3
Otitis media	10.8	9.4	3.7
Pneumonia, unspecified	6.1	10.9	3.1
Acute pharyngitis	5.8	9.4	7.5
Acute upper respiratory infection	4.3	10.0	7.0
Diarrheal disease	3.0	11.7	3.6
Chronic bronchitis	2.8	9.9	4.9
Acute tonsillitis	2.8	9.8	6.6
Eczema/dermatitis	1.6	8.8	6.6
Acute laryngitis/tracheitis	1.6	9.9	4.4
All other	35.7	–	–

Source: University of Southern California, 1978.

enced a fall in income of about 20%, again reflecting an increase in their number in contrast to a relatively stable child population.[10]

Income of pediatricians varies with practice location and age[10] (Table 19.17). An advantage of practicing in larger areas may be the higher income earned in metropolitan than in smaller communities. Earnings reach a peak in the age bracket 46 to 55 years and fall off sharply after age 65.

Pediatricians earn the least of all specialists, as my wife is well aware, although only slightly less than psychiatrists and family practitioners and about half or less as radiologists and some surgical subspecialists[11] (Fig. 19.5).

TABLE 19.16. Leading primary problems presented to pediatricians by type of care, 1977 (hospital care).

Primary problem/diagnosis	Percent	Mean length of encounter (min)	Mean patient age (years)
Medical or special examination	23.0	11.5	0.1
Single-born, w/o immaturity	11.8	12.9	0.0
Pneumonia, unspecified	4.1	13.3	2.9
Single-born, immature	3.8	15.2	0.0
Immaturity, unqualified	3.4	13.8	0.0
Anoxia/hypoxia	3.3	40.2	0.2
Diarrheal disease	3.1	12.9	5.2
Other conditions fetus/newborn	2.2	13.0	0.1
Diabetes mellitus	1.9	22.8	10.2
Meningitis	1.9	18.7	1.3
All other	41.6	–	–

Source: University of Southern California, 1978.

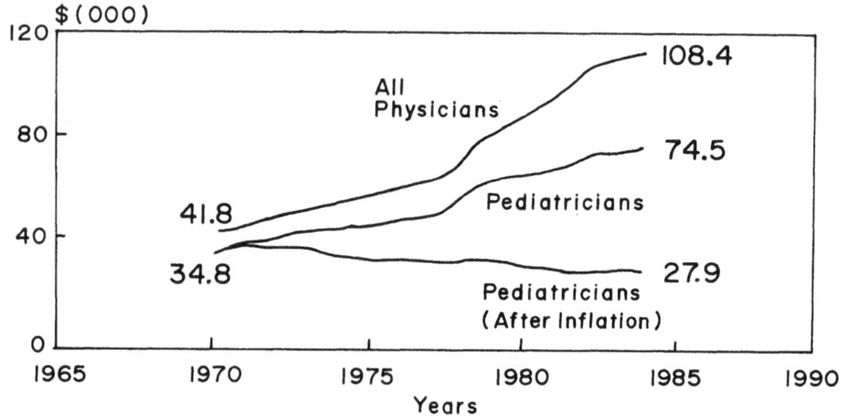

FIGURE 19.4. U.S. physicians' mean net income before taxes, 1970–1984. From *JAMA* 258:240–245. Copyright © 1987, American Medical Association.

Physicians have been criticized often for earning excessive incomes. This may be so in a minority of instances, but it has been pointed out that there are no $2.5 million fees in medicine like those charged by Ralph DeLorean's lawyers for saving him from a lifetime in jail. Further, doctors do not customarily ask a patient how much his life is worth to fix their fees before beginning treatment. Doctors as a group do have one of the highest annual pretax earnings[12] (Table 19.18). This is offset to some extent by their longest work week and most years of pre-practice educational preparation.

TABLE 19.17. Median pediatrician net income after expenses before taxes (in thousands of dollars), 1984.

All pediatricians	68.0
Type of practice	
Solo	67.5
Nonsolo	68.0
Location	
Nonmetropolitan	46.5
Metropolitan	
less than 1,000,000	70.5
1,000,000 and over	67.0
Physician age	
Less than 36 years	35.5
36–45 years	65.0
46–55 years	90.0
56–65 years	81.0
66 or more years	55.5

Source: AMA, 1985.

Neurosurgeons	Net $ 203,570
Orthopedic surgeons	$ 182,640
Plastic surgeons	$ 180,210
Thoracic surgeons	$ 156,480
Ophthalmologists	$ 148,000
Radiologists	$ 147,500
OBG specialists	$ 137,780
General surgeons	$ 122,370
Internists	$ 95,630
Psychiatrists	$ 86,670
FPs	$ 86,430
Pediatricians	$ 84,340
GPs	$ 72,840
All surgical specialists	$ 146,430
All non-surgical specialists	$ 106,460
All M.D.s	$ 112,790

FIGURE 19.5. U.S. Physicians' annual practice earnings by specialty. Copyright © 1987, Medical Economics Company Inc., Oradell, NJ 07649.

TABLE 19.18. Pretax earnings by profession.

	Income	Hours/week	$/hour	Years of education
Office-based MDs	$86,000	61	29	23
COs, small manuf.	96,000	50	40	17
Corp. attorneys	76,000	39	40	19
Cockpit crews	69,000	57	25	16
Private dentists	55,000	36	32	20
College professors	34,000	55	16	20
PhD chemists	33,000	45	15	21
Crane operators	33,000	40	16	12

Source: Medical Economics Company Inc., Oradell, NJ 07649, © 1983.

The sources of physicians' incomes reveal that pediatricians are at a disadvantage compared to other physicians[13] (Table 19.19). More of their patients have Medicaid as the payor, and twice as many are personally responsible for meeting their own bills. Medicaid, in Pennsylvania, reimburses the doctor $18 for an office visit, somewhat less than the usual charge. Pediatricians as a group have been commendably altruistic in accepting Medicaid patients, but it is understandable that some have limited the number for economic reasons. Parents of young children, the mainstay of pediatric practice, are often at the low end of their earnings potential and find it difficult to pay specialists' fees, especially when the services involved are often regarded as discretionary and attainable more cheaply from other physicians.

The prevalence in pediatric practice of well-child care and the unanticipated demand for behavioral interventions have led to some disenchantment with practice by physicians whose training had emphasized management of complex and life-threatening illnesses. This has stimulated a number of efforts, including those of the Task Force on Pediatric Education, the American Board of Pediatrics, and groups of pediatric educators, to modify residency training to make it more compatible with pediatric life.

Summaries of two recent conferences dealing with pediatric residency programs of the future will soon be published. One reports the deliberations of a

TABLE 19.19. Percentage of physicians' patients by type of principal payor, pediatricians and all physicians, 1983.

	All physicians	Pediatricians
Medicare	25.7	2.5
Medicaid	10.7	16.6
Blue Cross/Blue Shield	26.1	25.4
Prepayment plans	3.5	6.1
Other health plans	22.7	26.9
Payor not indicated	11.3	22.6

Source: AMA, 1983.

group of pediatric educators convened by the American Board of Pediatrics.[14] A proposal that appears to have merit is to establish three residency tracks for trainees with differing career goals: (1) a primary-care program emphasizing ambulatory activities with continuous supervision of a panel of patients, increased experience with community and school child health services, and psychosocial problems; (2) a program for hospital-based generalists who would function in a consultative role. Trainees would develop special competence in one or more subspeciality areas during a training period extended 1 or more years beyond the current 3-year residency; (3) a program for academic pediatricians, with a postresidency fellowship of 3 or more years, emphasizing research training in preparation for a productive investigative career. These proposals were not accepted by the conference participants, who supported continuing the present mode of residency training.

Some recent developments that have affected pediatric practice are likely to become increasingly significant in the future.

We are all familiar with the cost consciousness that has been directed at medicine in our country. This began in 1965 with the enactment of Medicare and Medicaid, making the federal government the largest purchaser of medical care. In the 1970s inflation pushed health care costs upward, abetted by a hospital reimbursement system based on costs and even charges. In 1960, total health care costs were $41 billion, rising to $458 billion in 1986, constituting 6% and then 10.9% of the gross national product.

It is not surprising that cost containment rather than quality or access to health care has become the major concern of the public, the government, insurance companies, hospitals, professional practice groups, and even academic medical centers.

The impact on child health services has been considerable. The Congressional Budget Office reports that the absolute dollar volume budgeted for Medicaid has not increased since 1975, while costs and the poverty ratio for children increased 38% from 1980 to 1985. A substantially greater portion of children are poor than any other age group. This is especially true of minorities, 48% for black and 40% for Hispanic children. As many as 25% of American children are uninsured for all or part of the year.

The current environment has generated DRGs, for-profit health care combines, HMOs, preferred provider organizations, and other responses to limit and redirect the flow of health care dollars, some of which go to private investors in for-profit health care facilities.

Indebtedness of medical trainees has influenced career choices away from primary care (a decrease in family medicine of 12%, pediatrics 18% and internal medicine 26%), to the more lucrative surgical specialities.[14]

The increase of malpractice suits has profoundly affected patient-doctor relationships and the style and cost of medical practice. In Philadelphia in 1948, the cost of malpractice insurance for pediatricians was $300 per year. Now it is more than $7,000 for those who do no invasive procedures and $17,000 for those performing such minor procedures as lumbar punctures.

Predictions of future physician surpluses have been challenged but appear to be valid.[14] Reduction in the numbers of medical students and residents in training is a likely outcome of this perception.

The problems we face are serious ones, but the practice of pediatrics with the purpose of assisting children and parents toward achievement of a healthy and productive life remains one of the most rewarding of all callings.

By focusing more on the health care needs of patients and less on the often conflicting interest of physicians, hospitals, corporate medicine, insurance companies, and government, we can alter the system in a direction characterized by quality, accessibility, and humaneness. All physicians should recall their assurances to medical school admissions committees that their choice of a medical career was based on their fascination with medical science and their desire to serve sick people. Pediatricians, who historically have the most concern for the physical, emotional, and socioeconomic conditions affecting their patients, are in the best position to lead this endeavor.

References

1. Roback G, Randolph L, Mead D, Pasko, T: *Physician Characteristics and Distribution in the U.S.*, 1984 Ed. Chicago: American Medical Association, 1985.
2. Brownlee RC: Personal communication.
3. American Board of Medical Specialties, 1985.
4. *The Future of Pediatrics.* Report of the American Medical Association Council on Long-Range Planning and Development in cooperation with the American Academy of Pediatrics.
5. U.S. Bureau of the Census, May 1984.
6. University of Southern California, Division of Research in Medical Education: *Pediatrics Practice Study Report.* Los Angeles: University of Southern California, 1978.
7. Hoekelman RA, Klein M, Strain JE: Who should provide primary health care to children: Pediatricians or family medicine physicians? *Pediatrics* 74:460–477, 1984.
8. Newhouse JP, Williams AP, Bennett BW, Schwartz WB: Where have all the doctors gone? *JAMA* 247:2392–2396, 1982.
9. Helfer RE: Primary care: Does it belong in pediatrics? *Am J Dis Child* 139:974–975, 1986.
10. Reynolds RA, Duann DJ: *Socioeconomic Characteristics of Medical Practice 1985.* Chicago: American Medical Association.
11. Owens A: *Medical Economics*, September 1987, p 219.
12. Owens A: *Medical Economics*, March 1983, pp 66–67.
13. American Medical Association: *Center for Health Policy Research*, annual core survey, 1983.
14. Cleveland WW, Brownlee RC: Future training of pediatricians: Summary report of a series of conferences sponsored by the American Board of Pediatrics. *Pediatrics* 80:451–457, 1987.
15. Hoekelman RA, Starfield B, McCormick C, DeChant H, Moynihan C, Radecki S, Mendenhall RC: A profile of pediatric practice in the United States. *Am J Dis Child* 137:1057–1060, 1983.

20
Pediatrics in Perspective

CHARLES C. LOBECK

Introduction

Assessments of the state of pediatrics have been frequent in recent years.[1-3] Most commentators see the discipline forced into new directions by its past successes, new problems, and societal demands, and are concerned by the immediate problems of the future. Few have analyzed the roles of pediatricians as they have changed or have recognized the growing behavior of pediatricians in contemporary society as major reformers of child health practices.

This paper addresses the several roles of the pediatrician and suggests that a dramatic change will occur in the functions that make up those roles. It also suggests that education for a career in pediatrics and the directions of pediatric research must change if pediatrics is to have a bright future.

Roles of a Pediatrician

It is evident, though not usually recognized, that pediatricians have roles other than that of personal caretaker of children. Every pediatrician is a reformer of child health practices and a public educator. Credibility and ability as a reformer and educator derive from both caretaker and scholar roles.

Scholarship is not only fundamental to function as a reformer and caretaker, but is also the basis for the creation of new knowledge through the process of research. At present, this is mostly the province of academic pediatricians. Thus, these three professional roles—caretaker, reformer, and scholar—are interdependent. The proportions of effort for each vary greatly between individuals, but all must be present for the pediatrician to have a complete professional identity. Administrative duties detract from or occasionally facilitate performance as educator, scholar, and caretaker, and indirectly have an impact on the time available for these roles.

From the Department of Pediatrics, University of Wisconsin School of Medicine, Madison, Wisconsin.
Presented in honor of Lewis A. Barness, MD, November 11, 1988.

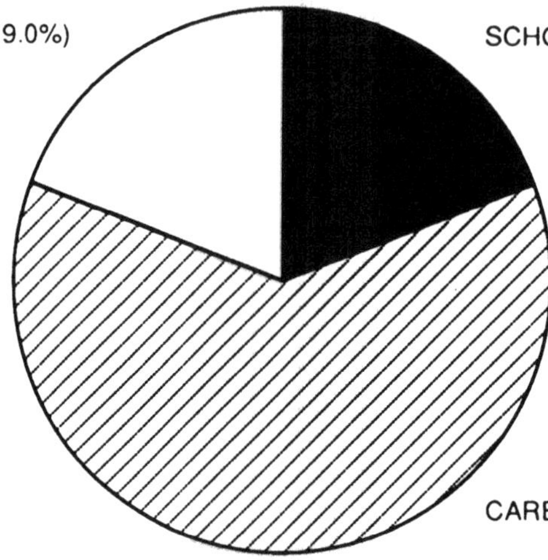

FIGURE 20.1. The functions of a pediatrician based on a 60-h professional work week. Times for reform and scholarly functions are shown at their maximum and may be reduced significantly by time required for administration and increase use of time for nonprofessional activities.

It is true that all physicians may have these characteristics, but they have been central to pediatricians for many decades. Pediatrics may be unique in that the proportions of these qualities in pediatric practice and academic pediatrics are less disparate than in other disciplines, and therefore there is less distinction between practice and the academy. Unfortunately, medical student education and graduate medical education in pediatrics focus almost completely on the caretaker function, truly the core mission of the pediatrician, but certainly not the only one.

Caretaker

Pediatrics has been a fast-growing specialty, but the number of pediatricians in practice will not grow as rapidly when the numbers of foreign-trained physicians admitted to practice in the United States are reduced.[1] The number of U.S. medical school graduates in pediatrics increased by 76% from 1970 to 1985, while the number of foreign medical graduates practicing pediatrics grew twice as fast. Still, the number of physicians practicing in the United States grew only 66% during this same period. The number of women practicing pediatrics more than doubled during this period so that in 1985, 35% of all pediatricians were women. Thus, it is clear that pediatrics is still an attractive discipline to medical students, particularly women.

Pediatric practice is almost never solo, and most pediatricians are members of corporate groups. Though much of practice is in the office, the proportion in non-

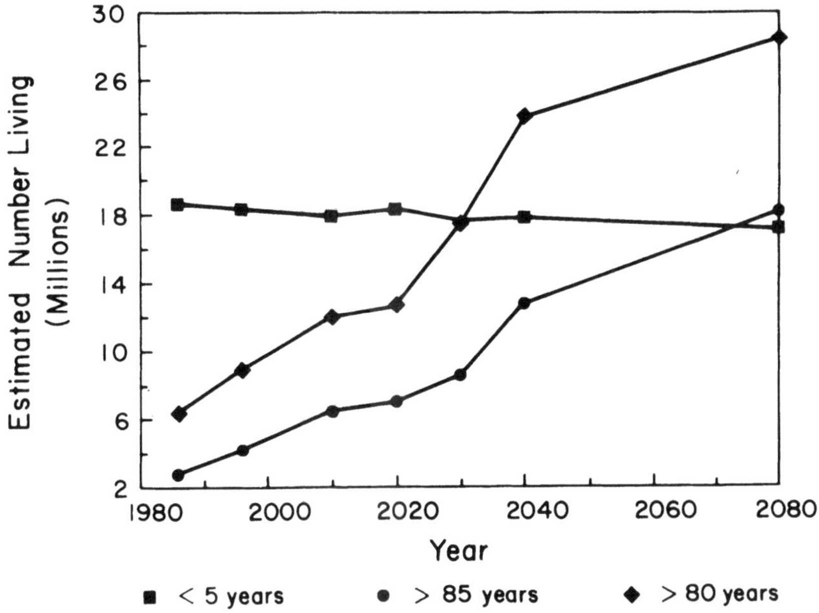

FIGURE 20.2. Estimate of number of children under 5 years during next 100 years compared to increase in the number of elderly.

traditional settings (schools, public clinics, etc) is growing. In the study by Wedum,[4] office hours were reduced, in the period from 1973 to 1984, from an average of 35 to about 30 h per week with about 7 h spent in the hospital. Thus, there was a decrease in total caretaker time per week. During this 10- year period, the time of a single office visit increased slightly, but the time required to make an appointment decreased dramatically from about 10 to 5 days, suggesting a lower demand for services.

Based on these data, Figure 20.1 shows the pediatric professional work week, assuming that about 60 h is spent in professional activity. The amount of time working on documentation, office management, and other administrative tasks cannot be estimated, but there still must be time available for other professional functions. Free time may also increase, but even this will not eliminate time available for professional activities outside of patient care.

The population of children in the United States is also undergoing change. Almost all estimates of population growth indicate that the number of children under 5 years will not increase, while the number of people over 80 and 85 years will increase dramatically (Fig. 20.2). The number of children in poverty has remained between 12 million and 13 million since 1981, while the number of aged in poverty has been slowly decreasing, from 3.8 million to 3.4 million during the same period.[5] A large increase in the poverty population of all ages has occurred among Hispanics, while the increase of poverty in blacks has not been as great. Most of this increase is in metropolitan areas. The 1974 prediction by Haggerty[6] that the new morbidities of children would be accidents, violent deaths by homicide and suicide, drug abuse, teen pregnancy, and increase in sexually transmitted diseases has become a reality.

These data suggest that the pediatrician will have a different role in the future and that the attractions to pediatrics have changed and will change further. The following are the most secure predictions of the future pediatric caretaker role:

1. There will be less time demanded of the pediatrician as a caretaker of children. The ratio of the number of pediatricians to the number of children will continue to increase.
2. More pediatricians will move into rural settings. There will continue to be a disparity between the location of pediatric services and that of large numbers of children in poverty, chiefly in urban areas, requiring those services. The care of these children will continue to be a major national problem without easy solution.
3. Income levels of pediatricians will not rise above increases due to inflation. Reimbursement for services per unit of primary care delivered may improve,[7] but the increase in number of pediatricians per child in the United States will reduce income potential.
4. At least 50% of pediatricians will be women.

These predictions require comment. The disparity between the location of children in need and the location of the pediatrician has no easy solution. It is much easier to predict that, as members of corporate groups, pediatricians will move to rural areas, providing competition with family physicians for the care of children. It is unlikely that without special inducements many pediatricians will practice in central urban areas. This leaves the care of children, particularly those in poverty in the inner cities, in question.

The aging of the population may draw more attention to the elderly than to children. Older Americans are politically active and instrumental in the development of policy concerning public health; children are not. Pediatrics must develop ways to appeal to the growing older segment of society. An active alliance of pediatrics and organized groups of older citizens could further child health in the United States.

The effect of the increased number of women in medicine, and particularly pediatrics, has not been sufficiently recognized in practice or academe.[8] A number of changes in the style of practice have already occurred that are at least partly due to the influence of women. The ethos of paternalistic professionalism has changed to one of cooperation. Much of this new, more sympathetic, informal style comes from the infusion of women into pediatrics. It is now more likely that families and physicians arrive at management decisions jointly. There is also less single-minded dedication to medicine by women and men. Acceptance of relatively less pay for more free time is becoming a reality. A major influence of women may be the increased role of the pediatrician as a social reformer.

Reformer

This function of a pediatrician is not widely understood by members of the profession. It is best described by example. Internationally recognized reformers are usually members of the academic community, but local examples of community pediatricians can be identified by the reader. A review by the author of the reformer role by pediatricians in Wisconsin revealed many who are active in this role. Two prominent pediatric reformers are illustrative: C. Henry Kempe (1922–1984), and Helen Taussig (1898–1986).

Henry Kempe, a well-known student of infectious disease, became increasingly concerned with high incidence of child abuse.[9] As chair of the program committee of the American Academy of Pediatrics in 1961, he organized a conference on the subject, and he and his co-workers produced the now famous book *The Battered Child*.[10] Largely through his efforts and those of his colleagues, including, not insignificantly, his wife, Ruth Kempe, national attention was drawn to the problem and frequency of child abuse. This problem is now in the differential diagnosis of suspicious signs or symptoms and is well recognized by the public. The result has been increased awareness by all segments of society of the prevalence of child abuse in the United States.

Helen Taussig, the founder of the specialty of pediatric cardiology and perhaps the most highly regarded woman physician of her age, teamed with Frances Kelsey in the successful effort to ban thalidomide from the American market.[11] She also testified repeatedly supporting the liberalization of abortion laws. Ironically, she was killed in an automobile accident in 1986 at the polling place where she had taken friends to be sure they voted in an election. The present concern of the public about the use of drugs in pregnancy is certainly an outgrowth of her social activism, as is the increased vigilance of the effect of drugs during pregnancy by the Food and Drug Administration.

Both of these famous pediatricians turned from their basic specialties to social reform. Though their stories are well known to pediatricians, the methods used in their reform efforts are not often considered. The processes used by both were similar and are used by other, less prominent pediatric reformers in local efforts. They are as follows:

1. The problem, usually one surrounded by emotion, is subjected to analysis. How is the injury or maladaptive behavior produced? Cause and effect are examined objectively in medical terms. This tends to make the problem medically understandable and strip it of some of its emotional content.
2. The etiology is identified and publicized. Publication of the etiological factors is usually made first to the profession but eventually must be made to the public. This requires social action on the part of the pediatrician and, in some cases, flamboyance.
3. The prevalence, usually much higher than suspected by the profession and the public, is publicized to both.

4. A system of management is devised, but prevention is recognized as being the only way to eradicate the problem.
5. Usually, after this sequence of events, the professional and public educational systems recognize the issue, and it is incorporated into the educational structure. Governmental action to facilitate prevention and management of the problem frequently results.

This process is not only the province of internationally recognized pediatric reform. Many practicing pediatricians and academicians have pursued these same efforts. Community pediatricians have reformed or begun the public reform of sports injuries, accidental injury, sexually transmitted disease, alcohol and drug abuse, teenage pregnancy, and many other problems. Pediatricians should be taught to recognize this as an important role for which they will have time in the future and one in which they can gain great satisfaction. The cornerstone of this reformer role is the scholar role, since it is central to objective examination of cause and effect.

Scholar

The scholar is a student. The method of scholars is scholarship—the discipline and use of techniques to learn about subjects in depth. This is not the exclusive process of the academic. The academic pediatrician uses the laboratory to do special scholarship—research. He or she is able to design experiments that test hypotheses and thus produce new knowledge. This form of scholarship is the farthest on the continuum from the caretaker role and the most difficult to incorporate into the role of the practicing pediatrician.

Pediatric research is the most successful form of clinical research. The conquering of acute infectious diseases of children is one of the happiest chapters in all biomedical scientific history. Obviously, more and more has become known about less and less. The remaining problems of children are for the most part chronic and extend into later life.

Fries and his colleagues[12] have stated an ideal for the human life span simply, in the rectangular curve of mortality shown in Figure 20.3. As this ideal is approached in the developed world, the goal of medicine becomes, more clearly, the maintenance of low mortality and reduction of morbidity until the end of the span. The ideal cannot be achieved without reduction of morbidity and mortality due to social causes and prevention or management of chronic disease produced during childhood. This objective view of the life span suggests that pediatric research should concern itself more with later life.

Indeed, the process of degeneration may be as orderly as that of development. The factors that drive it are unknown but may have their origins in childhood. Pediatric research must address these questions. Study of the effect of infant and child nutrition on the production of cardiovascular disease later in life is an example of this kind of research already under way.[13] Attempts have been made to assess the impact of pulmonary events in early life on the later development of

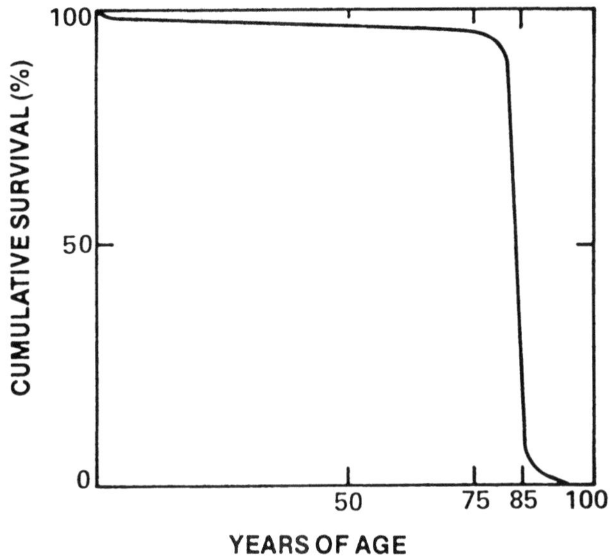

FIGURE 20.3. The rectangular survival curve assumes minimum mortality during life span until average age of 85 years.

chronic lung disease and reduced lung function.[14] The expression of genetic effects in later life must also be explored.[15] All of these studies and others should be recognized as the new frontiers of pediatric research.

Diseases of children are increasingly chronic and extend beyond childhood. Development of methods of prevention becomes as important as cures in many of these problems. These diseases, coupled with social problems, now described as "new morbidity," require objective analysis and research. Pediatric research and scholarship should be increasingly applied to these issues. The techniques of biostatistics and epidemiology are central to this kind of research.

While much of this effort will occur in academic pediatrics, research by the practicing pediatrician can be productive and rewarding, particularly with the growing number of problems amenable to social reform. The practicing pediatrician, by virtue of access to populations, should be able to study the effectiveness of preventive measures and novel forms of management better than the academician, if the time is clearly set aside for this purpose.

Summary

Pediatrics will change more dramatically in the next decade than in any time in the past. The attractiveness of the profession is high, particularly to increasing numbers of women. There will be much more time for the pediatrician to spend in the rewarding roles of public reformer and scholar and less time as a caretaker of children. The role as reformer may become one of the more attractive aspects of the discipline, particularly to women.

A problem of national magnitude will be the increasing disparity between the locations of pediatricians and the large number of children in poverty. Pediatricians are already beginning to move to rural areas, and some may even enter international child care. Both locations appear to be more attractive than practice in the inner city.

The population of the aged will grow much faster than that of children. This will increase the need for pediatricians to recognize the political impact of the aged.

The reformer role of the pediatrician is an important, often unrecognized function of the pediatrician. It rests on the objective analysis of the growing number of social issues affecting children and the publicizing of the causes and effects of these problems. Many practicing pediatricians function effectively as reformers.

Scholarship is central to all roles played by the pediatrician. Pediatric research, a special kind of scholarship, will increasingly turn its attention to the prevention and amelioration of the problems of later life.

Conclusions

1. National programs to induce corporate medicine to establish care facilities for poor children in urban areas will be required to put pediatricians in contact with these populations.
2. Pediatrics should enlist the support of the growing politically active, elderly population by demonstrating the importance of control of child health problems to the health of older people.
3. Formal medical student and resident education should emphasize the other noncaretaker functions of the pediatrician, those of reformer and scholar, and inform the student of the changes in pediatric practice that can be securely predicted for the future.
4. Pediatric research should recognize the importance of its research effort to the maintenance of health in later life. The support of the growing older segment of the population should be an important stimulus to this effort.
5. Practicing pediatricians will be in an excellent position to perform the studies required of the growing social issues in child health. The recognition of this scholarly role and acquisition of the research techniques necessary to produce solutions to these problems can make the practice of pediatrics more rewarding.

References

1. Council on Long Range Planning and Development, American Medical Association: The future of pediatrics. Implications of the changing environment of medicine. *JAMA* 258:240–245, 1987.

2. Garfunkel JM: The pediatrician of the future. *J Pediatr* 107:911, 1985.
3. Nadler HL, Evans WJ: The future of pediatrics. *Am J Dis Child* 141:21–27, 1987.
4. Wedum E: Trends in physicians services. Johns Hopkins School of Hygiene and Public Health 1986. In: *Conference Proceedings. The Medical Profession: Enduring Values and New Challenges*. Chicago: American Medical Association, 1988, pp 53–55.
5. U.S. Bureau of the Census, Current Population Reports, Series P-60, No. 161: *Money Income and Poverty Status in the United States: 1987* (Advance Data from the March 1988 Current Population Survey). Washington: U.S. Government Printing Office, 1988, pp 713–717.
6. Haggerty RJ: The changing role of the pediatrician in child health care. *Am J Dis Child* 127:545–549, 1974.
7. Hsiao WC, Braun P, Dunn D, et al: Resource-based relative values, an overview. *JAMA* 260:2347–2353, 1988.
8. Morantz-Sanchez RM: *Sympathy and Science, Women Physicians in American Medicine*. New York: Oxford University Press, 1985.
9. Kempe CH, Silverman FN, Steele BF, et al: The battered child syndrome. *JAMA* 181:17–24, 1962.
10. Helfer RE, Kempe CH (eds): *The Battered Child*. Chicago: University of Chicago Press, 1968.
11. Nuland SB: *Doctors, The Biography of Medicine*. New York: Alfred A. Knopf, 1988, pp 422–456.
12. Fries JF, Crapo LM: *Vitality and Aging, Implications of the Rectangular Curve*. San Francisco: W.H. Freeman, 1981.
13. Cardiovascular risk factors from birth to 7 years of age: The Bogalusa Heart Study. *Pediatrics* 80(5) Part 2:767–816, 1987.
14. Burrows B, Taussig LM: As the twig is bent, the tree inclines: Perhaps. (Editorial.) *Am Rev Respir Dis* 122(6):813–816, 1980.
15. Childs B, Scriver CR: Age at onset and causes of disease. *Perspect Biol Med* 29:437–460, 1986.

21 Diagnostic Process in Hospitalized Pediatric Patients

BARBARA E. STRASSBERG, CELESTE M. MADDEN, FRANK A. OSKI

Introduction

Although much emphasis is placed on the need to establish a diagnosis, both in undergraduate and graduate education, very little information is present in the medical literature concerning the outcome of the diagnostic process, particularly among a group of consecutive hospital admissions.

How many patients are, in fact, admitted with a previously established diagnosis? How many patients are correctly diagnosed at the time of admission or during the hospital stay? What percent of patients are discharged from the hospital without a diagnosis or with an incorrect diagnosis? What contributes to the failure to establish a precise diagnosis?

In an effort to answer some of these questions and provide results for others to use as a basis for comparison, we reviewed our experience with a group of pediatric hospital admissions.

Methods

Study Population

The Upstate Medical Center (UMC) is located in Syracuse, New York, in Onondaga County (population 480,000). The Pediatric Department is based in two adjoining hospitals: the State University Hospital and the Crouse-Irving Memorial Hospital, with a total of 75 inpatient beds. There are only three hospitals in the county with inpatient pediatric services, with approximately 90% of all pediatric medical admissions being admitted to the Pediatric Service of UMC. The UMC also serves as a referral hospital for a 17-county region with a popula-

---

From the Department of Pediatrics, State University of New York, Upstate Medical Center, Syracuse, New York. Dr. Strassberg is currently in the Bronx, New York City. Dr. Oski is currently at the Johns Hopkins University School of Medicine, Baltimore.
Presented by Dr Frank A. Oski in honor of Lewis A. Barness, MD, November 12, 1988.

TABLE 21.1. Classification instrument.

- I. Patients discharged with a diagnosis
  - A. Diagnosis established prior to admission
    - 1. Correct
      - a) Complication
      - b) Maintenance
    - 2. Incorrect
  - B. Diagnosis at time of admission
    - 1. Correct
      - a) Presumed
        - i) Investigation attempted
        - ii) No investigation attempted
        - iii) Investigation attempted without completion
      - b) Specific cause identified
    - 2. Incorrect
  - C. Diagnosis made during the hospital stay
    - 1. Correct
      - a) Presumed
        - i) Investigation attempted
        - ii) No investigation attempted
        - iii) Investigation attempted without completion
      - b) Specific cause identified
    - 2. Incorrect
- II. Patients discharged without a diagnosis
  - A. Delayed diagnosis
  - B. Never diagnosed

tion of 2.2 million. Thus, UMC admissions provide a representative cross section in which to assess the diagnostic process.

In choosing the sample population for this study, pediatric medical admissions only, during a 1-year period were considered. Within each of the seasons a month was arbitrarily selected in an effort to provide a more representative sample of the various disease processes. These four months were August 1979, October 1979, January 1980, and May 1980.

Materials

A classification system was constructed and is presented in Table 21.1. Basically, the instrument divides all cases into two major categories depending on whether the patient was discharged with or without a diagnosis (categories I and II, respectively). As can be seen, category I (patients discharged with a diagnosis) is further divided into cases in which a diagnosis was established prior to admission (IA), cases diagnosed at admission (IB), and cases diagnosed during the course of the hospital stay (IC). For purposes of this study, the category of previously established diagnosis is restricted to established chronic disease states. Diagnosis at time of admission includes all diagnoses considered in the

TABLE 21.2. Representative examples of classification into categories IA and IB.

Patient	Classification	
4–4/12-year-old black male with known sickle cell disease admitted in sickle cell crisis	IA1a	(complication of a previously established chronic disease)
5–10/12-year-old white male with known ALL admitted for maintenance chemotherapy	IA1b	(maintenance care of a previously established chronic disease)
10–5/12-year-old white male with aortic stenosis demonstrated by prior catherization admitted for recatherization in anticipation of corrective surgery	IA1b	(maintenance care of a previously established chronic disease)
19-month-old black male with presumed ventricular septal defect by history and physical exam admitted for cardiac catherization to confirm diagnosis	IB1	(patient discharged with correct diagnosis which was made at time of admission)
2–6/12-year-old white male with history of easy bruisability and abnormal peripheral smear admitted through hematology clinic for confirmation of presumptive diagnosis of ALL by bone marrow aspiration and initial chemotherapy	IB1b	(patient discharged with correct diagnosis which was made at time of admission – specific cause identified)

physician's office and for which the patient was admitted, as well as those diagnoses made in the emergency room or in the initial admission note. Table 21.2 gives representative examples of the way we classified cases into categories IA and IB.

Within the categories, further classification was performed. Diagnoses were classified into those in which a specific diagnosis was established as contrasted with those in which the etiology was "presumed." For example, when a patient was admitted with a pulmonary infiltrate and when cultures obtained from either blood or lung resulted in the isolation of a bacterial organism, and appropriate antibiotic therapy produced a therapeutic response, the patient was classified in the category of specific disease established. In contrast, when a child was admitted with croup or bronchiolitis and improved without antibiotic therapy, the etiology of the illness was "presumed" to be of viral origin.

The thoroughness of the diagnostic process in patients with "presumed" etiologies was also reviewed. Complete evaluation was defined as a rigorous attempt to identify the responsible agent. Most specifically this would require evidence of attempts at viral isolation or requests for pre- and post-convalescent antiviral antibody titers. No attempt at diagnosis includes those instances in which efforts were solely directed at the exclusion of bacterial diseases although a viral etiology for the illness was seriously considered by the physicians.

The available inpatient hospital charts for the given months were reviewed by two of the investigators. One (C.M.) had a knowledge of the diagnostic thinking behind each admission, having been chief resident for the sampled period. UMC uses a problem-oriented record. Classification category was decided on by review of the house officers' and attending physicians' admission problem list, assessments, and orders to assure that assessment paralleled actual thinking as illustrated by laboratory tests and procedures chosen. Accuracy of diagnosis was determined by reviewing the entire inpatient chart to reveal any changes in thinking, laboratory results, or clinical findings in support of or against the original diagnosis or a diagnosis made during the hospital stay.

Categories were also compared by length of stay in an attempt to ascertain if a relationship existed between time of diagnosis and length of hospital stay.

In addition, all subcategories were analyzed by body system involved in an effort to better understand the types of illnesses that tended to be specifically diagnosed, "presumed," or not diagnosed. The body system classification was chosen because it is consistent with the United States Department of Health model.[1]

Results

The four months chosen for this study yielded a total sample size of 543 for whom 450 (82.8%) of the in-hospital charts were available and suitable for review. An additional eight charts were not used because these patients were admitted for purely social reasons. Thus, the final sample size for this study was 442.

As seen in Table 21.3, 408 (92.3%) of the 442 patients were discharged with a correct diagnosis while 33 (7.5%) were discharged without a diagnosis, and one patient (0.2%) was discharged with a diagnosis that ultimately proved to be incorrect.

Of the 408 patients discharged with a correct diagnosis, 119 (29.2%) had a previously established diagnosis, 164 (40.2%) had a diagnosis made at time of admission, and 125 (30.6%) had a diagnosis made during the hospital stay.

Eight (24.2%) of the 33 patients discharged without a diagnosis were subsequently diagnosed on the basis of laboratory results received after discharge for tests performed during the hospital stay. Thus, a total of 416 patients or 94.1% of our sample were ultimately correctly diagnosed on the basis of history, physical examination, laboratory tests, or procedure performed during the sampled hospital period.

A total of 159 patients were admitted without a previously established diagnosis or a diagnosis made at the time of admission. Of this group of 159, 25 patients, or 15.7%, were never diagnosed.

It can be noted in Table 21.3 that 18 (3 in category IA and 15 in category IB), or 4.4%, of the 409 diagnosed patients were discharged with a correct diagnosis following a misdiagnosis on admission.

Of the 147 patients discharged with a "presumed" diagnosis, 30 (20.4%) had a complete but inconclusive investigation attempted, 80(55.4%) had no investigation or only bacterial cultures attempted, and 37 (25.2%) had an incomplete investigation attempted. In 22 of the 37 patients (59.5%) with an incomplete

TABLE 21.3. Diagnostic subclassification of pediatric admissions (N = 442).

I. Patients discharged with a diagnosis	409						
A. Diagnosis established prior to admission		119					
1. Correct			116				
a. Complication				65			
b. Maintenance				51			
2. Incorrect			3				
B. Diagnosis at time of admission		164					
1. Correct			149				
a. Presumed				70			
i. Investigation attempted					18		
ii. No investigation attempted					30		
iii. Investigation attempted, without completion					22		
b. Specific cause identified				55			
c. No further subclassification				24[a]			
2. Incorrect			15				
						b	c
C. Diagnosis made during hospital stay		126					
1. Correct			125				
a. Presumed				77			
i. Investigation attempted					12		
ii. No investigation attempted					50		
iii. Investigation attempted, without completion					15		
b. Specific cause identified				48			
2. Incorrect			1				
II. Patients discharged without a diagnosis	33						
A. Delayed diagnosis		8					
B. Never diagnosed		25					

[a] Of these 24, 18 and first catheterizations, 3 are first diagnosis of asthma, 3 are drug ingestions for which no laboratory tests were available.
[b] Total presumed, 147; total investigation attempted, 30; total no investigation attempted, 80; total incomplete investigation attempted, 37.
[c] Total ultimately correctly diagnosed, 416.

investigation, investigation was considered incomplete as a result of the fact that only an acute viral titer sample was drawn.

As seen in Table 21.4, patients for whom a diagnosis was not made by the time of discharge had a significantly longer mean stay than when a diagnosis was made by discharge. The wide range of stays should also be considered when interpreting these data.

Table 21.5 illustrates classification of cases by body system within each diagnostic category. As seen in Table 21.5, 130 (88.4%) of the 147 patients categorized as having a "presumed" diagnosis had an apparent infectious disease, and 46 of 103 (44.6%) having a specific diagnosis had an infectious disease. None of the 19 incorrect diagnoses were of infectious origin.

TABLE 21.4. Length of hospital stay by diagnostic category (N = 442).

Category		N	Range (in days)	Mean (in days)				
I. Patients discharged with a diagnosis		409	1–40			4.4		
Diagnosis previously established	IA1a	65	1–40	5.7	4.9			
	IA1b	51	1–34	3.9			4.8	
	IA2	3	2	2.0				
Diagnosis at admission	IB1	24	1–5	2.0				
	IB1ai	18	2–22	5.9				
	IB1aii	30	1–9	2.8	4.0	4.7	4.6	4.4
	IB1aiii	22	2–14	3.9				
	IB1b	55	1–21	6.9				
	IB2	15	2–10	2.7				
Diagnosis made during the hospital stay	IC1ai	12	1–13	4.2				
	IC1aii	50	1–6	3.2	3.5	4.2	4.2	
	IC1aiii	15	2–9	3.9				
	IC1b	48	1–17	5.3				
	IC2	1	1	1.0				
II. Patients discharged without a diagnosis		33	1–169			14.4		
Delayed diagnosis	IIA	8	2–21	6.0				
								14.4
Never diagnosed	IIB	25	1–169	17.0				

Discussion

Our study suggests that, in a university hospital pediatric service, slightly more than 9 of every 10 patients are discharged with a correct diagnosis. Approximately 3 of every 10 patients are admitted with a previously established diagnosis. In an additional 4 of every 10 patients the diagnosis is readily apparent at the time of admission. When a diagnosis has not been made at the time of admission, approximately 15% of patients will be discharged without a correct diagnosis ever having been established.

Unfortunately, very few data are available in the literature that can be used to serve as a basis for comparison. Bongiovanni,[2] in an attempt to describe pediatric medicine in the United States, used Blue Cross reimbursement data collected in Philadelphia and the southeastern Pennsylvania area based on pediatric inpatient populations. He found that 37% of the children in community hospitals and 14% of children in two large children's hospitals were undiagnosed at the time of discharge. He speculated that this difference in percentage of undiagnosed or "not defined" cases represented failures of diagnosis and was therefore greater in general hospitals than in specialized children's hospitals.

Wexler and co-workers[3] found that 8.2% of pediatric admissions did not have a clearly established diagnosis at the time of admission. They demonstrated that

TABLE 21.5. Classification of cases by body system within diagnostic category (N = 442).

Classification category		Body system												Infections									
		Respiratory	Cardiovascular	GI	GU	Neuromuscular	Heme/onc	Endocrine	Psychiatric	Congenital	Ingestion	Trauma	FTT	Other	Respiratory	Cardiovascular	GI	GU	CNS	Sepsis	Viral syndrome	Soft tissue	Parasitic	Total
I.	Patients discharged with a diagnosis																							
IA1a.	Complication of a correct diagnosis established prior to admission	26	4	6	1	13	10	2	1	2	–	–	–	–	–	–	–	–	–	–	–	–	–	65
IA1b.	Maintenance care of a correct diagnosis established prior to admission	–	22	2	1	–	24	1	–	1	–	–	–	–	–	–	–	–	–	–	–	–	–	51
IA2.	Incorrect diagnosis made prior to admission	–	3	–	–	–	–	–	–	–	–	–	–	–	–	–	–	–	–	–	–	–	–	3
IB1.	Correct diagnosis made at time of admission	3	18	–	–	–	–	–	–	–	–	–	–	3	–	–	–	–	–	–	–	–	–	24
IB1a.	Correct presumed diagnosis made at time of admission	–	2	–	–	–	1	–	–	–	1	–	–	2	40	–	4	–	10	–	–	10	–	70
IB1b.	Correct specific diagnosis made at time of admission	–	–	2	–	3	2	1	–	–	12	4	–	–	6	–	1	2	10	4	–	7	1	55
IB2.	Incorrect diagnosis made at time of admission	–	12	–	2	1	–	–	–	–	–	–	–	–	–	–	–	–	–	–	–	–	–	15
IC1a.	Correct presumed diagnosis made during course of hospital stay	–	–	2	–	4	1	–	–	–	–	–	–	4	16	–	17	–	2	–	31	–	–	77
IC1b.	Correct specific diagnosis made during course of hospital stay	–	2	8	1	9	2	–	–	–	–	–	7	4	5	–	–	2	2	2	–	4	–	48
IC2.	Incorrect diagnosis made during course of hospital stay	–	–	–	–	1	–	–	–	–	–	–	–	–	–	–	–	–	–	–	–	–	–	1
II.	Patients discharged without a diagnosis																							
IIA.	Delayed diagnosis	–	3	–	–	1	1	–	–	–	–	–	–	1	2	–	–	–	–	–	–	–	–	8
IIB.	Diagnosis never made	1	2	7	–	6	1	–	–	–	–	–	–	8	–	–	–	–	–	–	–	–	–	25
Total		30	68	27	5	38	42	4	1	3	13	4	7	22	69		22	4	24	6	31	21	1	442

diagnosis is delayed when the physician does not include the correct diagnosis among the initial considerations, a finding our study corroborates.

We found that a large number of patients with "presumed" diagnoses showed a lack of thoroughness of attempts to prove this diagnosis. As noted in Results, 88.4% of the presumed diagnoses were of infectious processes, and a large majority were believed to be of viral etiology. In many instances viral isolations were not attempted. In others, either the acute or convalescent serum was not obtained in order to make a retrospective serologic diagnosis of a viral infection. These data may reflect the limitations of our own hospital's viral diagnostic capabilities. They also reflect, in part, the fact that physicians made little attempt to diagnose specific viral illnesses for which no therapy is available and the disease is believed to be self-limited. This widely held impression appears to be confirmed by our findings.

Although our classification scheme is arbitrary, it has provided insights into the nature of the diagnostic process in hospitalized pediatric patients and highlights the need for improved viral laboratory services if more precise diagnoses are desired. We hope this analysis will stimulate others to review their experience. In view of the effort and attention directed to diagnosis, it seems only appropriate that the success of the process should be periodically evaluated.

References

1. USDHEW: *Health United States, 1978*. Publication No. (PHS) 78-1232, Dec. 1978, pp 48–65.
2. Bongiovanni AM: Hospitalization of children in the United States. *Mod Prob Pediatr* 9:113, 1965.
3. Wexler JR, Swender PT, Tunnessen WW, Oski FA: Impact of a system of computer-assisted diagnosis. *Am J Dis Child* 129:203, 1975.

22
The Pediatric Diagnostic Referral Service: Filling in the Subspecialty Cracks

WALTER W. TUNNESSEN, JR.

In a large academic tertiary-care center with scores of pediatric specialists and subspecialists, it is hard to imagine that there is not a "consultant" available to receive all patients referred for evaluation. Many centers, large and small, have a few clinically oriented or interested physicians who are willing to see patients referred with problems not clearly related to one organ system or specialty area. Some centers have long-established mechanisms for referrals and consultations, utilizing hospital-based generalists who are heavily involved in both the inpatient and outpatient services.[1] In other centers ambulatory pediatric faculty assist resident physicians who see patients referred by other physicians or self-referred by parents seeking a second opinion. Not uncommonly children are seen by subspecialists in a "best of fit" mode, hoping that the problem corresponds to their area of expertise. If the problem does not appear to be in the realm of the subspecialist, the patient may be referred to another subspecialist or simply returned to the referring physician.

A Pediatric Referral Office was recently reorganized at Johns Hopkins Hospital to coordinate consultative services for physicians and parents inquiring about entry into the system. Calls from physicians and parents unfamiliar with the hospital's services and the specialists offering them are channeled through this office. Not all referred problems are clearly in the dominion of pediatric subspecialists. The problems may be vague or the symptoms may overlap in the arenas of a number of specialists. For these reasons the Pediatric Diagnostic Referral Service (PDRS) was established, to tackle the ill-defined problems or complaints, or to offer second opinions to parents wishing to use the tertiary center for reassurance.

What kind of problems are seen by a diagnostic referral service? What are the characteristics of the patients seen? How does the service function in a land of subspecialists? The information to be reported was accumulated from a review of records of the first 150 patients seen by the PDRS.

From the Department of Pediatrics, Johns Hopkins University School of Medicine, Baltimore, Maryland.
Presented in honor of Lewis A. Barness, MD, November 11, 1988.

Background and Methods

The PDRS at Johns Hopkins Hospital was established in October 1986. Patients were initially referred by word of mouth primarily via faculty and house staff. Eventually information about the service was included in mailings to area physicians and in a brochure which provided a description of the service and the appropriate telephone numbers to contact. The multitude of calls the Children's Center receives each day with questions about services and referrals are coordinated with the Pediatric Referral Office. The PDRS complements the activities of this office.

Most of the PDRS referral calls or inquiries by parents are forwarded to the director of the service, who personally contacts the caller. If the suspected problem seems to fit best in the arena of a particular clinical specialist, the caller is referred to that specialist. If the problem seems to be best served by the PDRS, an appointment is made. Most appointments are allotted 1½-h time period, although some patients require more time and some less time. The patients are seen in the specialty clinic, an area housing 17 examining rooms utilized by various subspecialists and supported by appropriate secretarial and nursing help. Initially the patients were seen by the director of the service alone. As the clinical activities of the service grew, assistant and senior assistant residents elected 1-month blocks of time in the PDRS, seeing patients with the director and accompanying him in his other clinical duties.

Physicians who refer patients for consultation receive a complete written report outlining the history and physical examination, discussing the likely possibilities for the problem, and suggesting a course of investigation and management. Patients who are seen on a self-referred basis are asked to provide the name of their primary care giver, and, with the parent's permission, a report is sent to the identified physician. The PDRS does not function as a primary care giver.

Data Review

Calls to the Pediatric Referral Office were recorded for an 8-week period during August and September 1988. An average of 63 calls per week were received. Almost 80% of the calls were for general information and did not entail patient referrals. Only 14 of the inquiries during the 8-week period were received from physicians. A total of 117 referrals were made by this office to 26 different specialty clinics during this period. The five specialty clinics most frequently referred to were cardiology (17), neurology (15), PDRS (9), dermatology (9), and gastroenterology (9).

Of the 150 patients seen by the PDRS (Table 22.1), 67 (45%) were referred by physicians, primarily pediatricians and family physicians, and 83 (55%) were parent referrals. Patients ranged in age from 1 month to 18 years. More than half the patients (56%) were less than 6 years of age, and 30% were less than 2 years of age. All but 28 patients were from Maryland.

Only 14 (9%) patients were seen for revisits, half of them once, 4 twice, and 3 for three or more times. Eight admissions resulted from the PDRS visits. Three

TABLE 22.1. Initial 150 patients seen by the diagnostic referral service.

Pattern of referral
67 (45%) physician-referred
83 (55%) parent-referred
Age
< 6 years–56%
< 2 years–30%
Range: 1 month to 18 years

children were admitted for more extensive evaluation of poor growth, and one each for Kawasaki disease, surgery for a retroperitoneal abscess, removal of a chest wall mass, rehydration for vomiting secondary to a somatization disorder, and the last for an in-depth evaluation of recurrent infections.

Consultations from or referrals to subspecialists were requested on 26 (17%) of the 150 patients. Four patients were referred for psychiatric, 4 for ophthalmolgic, and 4 for allergic evaluations. Two children each were referred for orthopedic, endocrinologic, pediatric surgical, genetic, and gastrointestinal evaluations.

Children Referred by Physicians

Sixty-seven children were referred to the PDRS by physicians (Table 22.2). Fifteen (22%) of these children had short stature and/or poor weight gain as the presenting complaint, and in seven of these children no cause for the problem has yet been identified. Some may represent genetic or constitutional delays in growth and adolescent development. None appeared acutely or chronically ill. In 4 of the 15 children a diagnosis of psychosocial "failure to thrive" was made. One child represented a normal shift in linear growth occurring during the first 15 months of life, and in another child the referring physician's suspicion of renal tubular acidosis was confirmed.

TABLE 22.2. Complaints and diagnoses of 67 physician-referred children.

Complaint	Diagnostic summary
Short stature/poor weight gain (N=15)	No Dx (N=7)
	Psychosocial (N=4)
Fever: recurrent/unknown origin (N=6)	No Dx (N=4)
Multiple complaints (N=6)	Somatization (N=4)
Recurrent infections (N=4)	Allergies (N=3)
Recurrent leg pain (N=3)	
Lymphadenopathy (N=2)	Normal (N=2)
Abdominal pain (N=2)	
Miscellaneous (N=29)	Migraine (N=3)

Six children were referred for evaluation of fever of unknown origin or recurrent fevers. In four of these children no diagnosis has been established, and the children remain well despite recurrent fevers. One child was found to have a retroperitoneal abscess, and another represented normal temperature variation.

Six children were seen with multiple complaints, including combinations of headache, stomach ache, lethargy, and dizziness. In four of these children the complaints were felt to be consistent with somatization disorders; in another they represented exaggerated maternal anxiety; and in the last, no cause has been found to explain the symptoms. Four children were evaluated for recurrent infections, three of whom were felt to have allergic disorders, while the fourth represented a normal range for numbers of infectious illness in children.

Three children were seen for recurrent leg pain. One of these children was found to have reflex sympathetic dystrophy, another had viral arthritis, and the last had a transient postinfectious complication. Both children referred for evaluation of adenopathy were found to have benign lymph node hypertrophy. Only two children were seen for evaluation of abdominal pain. In one child the apparent "pains" were actually episodic myoclonic seizures; no apparent cause was found in the second patient.

The remaining 29 physician-referred patients had various reasons for consultation. Three children were felt to have migraine—one because of recurrent headaches, one with recurrent episodes of vomiting, and the last with recurrent episodes of transient hemiplegia. Two children were seen for second opinions—one regarding the need for adenoidectomy for recurrent otitis media, and the other regarding the need for scoliosis surgery in a severely retarded adolescent.

Although many of the diagnoses are by necessity based on clinical judgment since there are no confirmatory laboratory tests, in 19 (28%) no definite diagnosis was reached. Seven of these were patients referred for evaluation of short stature or poor growth, and four for evaluation of recurrent fever. In 12 children (18%), the referring physician's suspected diagnosis was confirmed, and in another 36 (54%) a diagnosis for the problem was offered by the PDRS.

Children Referred by Parents

Eighty-three (55%) children were seen for evaluation at the parent's request without a physician referral (Table 22.3). All of these children had been seen by other physicians, often their primary care giver, but the parents desired another opinion because they had not been given a diagnosis, because they wanted confirmation of the suspected diagnosis, or because they were unhappy with the explanations they received. The most common reason for referral was recurrent colds or coughs. Eighteen children (22%) presented with these complaints, 12 of whom were felt to have allergic disease, and 5 others were shown to have reactive lower-airway disease. The last child had upper-airway obstruction secondary to hypertrophic tonsils and adenoids and was referred for removal of this tissue.

Five children were seen because of parental concern about recurrent fevers. In two cases the "fever" was actually a normal variation in temperature. Another

TABLE 22.3. Complaints and diagnoses of 83 parent-referred children.

Complaint	Diagnostic summary
Recurrent colds/cough (N=18)	Allergic upper-airway disease (N=12)
	Reactive airway disease (N=5)
Recurrent fever (N=5)	Normal variation (N=2)
Headaches (N=5)	Migraine (N=2)
	Tension (N=2)
Lymphadenopathy (N=4)	Normal reactive (N=4)
Chronic lethargy (N=3)	Somatization (N=3)
Recurrent abdominal pain (N=2)	Somatization (N=2)
Nausea and vomiting (N=1)	Somatization (N=1)
Fainting spells (N=1)	Somatization (N=1)
Multiple complaints (N=1)	Somatization (N=1)
Multiple parental concerns (N=2)	Normal children(N=2)
Poor appetite (N=2)	Normal children (N=2)
Passing out (N=2)	Breath holding (N=2)
Short stature (N=2)	
Miscellaneous (N=35)	

child was recovering from a viral illness which the parents felt had been present too long, and the fourth appeared to have cyclic neutropenia. No diagnosis was established in the fifth child, and he will be followed.

Headaches were the presenting complaint of five children. Two of the children were felt to have migraine headaches as the cause, while in two others "tension" headaches seemed likely. One child had headaches with febrile episodes, and this complaint was felt to be a physiologic response.

Lymphadenopathy was the main concern of four parents, and each of their children had normal reactive lymph node enlargement secondary to allergies or infections. Chronic lethargy in three teenagers was felt to be a somatization disorder. Two with recurrent abdominal pain, one with nausea and vomiting, one with fainting episodes, and one with multiple complaints were also given this diagnosis. In two children with multiple parental concerns and normal examinations, the parents were reassured that their child was healthy, as were the parents of two children with "poor appetite." Breath-holding episodes were responsible for loss of consciousness in two children. Only two children were seen with the complaint of short stature, one of which was familial while the other was a discordant twin.

In four (5%) of the self-referred children no definitive diagnosis was reached, while in 66 a diagnosis for the presenting complaint was given to the parents. In 13 cases seen for second opinions, the original physician's diagnosis was confirmed.

Discussion

The majority of problems seen by the Pediatric Diagnostic Referral Service do not "fall between the subspecialty cracks." This is clearly true of children referred by their parents. In most of these cases the presenting complaint was vague or so general that it was difficult to determine in whose area of subspecialization the child fit. A generalist, however, is most appropriate for referral of these patients. Most of these problems should have been handled by the primary care physician since the diagnoses were not obscure and the management not complicated.

There are, however, a number of reasons why parents seek consultation. They may be dissatisified with the explanation they receive from their primary care giver, or they may have "hidden agendas" that have not been addressed. The parents may perceive that their child's physician has not spent enough time discussing the diagnosis and management of the problem, or the actual diagnosis may have been missed. In addition, some parents may need the reassurance of hearing the diagnosis from another source, especially a medical center. The PDRS has the luxury of time to uncover and address parents' concerns.

Children referred by physicians often have presenting complaints or problems that do not clearly fit into the realm of a subspecialist. This is true of problems like short stature/poor weight gain, fever of unknown origin, and the child with multiple complaints. As might be expected, these patients present greater diagnostic challenges since most have been thoroughly evaluated before referral. The 28% PDRS failure rate in establishing a diagnosis is indicative of the challenge. Not all referrals are made without a diagnosis. The referring physician may have a working diagnosis for which he desires confirmation, or, on occasion, the diagnosis is clear but a second opinion is sought to solidify the parents' acceptance.

Are there specific areas of vulnerability or weakness in the diagnosis or management by physicians that are reflected in these data? Recognition of somatization disorders seems to be one such area of weakness. Almost all of the children with these problems were adolescents with multiple general complaints who had extensive and expensive evaluations before referral. Management of these problems is difficult, frequently requiring a team approach, working with child psychiatry. Rarely was a psychiatric diagnosis one of inclusion in the primary case assessment. It is interesting to note that 11 of 31 adolescent patients seen in the PDRS were felt to have somatization disorders as the basis for their complaints.

A failure of recognition of allergic disorders is the second area that reflects a weakness in diagnosis by physicians. More than one fifth of children referred by parents had underlying allergic problems, all of whom were treated with repeated courses of antibiotics for colds and coughs.

A PDRS should be available in referral hospitals to provide a service to physicians and parents. It would be impractical to organize such a service solely around subspecialists since referred problems are often vague. A pediatric generalist should be able to sort out most of the referred problems and direct subsequent investigation as necessary. In centers with pediatric training programs a PDRS can provide experience in consultative general pediatrics, an area training programs seem to be neglecting.

Reference

1. Gartner JC Jr, Zitelli BJ, Malatack JJ, et al: Consultative pediatrics: A role for the generalist in an academic setting. *J Pediatr* 112:1035–1038, 1988.

23
Research in General Academic Pediatrics

MARIE C. MCCORMICK, DAVID CORNFELD

Introduction

The evolution of the academic generalist can be viewed either as a relatively recent phenomenon or as reincarnation of an older clinical model.[1] The latter individuals can still be found in most medical schools as a small number of faculty whose status derives from extensive clinical experience and who are respected for their clinical expertise in diagnosing or managing the individual patient. Their contribution to the intellectual content of medicine evolves from thoughtful, questioning observation more often than for formal research endeavors.

The new academic generalist who has emerged is less a reflection of this older clinical model and more the product of a reaction to the shift toward subspecialization and laboratory-based research that followed World War II.[2,3] As a result of the changes that led to a lessening of the role of the clinically-based practitioners, most clinical academicians functioned at an intensive level within a fairly narrowly defined subset of health problems which were generally organ-based. Much of their status and prestige derived from contributions to new knowledge through application of biological science theories and techniques to problems. This clinical model contributed significantly to the elucidation of the etiology and pathogenesis of disease and to the development of sophisticated management techniques.[4]

However, the limits of an educational model based on such subspecialists also has come to be recognized. While suitable for training future subspecialists in a hospital, caring for a relatively small group of sick patients, the subspecialist model is less applicable to the training of the majority of physicians, who see large numbers of patients primarily within an office setting. Concern about providing a more appropriate educational experience, as well as pressures to provide more care in outpatient departments of teaching hospitals, has led to the rapid expansion of divisions of ambulatory and primary care pediatrics. These programs

From the Department of Pediatrics, University of Pennsylvania School of Medicine, Philadelphia. Dr McCormick is currently at the Brigham & Women's Hospital, Boston.
Presented by Dr David Cornfeld in honor of Lewis A. Barness, MD, November 12, 1988.

have relied on, and incorporated the teaching and service experience of, several model programs for the 1950s and early 1960s.[5-8]

The initial focus of these academicians was the strengthening of the teaching and service components of the outpatient experience. The generic theme in these educational and service activities was to reduce the reliance on "high-tech" inpatient management, and increase reliance on the development of a continuous long-term relationship with a patient/family to foster health, to treat acute problems in their early stage, and to develop a better idea of the normal processes of growth and development in the healthy and the chronically ill individual.[5,8,9]

In contrast to their predecessors, however, the new academic generalists operate and must compete in a milieu in which prestige and status (not to mention promotions) are more tightly linked to research productivity.[1] This situation has created a dilemma for the faculty of these relatively new divisions. Although they are often recruited for their clinical expertise and ability to teach, academic promotion may be dependent on other skills for which they may have had little or no training. The dilemma is highlighted in a recent survey of heads of departments of internal medicine,[10] who report that a high priority for establishing divisions of general internal medicine continues to be the education of medical house officers and medical students in ambulatory care with research as a much lower priority. However, they also consider lack of research productivity to be the major threat to the academic viability of such divisions and to the careers of individual faculty.

Thus, academic generalists may often be viewed as second-class citizens.[10] Several factors contribute to this perception. The first is that the generalists are often considered as "jacks of all trades" with the unspoken implication of "masters of none"– ie, without focus to their teaching or research, and with no specific contribution to new knowledge that does not overlap or duplicate subspecialty research. Second, they are often considered less "productive" than their subspecialty colleagues. In part, this reduced academic productivity may result from often disproportionate patient care, teaching, and administrative activities. These nonresearch activities may also reflect different roles that have emerged in generalist divisions.[3] The limited research grants available for generalist research may also contribute to the cycle of lower research effort. However, the perceived lack of productivity may be more a lack of awareness of the length of observation time needed to obtain results in studies with humans as compared to those conducted with white rats, Sephadex columns, or tissue culture. In addition, the research problems and approaches may attract less attention from trainees and peers when compared to the "high-tech" excitement of the intensive care unit or the laboratory bench.

This external pressure to strengthen and expand the research activities of academic generalists has been reinforced by a more positive one. The development of curricula and other educational experiences has led to the identification of the need for new inquiries into the quality and content of the teaching experience. These inquiries include investigations in diagnostic and management approaches appropriate to the ambulatory setting, the most efficient organizational arrangements for delivering these services, and educational techniques appropriate for both patients and professionals.[11-14]

The need to strengthen the scholarly activities of generalists has stimulated the recent development of divisions/sections of general pediatrics (with parallels in internal medicine).[1,3] The initial success of these divisions is evident from the fact that they have attracted capable faculty and highly qualified fellows, identified a patient-care role that is complementary to that of subspecialists, achieved recognition and respect by trainees and peers, and enhanced the quantity and quality of generalist research. Now it is important for general pediatric divisions to move into a more "mature" phase in which they become self- sustaining units capable of making cumulative contributions to medical education, to training of new generalists, and to fostering the development of such generalists within the academic setting.

The familiar model of subspecialty divisions offers one approach for this evolution. It involves (1) development of a "theme" which provides cohesion and direction to research and teaching activities, (2) specification of the appropriate "basic science" support required to carry out these activities, and (3) development of the "laboratory" and "models" appropriate to activities of the division.

Developing the Theme

While providing broad clinical expertise, most successful subspecialty divisions have narrower, well-defined research interests. Thus, a division of hematology may do research in specific hemoglobinopathies; a division of metabolism, in specific classes of metabolic disorders. This focused research effort enhances productivity in several ways. A shared commonality in research endeavors encourages a synergistic "division of labor" in maintaining currency in the relevant literature and methods; increases the efficient use of resources including space, materials, and support personnel; is more likely to produce a cumulative addition to new knowledge; and provides a clearer signal to trainees and funding agencies regarding the strengths of the group.

Two approaches have emerged to identify an appropriate research theme for general pediatrics. One is the selection of a clinical problem of sufficient importance to warrant a multiproject research effort. This type of approach has been used successfully to generate research and teaching programs in areas such as behavioral and developmental problems[15] and the identification of serious illness in young febrile children.[16] Because it is analogous to the subspecialty model, this approach offers the potential for greater understanding, acceptance, and clinical applicability within the hospital setting. However, there are several potential disadvantages. Among these are the limited number of questions broad and important enough for the research efforts of a significant group of investigators and fellows. This second is a risk of being seen as duplicative or competitive with subspecialist activities. Perhaps most importantly, such an approach may not foster an image or a role of a "generalist."

An alternative approach involves the identification of issues that may cross clinical problems and the examination of processes basic to the practice of medicine.[17] It has the advantage of (1) reinforcing the "generalist" approach, (2) providing a breadth of problems sufficient to support a research program tailored to a variety of interests of researchers, and (3) maintaining the potential to develop a cumulative body of new knowledge. The identification of these processes is straightforward, and includes activities such as (1) well-person care—health maintenance, prevention; (2) screening for presymptomatic or early disease; (3) diagnosis of illness; (4) treatment and management of illness; and (5) referral and rehabilitation.

The delineation of the specific research questions is more difficult. The charge to the practitioner is to prevent illness or ill health when possible, and otherwise to diagnose and manage health problems so as to minimize their adverse effects. Thus, the questions must not only be generic to a number of diseases, but also deal with the patient as a member of a community. A critical element in this process is the application of interventions of demonstrated efficacy in the least costly fashion to maximize health. Thus, one mission for the research for academic generalists is the characterization of effective modes of practice for the practitioner.

For several reasons, the identification of optimal modes of clinical practice has different emphases from those required of subspecialist investigators.[18] The latter must be knowledgeable about the basic sciences that explain normal processes and be competent in the formulation and testing of alternative hypotheses concerning pathophysiology. They must also be able to translate this knowledge into the development and assessment of the efficacy of interventions in randomized controlled trials. Intellectual rigor is determined by the quality of the underlying hypotheses and the experimental purity of the trial.

Clinical practice depends less on the power to explain and more on the power to predict.[18] The generalist is confronted with the necessity of characterizing patients as to their status (well vs ill), severity and duration of their problems, utility of diagnostic strategies, and potential sensitivity to a variety of potentially prophylactic and therapeutic agents. Moreover, the practitioner must attempt to enhance health outcomes as defined by function (not just biological control). In other words, the generalist must translate what is known about pathophysiology into measures and observations of functional status relevant to individuals and groups, and assess the "real-world" effectiveness of therapeutic interventions. The intellectual rigor rarely involves explanation or hypothesis testing. In fact, statements of "hypotheses" in much of this research appear self-evident or naïve. What is more difficult and requires more scientific imagination is the development of measures to delineate the characteristics of patients and the processes of care that produce better or worse functional outcomes. Since such investigations may be less amenable to randomized trials because of ethical or logistic constraints, establishing effective modes of practice relies on different measurement techniques and a range of experimental/observational strategies.

Research Methods and Appropriate Basic Sciences

The research approaches that lead to the delineation of basic pathophysiologic mechanisms of disease and to the development of effective, specific theories derive from the physical sciences. The translation of these disease-specific findings to clinical practice for general populations relies heavily on social-science theories and methods.

Conceptual or theoretical contributions of these sciences to academic generalist activities are obvious.[19] For example, if one is to maximize the effectiveness of medical care, then knowledge about factors affecting access to, utilization of, and compliance with medical care is critical. If enhancing the potential of normal development is a goal, then knowledge about the factors affecting development and elucidation of the potential effect of illness is important. The training of practitioners and the tailoring of clinical practice to specific groups depend on information about the cultural interactions of these groups with each other and with formal social organizations and appropriate educational techniques.

Fluency in social-science research methods is perhaps equally or even more important for the generalist. As noted earlier, a critical element in generalist research is the ability to quantitate the patient's status before and after therapy along functional domains and to characterize the processes that might contribute to change. Just as the "wet lab" scientist may rely on replication or genetically identical laboratory animals to test hypotheses, the generalist must be able to select research designs that minimize the threats to experimental validity and ability to generalize appropriate to a variety of human situations, including those where true experiments with randomization may not be possible. Lacking the ability to control for threats to experimental validity provided by replication or homogeneity of inbred lab animals, the academic generalist must be conversant with statistical techniques for examining or "controlling" for confounding variables, as well as estimating the probability of an experimental effect (ie, the statistical significance).

The "Laboratory"

The fact that much of their clinical work involves essentially healthy patients can pose a difficult problem for academic generalist pediatricians. Research aimed at establishing the effectiveness of clinical maneuvers to improve functional status may require large numbers of subjects or long periods of observation to measure outcomes using currently available techniques or instruments. Greater attention to the development of health status measures appropriate to relatively healthy children, which has lagged behind that available for adults,[20] might expand the range of outcome measures available.

While development of appropriate measures is an important research priority for the academic generalist, assessment of current practices and development of appropriate training approaches cannot await such developments. Thus, the academic generalist must identify situations in which such research is feasible. Characteristics of such "laboratories" include the following:

1. The prevalence of the factor under study is sufficiently high that adequate sample sizes can be collected and observed within a reasonable time.
2. The range of severity of illness is such that there is a reasonable chance of documenting improvement with interventions.
3. The characteristics of the situation are such that the results can be argued to apply to more general populations.
4. The conduct of research is an accepted part of the process of care.

Four examples of patient groups meeting these criteria can be identified.

The Low-Birth-Weight (LBW) Infant

Much of the interest in LBW infants reflects concern about application of cutting-edge technology for extremely premature infants. It is less well appreciated that birth weight can be used as a "screen" to identify 5% of the population at substantially increased risk for health problems which encompass a broad range of pediatrics. Such infants are at increased risk for difficulties in physical and psychosocial development, congenital malformation, and lower respiratory tract disorders, among others. The management of these problems is complicated by higher levels of socioeconomic disadvantage, prolonged and recurrent separations, and poor maternal health, thus illustrating the interplay of child health with the environment. Finally, providing care for these children illustrates the kinds of financial, organizational, and educational stresses and other societal concerns that may accompany childhood illness.[21]

Children with Chronic Illness

With the exception of asthma, most chronic illnesses in children are not frequent enough to satisfy the conditions noted previously, and many of the children require subspecialty management. As a group, these children constitute 3% to 5% of the population and present a common set of problems of importance to the generalist. For one thing, they are most likely to exhibit functional impairments for which measures are currently available, such as limits in activities of daily living due to health.[17,22] Thus, studies of these children can be used to assess the relevance of measures of dysfunction, to ascertain the predictors of dysfunction, and to evaluate interventions designed to prevent specific problems.

Children with chronic illnesses present some generic management challenges as well. For example, almost all such conditions require compliance with longer-term therapeutic regimens, such as diets, medication, or physical therapy. In addition, many present opportunities for implementing selective screening or diagnostic programs, and for assessing the effectiveness of such techniques. The quality of routine care may also be reflected in the use of emergency/inpatient services, and thus changes in the use of hospital services by chronically ill children may be useful for examining primary care. Finally, since chronic conditions vary in severity both within diagnosis and over time for a given individual and may require multiple therapies, they should prove useful in examining the effectiveness of referral and coordination strategies for primary care practitioners. Conversely, since the needs of such children may be relatively intense, they and their families prove more vulnerable to financial and organizational changes in the practice of medicine and serve as a target group for observing the effects of such changes in access to care and family functioning.[23-25]

Childhood Injuries

The study of childhood injuries is important if for no other reason than because of their magnitude as a health problem. As a model for the academic generalist, injuries offer an opportunity to define the risk factors for, and functional sequelae of relatively acute problems in, otherwise healthy children, as well as to examine the potential for prevention of either the event itself or unnecessary subsequent dysfunction. Injuries and their management also illustrate the issues related to the provision of acute emergency services for children, assessment of the diagnostic approaches to specific problems, and the necessity to consider the social milieu when dealing with such problems as sports injuries in organized athletics, child abuse, and specific environmental hazards (eg, dangerous toys, inadequate construction).[26]

Disadvantaged Children

Many medical centers are located in inner cities and serve a largely indigent population, especially in the ambulatory arena.[27] Such populations have higher levels of common and potentially preventable illnesses.[26] The management of these problems is made difficult by factors that range from the lack of financial and other resources in the families to total disorganization and psychosocial pathology. Such populations offer the opportunity to examine the efficacy of interventions suitable to demanding situations, as well as providing the experience in team management (medical, social, educational) in addressing the problems of these children.

The enumeration of these potential "laboratories" suggests another external pressure for development of active generalists research programs: the pressure to employ one or more cost containment strategies in the delivery of medical care.[23] Each of these groups illustrates the types of children who may be adversely affected by increased parental burden for paying for care or by restriction in access to needed subspecialty services.[25] Without solid, empirically derived evidence of the importance of management strategies for improving the function of those with health problems, cost-containment policies may adversely affect the health of the most vulnerable.

Faculty and fellows in the Division of General Pediatrics at Children's Hospital of Philadelphia have started to emphasize certain themes for their scholarly activities. The clinical arenas have included the Emergency Medicine Program, a primary care office practice, the low-birth-weight neonatal follow-up clinic, the communitywide injury prevention program, and the adolescent program. The Emergency Medicine Department has provided a locale for studies of a variety of risk factors which might produce poor health status including a definition of risk for sepsis in the febrile infant; the effect of oral antibiotics on febrile infants at risk for bacteremia; the effect of a smoke detector giveaway program in an ambulatory setting; assessment of the risk for respiratory compromise in infants with bronchiolitis; and epidemiologic studies of chest pain, bicycle injury, and household falls.

The primary care office practice has lent itself to similar studies. Issues such as compliance and patient education have been emphasized. Studies have included impact of educational intervention on compliance of patients with otitis media; intervention to reduce functional morbidity following minor head trauma; evaluation of educational intervention to improve management of fever by patients; and study of the impact of a prenatal interview on compliance.

As noted, low-birth-weight infants represent a population group in which health problems are more prevalent than in the general population. In the high-risk newborn follow-up program, studies have been undertaken to define temperament and neurologic development; to evaluate effects of regionalization on perinatal care and health outcome, including a study of costs and health status; to evaluate immunologic responses in high-risk neonates following immunization; and to determine nutritional requirements of the premature with severe pulmonary disease.

Interest in injury research has been promoted in a multiinstitutional program with the Centers for Disease Control (CDC), the City of Philadelphia Health Department, and the Clinical Epidemiology Unit at the University of Pennsylvania. A collaborative project has been initiated to evaluate epidemiologic factors important in the pathogenesis of injuries in a large urban population in the immediate neighborhood of the hospital. This study extends those that have already looked at risk factors for injury in adolescents and in the undergraduate college population. The next phase will include development, study, and evaluation of an intervention on the injury problem.

In addition to providing an opportunity to extend the injury research, the adolescent age group has been the subject of studies of other risk-taking behaviors. These have focused on the suicide issue, self-esteem, and the related drug and alcohol problem.

These activities emphasize the common themes (eg, identification of clinically relevant risk factors for common problems, and intervention modalities appropriate to the ambulatory setting). Less evident from this description is that these efforts have also begun to incorporate similar conceptual and measurement approaches and other common methodologies that foster comparisons across different health problems and that begin an empirically based generic approach to ambulatory care.

Constraints and Challenges

Feinstein[18] has identified four basic constraints to the recognition and acceptance of generalist research of this type. First is the perception of the basic goals of science. As noted earlier, much of physiologic medical research is aimed at explaining phenomena through experimental testing of alternative hypotheses. The basic goal of the generalist is prediction–ie, making a probabilistic statement concerning the functional outcomes and the potential effect of interventions for groups of patients characterized by various sociodemographic factors and dimensions of disease. This goal relies less on the ability to generate hypotheses than on the ability to define as precisely as possible the initial and final status of the patient, and the processes that contributed to the change.

The second constraint is the perception of what constitutes scientific data. Much of subspecialty research depends on data derived from specimens or by machine and thus considered "hard." Generalists must use data on patient condition, the processes of care, and familial and environmental factors relating to the patient and outcome. As noted earlier, the social sciences have developed applicable theories and techniques to address these issues, such data are still often considered "soft."

Third, different goals require different skills: hypothesis-testing in the subspecialties; measurement in the generalist realm. Finally, the generalists' choice of appropriate experimental strategies may have to be broader than those relevant to hypothesis-testing.

Despite these and other difficulties in developing and describing research in generalist divisions, this type of research also presents a timely and exciting challenge. As Ellwood argued in his recent Shattuck lecture,[29] changes in medical services, and how they are organized and paid for over the past decade, emphasize the urgent need for "outcomes management." He defines this as a technology of patient experience designed to help patients, payers, and providers make rational choices based on the effect of these choices in the patient's life. For the pediatric patient, many of the specific activities that would underlie such an outcomes-management approach will be conducted by the office-based practitioner. By characterizing the generic problems confronting these patients and generic management approaches to enhancing functional status, the academic generalist who resides at the interface between the hospital-based subspecialist and the office-based primary care practitioner is well placed to help the practitioner take on this exacting and exciting role.

Acknowledgments. We thank Dr Margaret Heagarty for her critique of previous drafts and ongoing support, the members of the Division of General Pediatrics of the Department of Pediatrics of Children's Hospital of Philadelphia for their comments, and Merceda Lafferty for technical assistance in preparing the paper.

References

1. Eisenberg JM: Sculpture of a new academic discipline. Four faces of academic general internal medicine. *Am J Med* 78:283–292, 1985.
2. Ebert RH, Brown SS: Academic health centers. *N Engl J Med* 308:1200–1208, 1983.

3. Eisenberg JM: Cultivating a new field: Development of a research program in general internal medicine. *J Gen Intern Med* 1(14):S8–S18, 1986.
4. Frederickson DS: Biomedical research in the 1980s. *N Engl J Med* 304:509–517, 1981.
5. Alpert JJ, Robertson LS, Kosa J, Heagarty MC, Haggerty RJ: Delivery of health care to children: Report of an experiment. *Pediatrics* 57(6):917–930, 1976.
6. Proger S: A career in ambulatory medicine. *N Engl J Med* 292:1318–1324, 1975.
7. McDermott W: General medical care. Identification and analysis of alternative approaches. *Johns Hopkins Med J* 135:292–321, 1974.
8. Alpert JJ, Charney E: The education of physicians for primary care. Washington: DHEW, publication No. (HRM) 74-3113, 1974.
9. Green M, Hoekelman RA: Trends in the education of pediatricians. *Adv Pediatr* 29: 325–350, 1982.
10. Friedman RH, Pozen JT: The academic viability of general internal medicine. The views of department of medicine chairmen. *Ann Intern Med* 103:439–444, 1985.
11. White KL: Teaching epidemiologic concepts as the scientific basis for understanding problems of organizing and evaluating health services. *Int J Health Serv* 2:525–529, 1972.
12. McKeown T: The direction of medical research. *Lancet* 2:1281–1284, 1979.
13. Feinstein AR: What kind of basic science for clinical medicine? *N Engl J Med* 283: 847–852, 1970.
14. Sevales J: What has happened to academic medicine? *Lancet* 1:1194–1196, 1986.
15. Levine MD: The high prevalence–low severity developmental disorders of school children. *Adv Pediatr* 29:529–554, 1982.
16. McCarthy PL, Sharpe MR, Spiesel SZ, et al: Observation scales to identify serious illness in febrile children. *Pediatrics* 70:802–809, 1982.
17. Stein REK, Jessop DJ: A non-categorical approach to chronic childhood illness. *Public Health Rep* 97(4):361–378, 1982.
18. Feinstein AR: An additional basic science for clinical medicine. I. The constraining fundamental paradigms. *Ann Intern Med* 99:393–397, 1983. II. The limitations of randomized trials. *Ann Intern Med* 99:544–550, 1983. III. The challenges of comparison and measurement. *Ann Intern Med* 99:705–712, 1983. IV. The development of clinimetrics. *Ann Intern Med* 99:843–848, 1983.
19. Donabedian A: *Aspects of Medical Care Administration*. Cambridge, MA: Harvard University Press, 1973.
20. Bergner M: Measurement of health status. *Med Care* 23:696–704, 1985.
21. McCormick MC: The contribution of low birth weight to infant mortality and childhood morbidity. *N Engl J Med* 312:82–90, 1985.
22. Eisen M, Donald CA, Ware JE, et al: *Conceptualization and Measurement of Health for Children in the Health Insurance Study*. Santa Monica, CA: Rand, 1980.
23. Luft HS: Competition and regulation. *Med Care* 23:383–400, 1985.
24. McCormick MC: The medically vulnerable child and the financially vulnerable family. Presented at a National Conference, Comprehensive Approaches to Disabled and At-Risk Infants, Toddlers, and Their Families, National Center for Clinical Infant Programs, Washington, D.C., December 14, 1984.
25. Hobbs N, Perrin JM, Ireys HT: *Chronically Ill Children and Their Families*. San Francisco: Jossey-Bass, 1985.
26. Pless IB, Stulginskas J: Accidents and violence as a cause of morbidity and mortality in childhood. *Adv Pediatr* 29:471–495, 1982.

27. Rogers DE, Blendon RJ: The academic medical center today. *Ann Intern Med* 100:751–754, 1984.
28. Egbuonu L, Starfield B: Child health and social status. *Pediatrics* 69:550–555, 1982.
29. Ellwood PM: Outcomes management. A technology of patient experience. *N Engl J Med* 318:1549–1556, 1988.

24
Parents' and Children's Rights in Conflict: The Religious Exemption to Treatment

THOMAS J. SCULLY

Public attention has recently focused on a number of instances in which parents have refused consent to medical care for their children, based on the parents' belief in "faith healing" and/or their rejection of the value of currently accepted medical treatment. The exact number of such cases nationwide is unknown and the underlying reasons for the increase in numbers are varied. But at a minimum they include a resurgence in the United States of fundamentalist religions, the primacy of the family in society, and the notion that government intervention into the private lives of citizens has gone too far.

In reported cases, treatment denials have been for correctable surgical conditions and curable infectious diseases such as meningitis and diabetes.[1] In those instances in which the child died as a result of treatment denial, the state has usually intervened, after the fact, and prosecuted the parents for manslaughter or felony child neglect, though not uniformly!

"Trial OK'd for Mom in Prayer-Cure Death" headlined the *Sacramento Bee* story[2] of the decision of the California Supreme Court to permit the Sacramento district attorney to prosecute Christian Scientist Laurie Grouard Walker for involuntary manslaughter in the death of her 4-year-old child of meningitis in 1984. The California court noted the 1944 U.S. Supreme Court decision in *Prince v Massachusetts*:

> Parents may be free to become martyrs themselves. But it does not follow they are free in identical circumstances, to make martyrs of their children before they have reached the age of full legal discretion when they can make that choice themselves.[3]

A month earlier the U.S. Supreme Court refused to review the involuntary manslaughter conviction of a Pennsylvania couple who relied on faith to heal their child, who died subsequently of an untreated Wilms tumor. In denying the review, the Pennsylvania court's ruling was affirmed:

From the Department of Pediatrics and the Program in Bioethics, University of Nevada School of Medicine, Reno, Nevada.
Presented in honor of Lewis A. Barness, MD, November 12, 1988.

Parents have natural-law duty that state statutes impliedly recognize to act to avert child's untimely death by seeking medical care for life-threatening illness; parents whose child's health was obviously deteriorating from presence and continuous growth of tumor in abdomen cannot claim not to have had notice that they were risking criminal liability for consciously disregarding risk of their child's death; where child's life is at stake, parents may not defeat criminal charges by relying on right to exercise religious tenets against seeking medical help.[4]

Two months later, a former deacon of a faith-healing sect, known as the No Name Fellowship, was sentenced in Spokane, Washington, to 41 months in prison for failing to seek medical help for his dying diabetic son.[5]

The prosecution of cases in which death occurs, however, seems to be uncommon. Recent articles and commentaries in the *New England Journal of Medicine* on the subject of "faith healing" point out that many states *do not* enforce laws related to child neglect when a religious exemption is claimed.[6] Furthermore, the Committee on Bioethics of the American Academy of Pediatrics in its *APA Statement on the Religious Exemption for Child Abuse* notes that there are now "statutes in 44 states which contain a provision stating the child is *not* to be deemed neglected merely because he or she is receiving treatment by spiritual means through prayer according to the tenets of a *recognized* religion"[1] [italics added].

In addition, the federal government, through Medicare, acknowledges Christian Science practitioners as healers and reimburses them as other practitioners, including physicians, are reimbursed,[6] despite the First Amendment prohibition that "Congress shall make no laws respecting the establishment of religion. . . ." How can it be that 44 state statutes speak of "recognized religion" and the federal government reimburses for "Christian Science healing"?

Could it be that the interests of government coincide more with parents' religious interests than they do with children's health interests? It would appear that the lobbying forces in Congress and state legislatures on behalf of parents' religious interests have been more influential than those on behalf of children's interests!

In commenting on two opposing views expressed in 1983 in the "Sounding Boards" section of the *New England Journal of Medicine*, editor Arnold S. Relman, MD, noted:

If the present Administration believes so firmly in parental discretion as to allow parents to choose prayer instead of medical therapy for a child with meningitis, how does it justify its attempts to interfere with parental choice in the management of infants born with major congenital defects, in whom indications for medical treatment are far more debatable?[7]

Justice Brandeis, in his famous dissent in *Olmstead v United States*, articulated the deeply held belief in the right to privacy cherished by all Americans and expressed in the Fourth Amendment when he wrote:

The makers of our Constitution undertook to secure conditions favorable to the pursuit of happiness. They recognized the significance of man's spiritual nature. . . . They sought to protect Americans in their beliefs . . . They conferred . . . the right to be let alone—the most comprehensive of rights and the right most valued by civilized men.[8]

The makers of our Constitution also undertook to secure conditions favorable to the pursuit of liberty when they wrote in the First Amendment that "Congress shall make no laws respecting the establishment of religion or prohibiting the free exercise thereof. . . ."[9]

But is this "freedom of religion" absolute? The answer is no! Chief Justice Waite, in delivering the opinion of the Supreme Court more than 100 years ago in *Reynolds v United States*, wrote:

Laws are made for the government of actions, and while they cannot interfere with mere religious *belief* and *opinions*, they may with *practices* [italics added]. Suppose one believed that human sacrifices were a necessary part of religious worship, would it be seriously contended that the civil government under which he lived could not interfere to prevent a sacrifice . . .? Can a man excuse his practices to the contrary because of his religious belief? To permit this would be to make the professed doctrines of religious belief superior to the law of the land and in effect to permit every citizen to become a law unto himself. Government could exist only in name under such circumstances.[10]

Thus, the Supreme Court of 1879 upheld an 1862 Congressional Act making "bigamy a crime," setting limits on a citizen's actions, based upon religion.

The right to refuse or consent to medical treatment arises from our fundamental notions of liberty, privacy, and autonomy—a principle first articulated by Kant—in which persons are equal and each "recognizes the other as equally a person as oneself."[11]

In *Schloendorff v Society of New York Hospital* (1914), Justice Benjamin Cardozo wrote for the New York Court of Appeals: "Every human being of adult years and sound mind has a right to determine what shall be done with his own body, and a surgeon who performs an operation without his patient's consent commits an assault for which he is liable in damages."[12]

This landmark decision became the definitive statement upon which most statutory and case law on informed consent stands. There is little argument that a competent adult has the absolute right to decide what shall and shall not be done to him or her in the diagnostic and treatment environment even if some would consider the decision foolish.

As noted in the *Bouvia v Superior Court*[13] decision, it mattered not what her motivation was even when the exercise of her right to refuse treatment created a life-threatening condition.

The right to refuse medical treatment is basic and fundamental . . . and is . . . recognized as a part of the right of privacy protected by both the state (California) and federal constitution. Its exercise requires no one's approval. . . . It is not a medical decision for her physicians to make. Neither is it a legal question whose soundness is to be resolved by lawyers or judges. It is not a constitutional right subject to approval by ethics committees or courts of law. It is a moral and philosophical decision that being a competent adult, is hers alone.[13]

There are many other court decisions in which an adult's refusal of treatment (ie, blood transfusion, immunizations, and surgery) has been upheld on religious grounds. In 1972, D.C. superior Court Judge Bacon upheld such a decision by "a man who did not wish to live if to do so required a blood transfusion, who viewed himself as deprived of life everlasting even if he involuntarily received the transfusion, and who had, through material provision and family and spiritual bonds, provided for the future well being of his two children." Judge Yeagley's concurrence was based on freedom of choice whether founded on religious beliefs or otherwise.[14]

Two years later, in the same jurisdiction, Judge Tim Murphy upheld Janet Pogue's right to refuse a postpartum blood transfusion for herself, on religious grounds, during an emergency hysterectomy, but ordered a transfusion for her newborn infant suffering from hyperbilirubinemia.[15] In so doing, Judge Murphy ruled that Janet Pogue was not competent to decide the best interest of her infant but was competent to decide her own best interest. The rights of adult parents and the rights of minor children came starkly into focus in this oft-quoted decision.

In his book *Parents and Children . . . The Ethics of the Family*, Jeffrey Blustein writes: "Caretakers must protect children's health" and prepare them "to take advantage of and responsibly exercise their rights and liberties as citizens. . . ."[16] There is little argument that parents have important duties to nurture, educate, house, and clothe their dependent children. But they also have important rights of custody to rear children in the religion of their choice and to consent to medical treatment for their children. "Under no circumstance should a child be subjected to any procedure that is not for his or her benefit *without* parental consent"[17] [italics added].

Statutory exceptions to parental consent for the treatment of minor children vary from state to state but usually include bona fide emergencies and treatment for such problems as drug abuse, mental illness, pregnancy, rape, abortion, sexual abuse, and sexually transmitted diseases. In addition, many state statutes recognize the emancipated minor and mature minor who can consent to medical treatment for himself or herself.[18]

These exceptions notwithstanding, there is "the strong presumption in our legal system in favor of parental autonomy and family privacy and *against* coercive state intervention. . . . In accord with fundamental notions of liberty, the law . . . presumes that parents . . . are qualified to decide how to meet the needs of their children until these children themselves become adults presumed competent to decide what is in their own and their children's interests."[19]

But when should the state override parental authority and intervene? Only, writes Yale Law Professor Goldstein, when the state can establish (1) that the medical profession is in agreement about what nonexperimental treatment is right for the child; (2) that the expected outcome of that treatment is what society agrees to be right for any child, a chance for normal healthy growth toward adulthood or life worth living; and (3) that the expected outcome of denial of that treatment would mean death for the child.[19]

Many courts and some legislatures have gone beyond the expected outcome of "death" and have considered the likelihood of severe disability as well. But courts have varied in their willingness to choose between different medical theories or treatments if the attending physician is a duly licensed practitioner and has assumed care of the child within limits set by the parents[20] or when the risks of treatment are significant and outweigh any potential benefits.[17]

When parents invoke their rights to religious freedom under the First Amendment and refuse consent for medical treatment for their child, courts have usually held that freedom of religion does "not extend to allowing their children to die or become disabled."[17]

In the 1984 Supreme Court ruling on the federal Baby Doe rules, the court wrote: "In broad outlines state law vests responsibility in the parents . . . subject to review in exceptional cases by the state acting as 'parens patria.' "

The court footnotes this statement with one taken from the 1983 report of the President's Commission for the Study of Ethical Problems in Medicine and Environmental Behavior Research as follows:

> The paucity of directly relevant cases makes characterization of the law in this area somewhat problematic but certain points stand out:
>
> *First*, there is a presumption strong but rebuttable that parents are the appropriate decision makers for their infants. Traditional law concerning the family buttressed by the emerging constitutional right of privacy protects a substantial range of discretion for parents.
>
> *Second*, as persons unable to protect themselves, infants fall under the "parens patria" power of the state. In the exercise of this authority, the state not only punishes parents whose conduct has amounted to abuse and neglect of their children, but may also supervene parental decisions . . . to be sure that the choices made are not so detrimental to a child's interest as to amount to neglect and abuse.
>
> *Third*, the courts have exercised their authority to appoint a guardian for a child when the parents are not capable of participating in the decision making or when they have made decisions that evidence substantial lack of concern for the child's interests.
>
> *Fourth*, societal involvement usually occurs under the auspices of governmental instrumentalities, such as child welfare agencies and courts, and
>
> *Finally*, the American legal system ordinarily relies upon the private initiative of individuals rather than continuing government supervision to bring the matter to the attention of legal authorities.[21]

The American Academy of Pediatrics through its Committee on Bioethics calls on its members to

> vigorously take the lead to (1) increase public awareness of the hazards to children growing out of religious exemptions to child abuse and neglect legislation; (2) support legislation in each state legislature to correct statutes and regulations that permit harm to children under the shield of religious exemption; (3) work with other child advocacy organizations and agencies to develop coordinated and concerted public and professional actions for recision of religious exemptions.[1]

It is unfortunate that we must relearn old lessons and revisit previously settled ground, but revisit we must!

References

1. American Academy of Pediatrics, Committee on Bioethics. Religious exemptions from child abuse statutes. *Pediatrics* 81:169–171, 1988.
2. *The Sacramento Bee*. Capitol/state news. Nov 11, 1988, p A3.
3. *Prince v Massachusetts*, 321 US 158, 166, 64 S Ct. 438, 88 L Ed 645 (1944).

4. *87-1722 Barnhart v. Pennsylvania* (Pa SuperCt, 345 PaSuper 10, 497 A2d 616); 57 LW 3212, *United States Law Week*, Oct 4, 1988.
5. Associated Press. Former faith-healing official sentenced in son's death. *Reno Gazette-Journal*, Dec 16, 1988, p 24-A.
6. Swan R: Faith healing, Christian Science, and the medical care of children. *N Engl J Med* 309:1639–1641, 1983.
7. Relman A: Sounding boards: Christian Science and the care of children. *N Engl J Med* 309: p 1639, 1983.
8. *Olmstead v US*, 277 US 438 at 478 (1928).
9. *Constitution of the United States of America*, 1791.
10. *Reynolds v U.S.*, 98 US 145 at 166, 167 (1879).
11. Jonsen R: *Encyclopedia of Bioethics*. New York: The Free Press, 1978, Vol 2, p 625.
12. *Schloendorff v Society of New York Hospital*, 211 NY 25, 105 N.E. 92, 93 (1914).
13. *Bouvia v Superior Court*, 179 Cal App 3d 1127, 225 Cal Reptr. 297; review denied (1986).
14. *In re Osborne*: 294 A 2d 372 (1972).
15. *In re Pogue*: *Washington Post*, metro edition, sec C; pp 1,5, Nov 14, 1974.
16. Blustein J: *Parents and Children, the Ethics of the Family*. New York: Oxford University Press, 1982, p 124.
17. Holder AR: Disclosure and consent problems in pediatrics: The silent world. *Law Med Health Care* 16:219–228, 1988.
18. Capron AM: The competence of children as self deciders in biomedical interventions. In Gaylin W, Macklin R (eds); *Who Speaks for the Child*. New York: Plenum Press, 1982, pp 92–114.
19. Goldstein J: Medical care for the child at risk: On state supervention of parental autonomy. In Gaylin W, Macklin R (eds): *Who Speaks for the Child*. New York: Plenum Press, pp 153–188, 163.
20. *In re Hofbauer*: 47 NYS 2d 648, 419 NYS 2d 936; 393 NE 2d 1009 (1979).
21. *Otis R. Bowen, Secretary of Health and Human Services, Petitioner vs American Hospital Association et al.*; 84 US 1529 at B2765, 1984.

25
Pediatric Care in the Era of the DRG: Who Are the Winners? Who Are the Losers?

JOHN S. CURRAN

Introduction

Both public and private regulatory programs have demonstrated an intense interest in the need to curb increasing hospital costs, related in part to the fact that health care expenditures now approximate 12% of the gross national product. Recent innovations attempting to curb health care expenditures include the development of prospective pricing systems. These were first proposed in 1975, and with various modifications they continue to the present.[1-10] The initial proposals were developed by investigators at Yale University/New Haven Hospital based on community hospital data that were later incorporated into a prospective payment plan utilized in the state of New Jersey. Under this prospective pricing system, hospitals were paid a fixed amount per discharge as dictated by the patient's diagnosis rather than the number of days of hospitalization and/or specific hospital services that were utilized.

Subsequently, the 1982 Tax Equity and Fiscal Responsibility Act (TEFRA) addressed three areas of cost containment for regulation of the expenditure of federal funds for health care services, which included three basic principles: (1) hospital cost limits were extended to include cost of inpatient hospital services; (2) a limit was to be required on the overall rate of operational costs per case; and (3) a prospective pricing method was to be developed calculating hospital charges for Medicare and Medicaid reimbursement.[11]

Prior to 1984, Medicare hospital reimbursement had been basically a cost-based per-diem method which included both capital costs and a pass-through of medical educational costs. The alleged objective of the Health Care Financing Administration in implementing TEFRA was to establish the federal government as a "prudent buyer" of health care services while maintaining patients' access to quality care.

From the Department of Pediatrics, University of South Florida College of Medicine, Tampa, Florida.
Presented in honor of Lewis A. Barness, MD, November 12, 1988.

The DRG system, as developed, classified all possible diagnoses in the ICD-9-CM system into 23 major diagnostic categories (MDCs) based on organ systems. These were further subdivided into 467 distinct groupings each of which was said to be "medically discriminative" in that patients within each DRG could be expected to utilize a similar set of clinical responses which, on a statistical average, resulted in an approximately equal use of hospital resources.

The initial application of this methodology to Medicare part A hospital inpatient services provided an exemption for the following types of inpatient care:

1. Children's hospitals—defined as hospitals whose patients are predominantly under 18 years of age
2. Psychiatric hospitals
3. Rehabilitation hospitals
4. Long-term care hospitals
5. Distinct psychiatric and rehabilitation units (free-standing)
6. Hospitals in states that had a waiver from the prospective payment system
7. Hospitals in the U.S. territories and the District of Columbia

With the exception of MDC 15 (newborns and other neonates with conditions originating in the perinatal period), the Medicare system of DRGs makes no provision for specific recognition of either pediatric medical or surgical services. Pediatric health care services, whether delivered in an acute-care general hospital or in a children's hospital, are, by nature of the intense personnel resources required, more expensive than those health care services provided to adults. Thus, there has been intense interest in the need to have a specific evaluation of the concepts that "children are different" and utilize a different pattern of services from those recognized from Medicare files, which utilized, in constitution of the original DRGs, an extremely limited sample of children provided care in community hospitals.

The implementation of the DRG system provided impetus to the development of hospital information systems (HIS) necessary to appropriately group patients into DRGs and to maximize the sequence of diagnoses to provide greatest reimbursement to hospitals. As information systems have proliferated, there has been a major effort to identify more accurately the costs of services by so-called product lines which are also applicable to children's inpatient health care services. As HISs have progressed in the ability to assign costs for each individual patient, there has arisen a new concept which distinctly threatens the economic viability of pediatric medical education and classic pediatric health care education as we view them today. Specifically, it is now possible through the HIS to evaluate the "relative worth" of the physician and the assignment of physicians to categories of "winners versus losers." Hospital management may then potentially utilize new perspectives in allocating resources to areas of pediatric care based on economic productivity regardless of need. There may be a perceived need for development of new incentives to evaluate efficiency of services delivered, which may affect access to less profitable areas of children's care. "Classic" surgical primacy, because of substantial charge generation, may no longer be valid; in fact, excessive use of operating room resources at high cost may render surgical care less competitive than pediatric medical care today. The incentives provided by HMOs and insurers to transpose "profit-making" types of pediatric surgery to the outpatient environment have increased the relative cost of inpatient pediatric surgery. By the unbundling of some types of surgery, pediatric surgical care as a group may be the most complex and costly inpatient service today.

The development of neonatal care groups (NCG) in the state of Florida by a collaborative group involving the Universities of South Florida and Florida for hospital, neonatal, and obstetric services, to provide prospective payment to physicians in both obstetrics and pediatric neonatal medicine, has been well described.[12-15] During the course of this development, the Florida Legislature mandated an audit of the *cost* of all neonatal care in the state of Florida. This promoted an evaluation of the total cost of care, the shifting of costs of care of the poor to paying patients, and a comparison of the acuity of care given in some 39 hospitals (self-identified) as providing neonatal intensive care. As part of that evaluation, there was rigorous review of the ratio of costs to charges (cost:charge conversion factor) by DRG occurring in those hospitals. From an evaluation of those data, there appeared to be promise for the use of cost-to-charge analysis as a useful tool for pediatric planning with the possibility that it might provide a more rational basis for the allocation of pediatric medical care services and costs.

Methods

General

The data presented were derived from the hospital information system and cost accounting module software provided by Shared Medical Systems (SMS) of Valley Forge, Pennsylvania, adapted to a large metropolitan teaching hospital. This software provides a DRG profile by cost center for pediatrics in the following areas: (1) pediatric medical/surgical inpatient wards (WARD); (2) pediatric intensive care unit (PICU); (3) newborn intensive care unit (NICU); and (4) newborn services (NSY). PICU and WARD services are usually aggregated; the remainder are maintained and reported separately. This software provides access to the following indices of performance:

1. Historical case mix data
2. Resource consumption profiles by cost center or by physician
3. Cost of services
4. Case mix profitability
5. Forecast case mix
6. Projected cost versus revenue

Assignment of direct and indirect costs were respectively divided into fixed and variable costs for each product code by cost center. These costs are heavily skewed by the contribution of personnel costs and reflect an allocation of time

TABLE 25.1. Components of costs of pediatric care.

1. Room and board—"the hotel cost"
2. Ancillary charges
a. Laboratory
b. Pharmacy
c. Radiology and imaging
d. Respiratory and pulmonary
e. Physical therapy
f. Nutrition support team, etc
3. Hospitalwide costs
a. Administration
b. Medical records
c. Social services
d. Communications and security
e. Personnel and programs
f. Marketing
g. Accounting/billing
h. Legislative lobbying
i. $$ etc
4. Medical education
a. House staff direct costs
b. Medical student direct costs
c. Nursing/allied health education
d. Medical library
e. Other costs
5. Capital expenditures
6. Indirect costs
a. Debt service
b. Funding of depreciation

and derivation of average costs. For the purpose of pediatric cost report analysis, the components of cost used in this study are shown in Table 25.1.

After resource consumption and inherent assumptions are analyzed, there is a final determination of the cost as the sum of room rate and ancillary consumption of services each with its own cost. Such a method applied to pediatrics in a general hospital must be considered semiobjective, at best. For example, many hospital procedures consume greater amounts of time in the area of procedures for each pediatric patient, and yet allocations are based on adult average time factors within an acute-care general hospital. In addition, there are controversial assignments of cost such as house staff equivalents and the allocation of the expense of nursing education. The assignment is potentially distortable if it must be made to appear more favorable for contracting with a payor with which the hospital intends to enter agreement. Finally, there is essentially no role for the physician "stakeholders" to critique recommendations that assign arbitrary decisions of cost allocation in most hospitals.

1. TOTAL PATIENTS = 4,331
   - SURGICAL 11.3% 1986/87
   - DATA PENDING 1987/88

2. TOTAL DAYS OF CARE = 26,212

3. AVERAGE LENGTH OF STAY (DAYS)
   - FY 87 5.7
   - FY 88 6.4

FIGURE 25.1. Patient population.

Specific

A proactive attempt to evaluate the distortions inherent to pediatric cost and charge descriptions in a HIS for pediatric care provided in an acute general hospital was undertaken for fiscal year 1987 and 11 months of 1988 (Oct 1, 1986, to Aug 31, 1988) for pediatric medical and surgical services at the Tampa General Hospital, a 1,000-bed teaching hospital affiliated with the University of South Florida. The hypothesis that cost-to-charge analysis possessed utility for pediatric planning was evaluated against the expectation that pediatric care services were relatively inexpensive as compared to those services provided in the operating suite.

To defend this hypothesis, all cost:charge data by DRG for pediatric services provided in the inpatient environment outside of MDC 15 (the newborn) were analyzed. The population was selected to utilize only those DRGs each of which provided greater than 10% of the total pediatric admissions during the 23-month period.

During this period, 4,331 patients were admitted to the pediatric services. The total days of care were 26,212; the average length of stay was 5.7 days and 6.4 days for FY87 and the 11 months of FY88, respectively (Fig. 25.1).

A summary of common pediatric diagnostic related groups that met the criteria for greater than 10% of all pediatric medical admissions is shown in Table 25.2.

It was not possible to utilize the same frequency of occurrence criteria for pediatric surgical DRG groups because of their diversity; therefore an arbitrary aggregation of them was performed into groups thought to be meaningful and related to pediatric surgical specialty practice (Table 25.3).

TABLE 25.2. Common pediatrics medical DRGs.

DRG number	Description
20	CNS infection
21	Viral meningitis
26	Seizure
30	Traumatic coma
44	Acute eye infection
70	Otitis and upper respiratory infection
91	Pneumonia
98	Bronchitis and asthma
184	Miscellaneous GI disorders
190	Other GI diagnosis
279	Cellulitis
296	Diabetes mellitus
298	Nutritional and metabolic conditions
322	Kidney and urinary tract infections
417	Septicemia
422	Viral illness and fever
451	Ingestions

Results

The charges and costs for all patients admitted to the pediatric medical and surgical services at the Tampa General Hospital during a 23-month period in FY87 and FY88 were evaluated. The total charges were $12,550,801 for FY87 and $13,653,122 for the 11-month period in FY88 (Fig. 25.2). The costs attributed to pediatric care services for FY87 were $8,038,922 and in FY88 (11 months) $8,826,903 (Fig. 25.2). For the respective periods of time, the total reimburse-

TABLE 25.3. Common pediatric surgical DRG groupings.

DRG number	Description
3	Craniotomy
36,37,39,42,43,47,48	Pediatric ophthalomogic procedures
52,54,55,56,58,59,60,62,72,74	Otorhinolaryngologic procedures
147–155,157–158	Miscellaneous gastrointestinal surgery
156	Upper GI surgery
163	Herniorrhaphy
165	Appendectomy, complicated
167	Appendectomy, uncomplicated
214,215,222–225,228–231,236,238, 239,244–246	Orthopedic surgical procedures
212	Hip and femoral procedures
220	Procedures of the lower extremity and humerus
235	Fractures of femur
255	Fractures of upper arm and lower leg
373	Vaginal delivery (less than 14 years old in study)
446	Multiple trauma

1. TOTAL CHARGES
   - 1986/87 = $12,550,801
   - 1987/88 = $13,653,122 (11 MTH)
2. TOTAL COST
   - 1986/87 = $8,038,922
   - 1987/88 = $8,826,903 (11 MTH)

FIGURE 25.2. Cost:charge study.

ment from all sources was $7,905,570 and for FY88 $7,938,091 (11-month estimate) (Fig. 25.3).

If it is assumed that the cost data were reflective of the "actual cost" incurred in the provision of pediatric medical and surgical services on an inpatient basis, the loss on cost (total collections less total cost) in FY87 was $133,352 and FY88 (11 months) $888,812; the marginal loss on cost (loss on cost divided by total cost) created loss margins of −1.69% and −11.20%, respectively. The financial case mix data presented in Figures 25.4 and 25.5 demonstrate the relatively unique attributes of a moderate pediatric service in an acute-care general hospital situated within the inner city and relatively dependent on governmental sources for support. The aggregate data by payor source by proportion of all patients both medical and surgical is shown graphically in Figure 25.6, again emphasizing the case mix relatively skewed to governmental sources for pediatric medicine. The relatively greater proportion of

1. TOTAL REIMBURSEMENT
   - 1986/87 = $7,905,570
   - 1987/88 = $7,938,091 (11 MTH EST)
2. LOSS ON COST
   - 1986/87 = $133,352
   - 1987/88 = $888,812 (11 MTH EST)
3. PERCENT MARGIN ON COST
   - 1986/87 = (-1.69%)
   - 1987/88 = (-11.20%)

FIGURE 25.3. Cost/charge study.

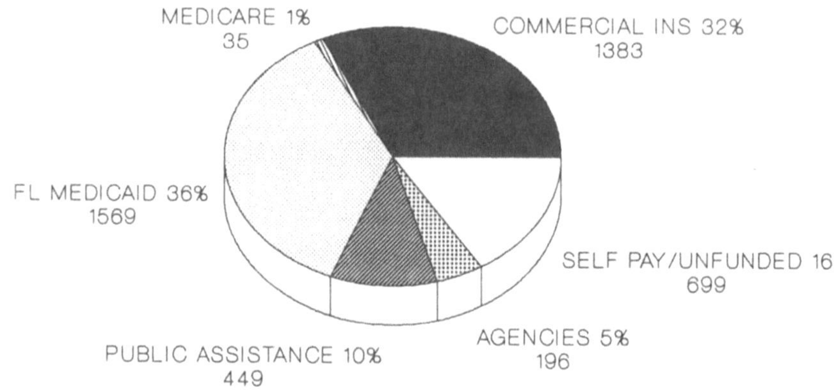

FIGURE 25.4. Financial case mix (all pediatric patients (non-newborn), USF/TGH FY86/87 and FY87/88.

commercial insurance for the surgical population reflects surgical physician selection of patients for surgery, particularly in the orthopedic area. The proportion of patients served as divided between medical and surgical (Fig. 25.7) demonstrated relatively low surgical volume as compared to inpatient medicine—a reflection on the current tendency to perform many classic high-volume procedures such as herniorrhaphy and ENT procedures in the outpatient environment unless there are significant comorbidities.

The distribution of patients by pediatric DRG in order of declining numbers is described by DRG graphically in Figure 25.8. The most common DRG was DRG-98 (bronchitis and asthma) followed by DRG-91 (pneumonia) and 184 (miscellaneous GI disorders). The least frequent DRG meeting the criteria was DRG-44 (acute eye infection). This distribution should be viewed as relatively typical for a general medical ward service without dominant subspecialty referral patterns. By compar-

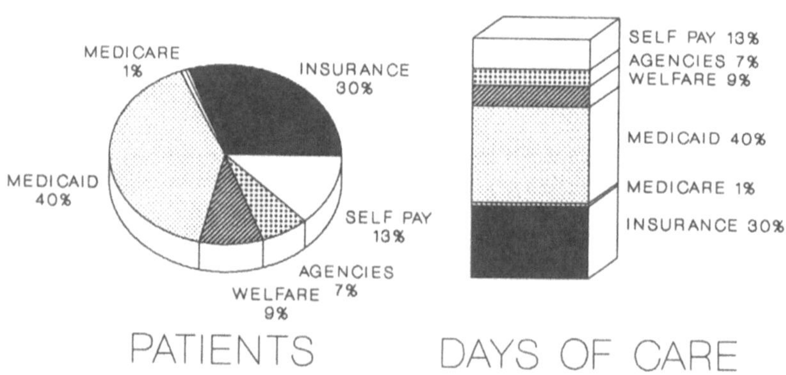

FIGURE 25.5. Admissions vs day distribution, USF/TGH FY86/87 and FY87/88.

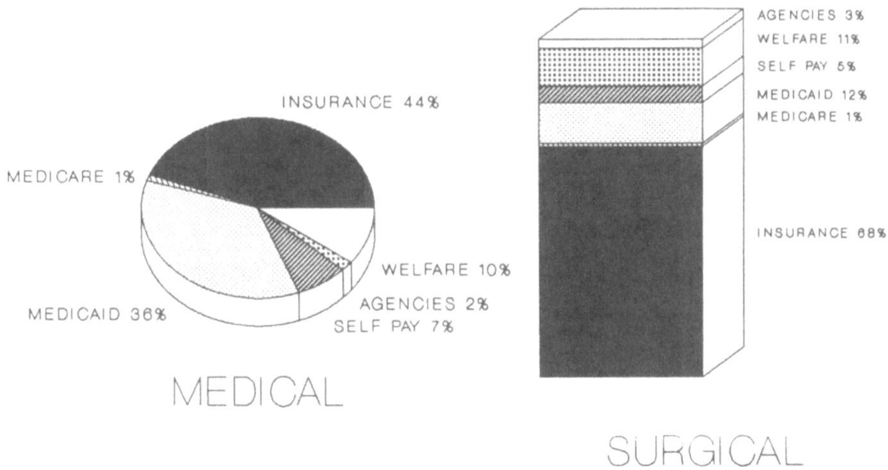

FIGURE 25.6. Financial case mix data, Medical vs surgical admissions.

ison, the patient-day distribution by DRG is given in Figure 25.9, with the most frequent in terms of number of days being DRG-20 (CNS infection) followed by DRGs 21 (viral meningitis) and 91 (pneumonia), and the least frequent being DRG-190 (other GI disorders) of the 17 most common groups.

The percent margin on charges (total charges less total collections) divided by total charges ×100) or percent margin on costs is calculated similarly for pediatric medical care for the 17 most common groups based on the financial case mix encountered at the Tampa General Hospital. Only DRG-295 (diabetes

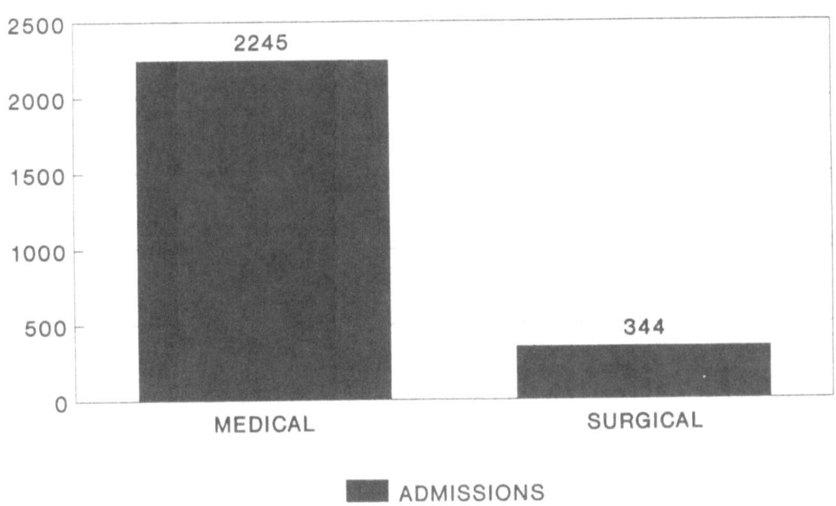

FIGURE 25.7. Distribution of patients, medical vs surgical admissions.

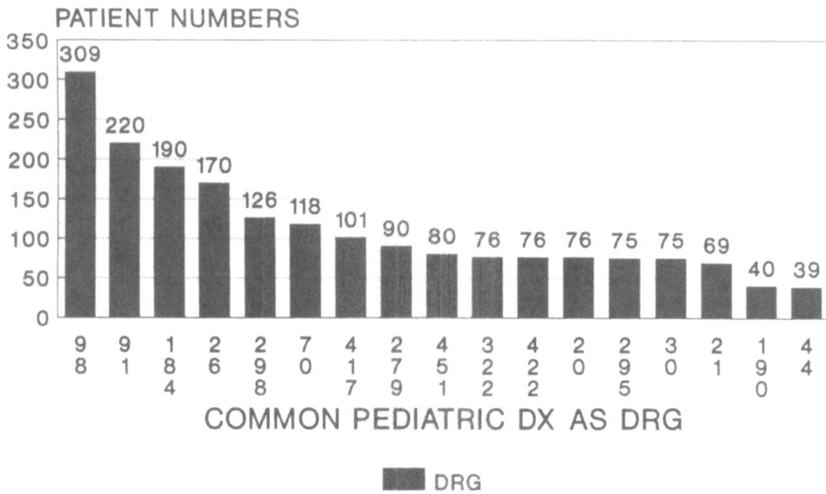

FIGURE 25.8. Distribution of patients by DRG, pediatric medicine.

mellitus) demonstrates relative profitability, with DRG-44 (acute eye infection) having the poorest experience from a hospital fiscal viewpoint (Figs. 25.10, 25.11). When pediatric surgery is evaluated with regard to the same or similar profile, the highest volume of patients admitted were in the categories of ENT surgery, orthopedic surgery, and burns. The least common was DRG-165 (appendectomy, complicated). Pediatric surgical patient days are heavily distributed to orthopedic procedures in this facility. The profit margins on charges for pediatric

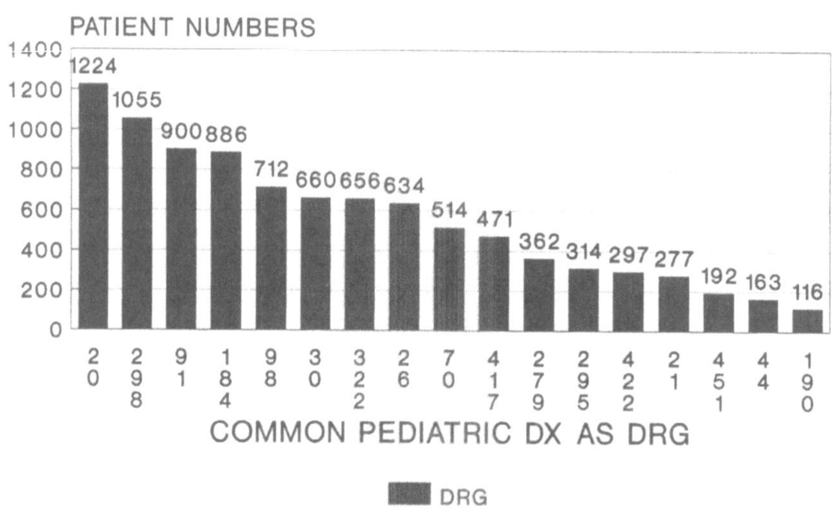

FIGURE 25.9. Distribution of patients by days, pediatric medicine.

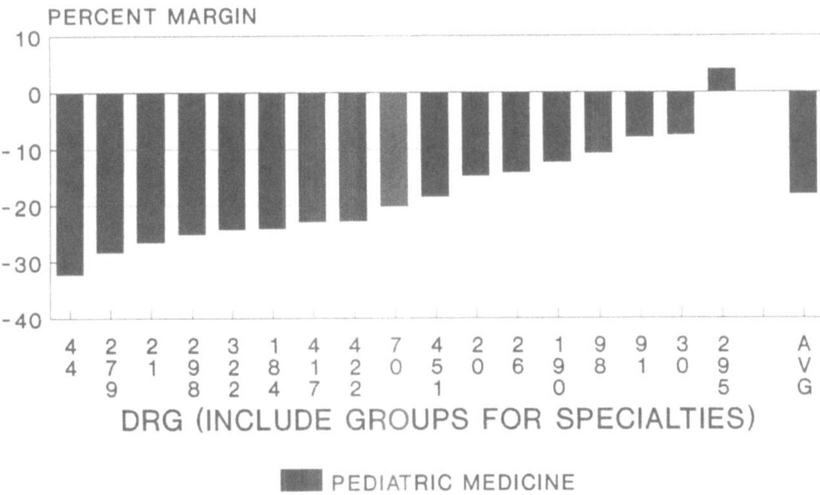

FIGURE 25.10. Percent margin on charges, pediatric medicine.

surgery included DRG-3 (craniotomy); DRG-165 (appendectomy, complicated); mixed orthopedic procedures; GI procedures; DRG-167 (appendectomy, uncomplicated); DRG-156 (upper GI surgery); and DRG-220 (procedures of the lower extremity and humerus), but the average margin on charges was negative. Similarly, when evaluated as margin on costs, DRG-220 (procedures of the lower extremity and humerus) was the most profitable. DRG-156 (upper gastrointestinal surgery), DRG-167 (appendectomy, uncomplicated), GI procedures, ortho-

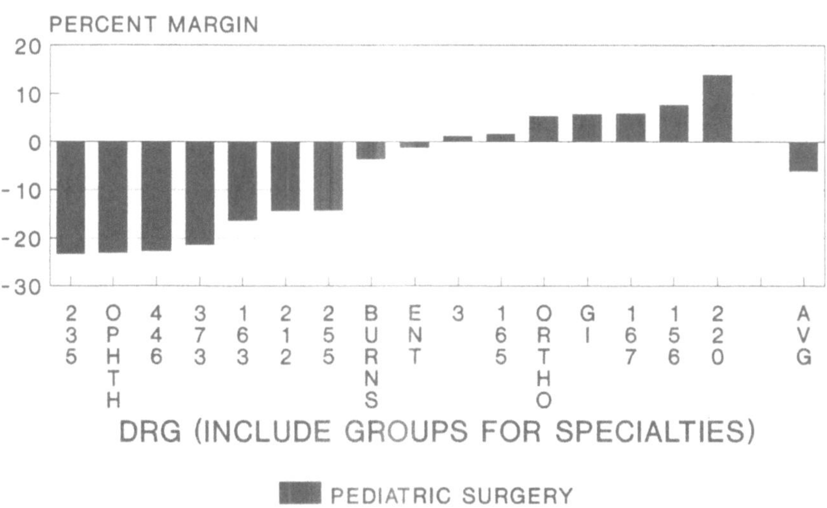

FIGURE 25.11. Percent margin on charges, pediatric surgery.

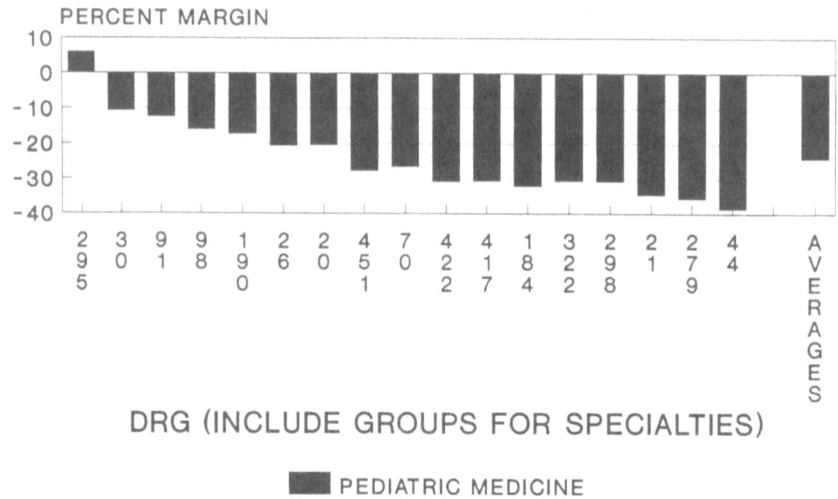

FIGURE 25.12. Percent margin on cost, pediatric medicine.

pedic procedures, and DRG-165 (appendectomy, complicated), and DRG-3 (craniotomy) follow. The average again was negative (Figs. 25.12, 25.13). Thus there is a relative paradox in that the net surgical fiscal benefit is negative performance by surgical specialties.

The usefulness of the cost-to-charge converter (C:C converter) was then evaluated for the same DRGs for both pediatric medicine and pediatric surgery. (The C:C converter is determined by dividing the costs by the charges and reporting

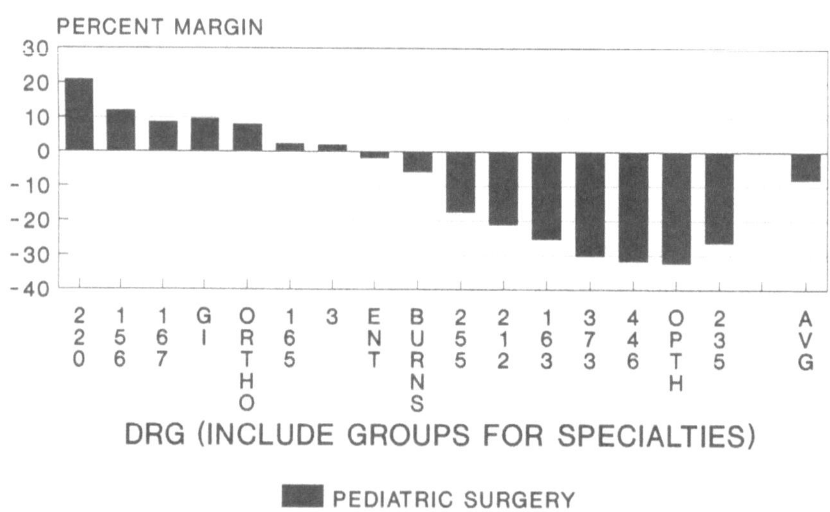

FIGURE 25.13. Percent margin on cost, pediatric surgery.

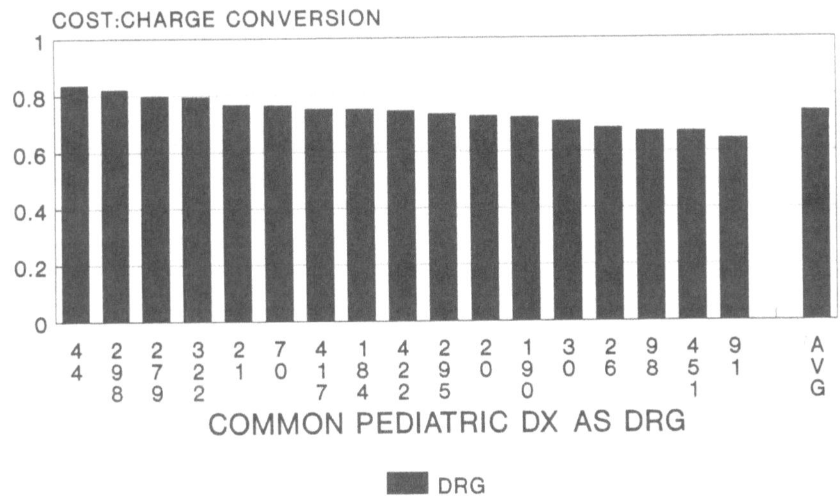

FIGURE 25.14. Comparative C:C conversion, pediatric medicine.

the result as a percent.) Those DRGs that utilize the fewest ancillary services have the highest cost-to-charge ratios. For example, DRG-44 (acute eye infection), DRG-298 (nutritional and metabolic conditions), DRG-279 (cellulitis), and DRG-322 (kidney and urinary tract infections) are all above average in C:C converter (Fig. 25.14). Surgical cost-to-charge data likewise demonstrate a similar C:C converter; however, DRG-235 and DRG-255 are well above the mean and reflect less ancillary service consumption (Fig. 25.15).

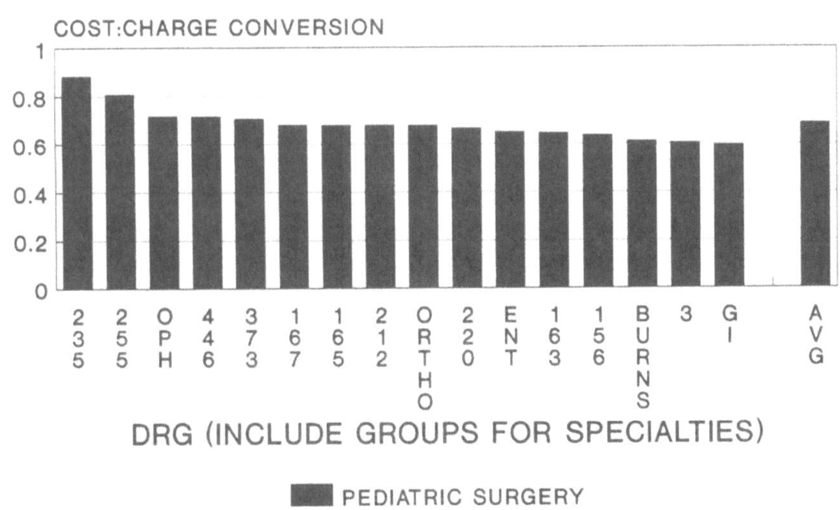

FIGURE 25.15. Comparative C:C conversion, pediatric surgery.

This relative paradox may well reflect the high use of ancillary services and utilization of operating room time in these DRGs. We were unable to rigorously evaluate this information from the data readily available from the HIS. Historically, there is a tendency for operating room charges to be falsely elevated because of the willingness of third-party payors to reimburse these services rather than room rate.

Future directions are not clear as long as commercial payors, governmental agencies, and others continue to pay on the basis of price of services and differentially reward ancillary consumption. It is likely that the C:C conversion inequity will continue. This is strongly discriminative against pediatric medicine in areas most crucial to medical education at the medical student and resident training level, as the inpatient teaching process has always taken time to learn with regard to a disease process. Since pediatric medicine generates relatively few extremely high ancillary charges except in the critical care area, this phenomenon of poor C:C converter experience will directly affect the willingness of hospital governing bodies and management to support the "losers" (general pediatrics) in the future unless a new method to differentially develop services based on efficiency indices is developed. The concerted movement by payors to reimburse on the basis of pediatric DRGs, as has been done by CHAMPUS and some state Medicaid programs, provides an avenue that may permit pediatric medical care to become more important than pediatric surgical care because of the inverse relationship between costs and charges attendant upon the relatively short stays and costs per patient.

Current information systems now make it possible to manage pediatric medical and surgical care to assess the efficiency of a pediatric resident's use of resources and stay. These may be linked to patients, their diagnoses, and the procedures utilized, and will provide cost/charge/diagnostic comparison with peers and national norms. Supervising faculty can be evaluated by their "profitability" and effectiveness in teaching trainees cost-effective medical care. Efficiency ratios for teams of physicians providing similar patterns of care can be developed that could provide incentive mechanisms to reward those who are most efficient in a DRG-type environment. It would appear that the new Harvard Resource Based Relative Value System (RBRVS)[16] would promote higher reimbursement for physicians for cognitive services.

This would only be of value in limiting health care expenditure if there were prospective payment mechanisms providing a cap of reimbursement for hospital care. Children's hospital DRGs developed with the input of NACHRI present an alternative method to represent the higher costs of children's hospitals; likewise, there is the same need for the development of efficiency indices and the development of incentives based on C:C converters. It would be apparent that those who can sustain a low cost/high charge in the presence of DRGs would be the "winners" in pediatric medicine in the future.

Discussion

These data readily demonstrate that there has been no alteration in the relative excess profitability of surgical services to the hospital as compared to pediatric medical services even though there have been major changes in surgical case mix with the in-hospital utilization transition to outpatient surgery, the new aspects of competition provided by alternative delivery services or systems, the trend to admit patients who are more consumptive of complex tertiary-care services, and the beginning evolution of quaternary care by university-associated services. It would appear that there is currently no mechanism for current hospital structures to reward the cognitive practice of inpatient pediatric medicine that uses relatively few laboratory ancillary services, because of the persistent policies established by third-party intermediaries of differentially rewarding change in ancillary charges. Hospital room rates have been kept at a subsidized level, subsidized in part by transfers from laboratory, radiologic, and other services. For example, the C:C converter merely perpetuates this relative inequity of reimbursement systems. As hospital information systems begin to evaluate physicians for relatively economic productivity for the institution, this type of information could be utilized in relatively punitive fashion against nonprocedural pediatric physicians who use very few ancillary services and do not generate large charges with high potential recoverability for the institution.

Conclusion

In order for pediatric medicine to have an effective voice in a competitive hospital industry for the development of new programs for children that are marginally economically effective, it is necessary to initiate institutional studies for comparison of resource consumption for similar groups of patients. These critical analyses for comparison should be carried out for both pediatric medical and surgical areas of care. There is a need to develop mechanisms to track the use of resources by pediatricians, residents, and their attending physicians as teams or groups. The adoption of a proactive role in securing methods of appropriate cost allocations for medical education is of paramount importance. If these are not developed, the aggressive procedures necessary for competition will have a direct effect on medical education with rewards only to those who provide the shortest inpatient stay. Such practices will make more difficult the teaching of medical students and resident physicians with regard to the longitudinal course of disease. Such an emphasis will provide stimulation for the development of alternatives in the outpatient environment and the care of an entirely new class of patients who are moderately ill in alternative care settings. Survival of pediatrics as a dynamic area of health care requires a careful understanding of the health care economics of today and proactive positions to assure that the children of tomorrow receive care that is at least the high quality that is practiced in this nation today.

References

1. Grimaldi PL, Micheletti JA: *DRG's, Diagnostic Related Groups: A Practitioner's Guide*. Chicago: Pluribus Press, pp 1–217.
2. AMA: *DRG's and the Prospective Payment System: A Guide for Physicians*. Chicago: American Medical Association, 1983.

3. National Association of Children's Hospitals and Related Institutions and U.S. Department of Health and Human Services: *The Use of Case Mix Based Prospective Payment for Inpatient Pediatric Hospital Care.* Merrifield, VA; Cardinal Printing, 1984, pp 1-25.
4. Caputi MA, Heiss WA: The DRG revolution. *Health Soc Work* 9:5–12, 1984.
5. Haley MJ: What is a DRG? *Top Health Care Finance* 6:5561, 1980.
6. Iglehart JK: Health policy report, New Jersey's experiment with DRG-based hospital reimbursement. *N Engl J Med* 307:1655–1660, 1982.
7. Iglehart JK: The new era of prospective payment for hospitals. *N Engl J Med* 307:1288–1292, 1982.
8. Fetter RB, Shin Y, Freeman JL, et al: Definitions by diagnosis related groups. *Med Care* 18(2):1–53, 1980.
9. Scott SJ: The Medicare prospective program. *Am J Occup Ther* 38:5, 1984.
10. Barnard C, Esmond T: DRG-based reimbursement: The use of concurrent and retrospective clinical data. *Med Care* 14:11, 1981.
11. Federal Register: Update of Code of Federal Regulations. Sept 1, 1983; 48(171): 39776; Chap. 42 CFR, parts 405, 408, 489.
12. Poland RL, Bollinger RO, Bedard MP, Cohen SN: Analysis of the effects of applying federal diagnosis-related grouping (DRG) guidelines to a population of high-risk newborn infants. *Pediatrics* 76:104–109, 1985.
13. Resnick MB, Ariet M, Carter RL, et al: Prospective pricing system for tertiary neonatal intensive care. *Pediatrics* 78:820–828, 1986.
14. Resnick MB, Ariet M, Carter RL, et al: Prospective pricing model for neonatologists and obstetricians in tertiary care centers. *Pediatrics* 82:442–446, 1988.
15. Resnick MB, Ariet M, Carter RL, et al: Prospective pricing system by diagnosis-related groups: Comparison of federal diagnosis-related groups with high-risk obstetric care groups. *Am J Obstet Gynecol* Mar:567–573, 1987.
16. Hsiao WC, Brown P, Dunn D, Becker ER: Resource-based relative values: An overview. *JAMA* 260:2347–2353, 1988.

26
Thoughts on the Modern Practice of Pediatrics

CHARLES D. COOK

Introduction

As chief of three pediatric services in three quite different cities—New Haven, Brooklyn, and Rochester, New York—I have been involved in studies related to quality assurance issues. Although the studies have been hospital based, some inpatient and some outpatient, I believe that extrapolations to the office practice of pediatrics are legitimate. A review of some of these and related studies by others of the quality of the medical care of children; some highlighting of major problems and thus challenges for future pediatric care; and some recommendations will be the subjects of this report. Major underlying theses will be (1) that there is a serious gap between what we know should be done for children and what we do, (2) that this has serious quality and cost consequences, and (3) that we are not using modern information processing and analysis techniques to assist in improving the quality of care in either hospital or office settings. Finally, I will make some suggestions about how the knowledge-performance gap might be reduced.

Study 1

The first study was done almost 20 years ago with Duff and others[1] in four Connecticut hospitals. We examined the appropriateness of hospital admissions of pediatric patients and the correctness and cost-effectiveness of their care. The data showed (Table 26.1) that in a teaching hospital inappropriate admissions to the pediatric and general surgical services were at an acceptably low level, about 7%, but that on at least one service, urology, and at community hospitals the rate was much higher. Calculations at that time indicated that, if these data were representative of the entire country, approximately $450 million in 1971 dollars was

---

From the Department of Pediatrics, University of Rochester School of Medicine and Dentistry, Rochester, New York.
Presented in honor of Lewis A. Barness, MD, November 12, 1988.

TABLE 26.1. Unnecessary admmissions by hospital and service.

Service	Hospital[a]									
	A		B		C		D		All	
Nonsurgical	21/50	(42%)	22/57	(39%)	12/42	(29%)	5/68	(7%)	60/217	(28%)
Surgery except urology	6/46	(13%)	5/41	(12%)	5/39	(13%)	2/40	(5%)	18/166	(11%)
Urology	3/4	(75%)	7/7	(100%)	17/19	(90%)	6/15	(40%)	33/45	(73%)
All	30/100	(30%)	34/105	(32%)	34/100	(34%)	13/123	(11%)	111/428	(26%)

Source: Reproduced by permission of *Pediatrics*, Vol 49, p 170, copyright © 1972.
[a] Hospitals A, B, and C are nonteaching community hospitals. Hospital D is a principal teaching hospital.

being wasted each year, to say nothing of the psychological and occasional physical harm being done to the inappropriately hospitalized children. An expanded study[2] done in 1974 confirmed the original findings. That unnecessary admission and hospital stays are still a problem is confirmed by a recent report of Kemper,[3] who showed that, even in the university hospital studied, 21% of children's hospital days were not necessary.

Study 2

I was involved in another study,[4] at Kings County Hospital in Brooklyn, again on an inpatient service. We found that the inappropriate hospitalization of pediatric patients dropped from 23% of all admissions to 6% and that the average length of stay decreased about 38% when some, even though minimal, criteria for admitting and keeping children in hospital were instituted. Clearly, many children were inappropriately admitted to the hospital, and reform resulted in the closing of about 50% of the pediatric beds.

Study 3

The largest study[5] in which I was involved concerned the 170,000 annual walk-in pediatric patients presenting for care to the Pediatric Emergency Room at Kings County Hospital. With variously trained, inadequately supervised physicians who were frequently overwhelmed by the sheer workload and who were working within an essentially financially bankrupt system, there was reason to believe that some method for quality assurance would improve both the quality and the cost-effectiveness of care. To give only one specific example of the challenges: because of the numbers involved, the choice between doing stool cultures on most patients with diarrhea or doing stool cultures only on selected patients would mean an approximately $50,000 annual difference in costs. I will return in a moment to a discussion of what we attempted to do at Kings County Hospital to improve the quality of ambulatory care.

Study 4

A more recent study,[6] this time at a hospital in Rochester, New York, was carried out in 1985 and 1986. Using well-established criteria for tonsillectomy and for adenoidectomy,[7] we found that 51% of the 157 tonsillectomies were inappropriate; indeed if more children with streptococcal sore throats had been treated with appropriate antibiotics rather than surgery after a therapeutic failure with penicillin, only about 27% of the tonsillectomies would have been justified. The study also showed that 31% of the adenoidectomies did not meet the generally accepted criteria. Thus, these studies confirmed those of others[8] that have consistently

TABLE 26.2. Pediatricians' knowledge of families.

Excellent	5%
Good	12%
Mediocre	14%
Poor	26%
Very poor	43%

Source: Duff et al.[9] Used with permission.

shown that even accepted criteria are not adhered to, and indicated that families and society are subjected to unnecessary costs and children to considerable trauma and at least some unnecessary risks. Although the excessive use of tonsillectomies and adenoidectomies is hardly confined to Rochester, the practice there is, at least in part, the legacy of George Eastman, Rochester's major 20th-century civic leader, who financed mass tonsillectomies in the misguided belief that this would produce healthier citizens.

Discussion

In an extensive study of the strengths and weaknesses of the practice of pediatrics in offices and clinics in New Haven carried out in the mid-1970s by Duff and coworkers,[9] deficiencies were found in the routine care of children. Since Duff et al looked at and beyond the management of physical problems, they were able to identify psychosocial conditions that were frequently inadequately cared for. For example (Table 26.2), pediatricians' knowledge of the families of their patients was rated as poor or very poor in 69% of cases. In addition, their knowledge of even severe psychologic problems, presumably the basis for practicing the "new pediatrics," was rated as poor in almost half the cases (Table 26.3).

Having cited a few examples of deficiencies in the practice of pediatrics, I offer some techniques for trying to improve the quality of care—ie, a system for quality assurance that we devised for the pediatric ambulatory clinic at Kings County Hospital. There were, of course, trials and tribulations involved in trying to impose such a system for quality assurance on the more than 100 physicians who

TABLE 26.3. Pediatricians' knowledge of children and families.

	Psychological problem	
Knowledge	None	Very severe
Good	37%	31%
Mediocre	29%	23%
Poor	34%	46%

Source: Duff et al.[9] Used with permission.

TABLE 26.4. Elements in quality assurance system.

Guidelines/optimal standards
Efficient data collection
Data processing/analysis
Motivated leadership

in any given year worked in the clinic at Kings County Hospital; but I will call your attention only to Machiavelli's comment on the process:

It must be remembered that there is nothing more difficult to plan, more doubtful of success, nor more dangerous to manage than the creation of a new system. For the initiator has the enmity of all who would profit by the preservation of the old institution and merely lukewarm defenders in those who would gain by new ones.[10]

The elements involved in our quality assurance system (Table 26.4) are fundamental components of almost all quality assurance efforts, and they all represent some of the challenges for us in academic pediatrics as well as for practitioners in primary care.

The most important, and at the same time most difficult, part of developing a quality assurance system is the establishment of guidelines – ie, criteria for diagnosis and guidelines for care. While guidelines, which should be based on decision analysis techniques, are becoming more readily available, not enough have been established, tested, and implemented. Indeed, there is an understandable reluctance on the part of physicians to establish standards of optimal (emphatically not average) care by which their management of patients can be evaluated. But both consumers and third-party payors, as well as regulatory agencies, are demanding accountability as judged by established guidelines, and certainly it is patently impossible to "referee the game" without rules.

The guidelines, though usually quite stable over relatively long periods of time, must nevertheless be subject to regular review and revision as necessary. Indeed, review of the results from applying the guidelines should contribute to the development of better guidelines.

Another essential element of quality assurance is the presence of adequate patient information for review. Except for the use of paper and a ball-point pen instead of a clay tablet and a stylus, patients' records today are about the same as those of Hippocrates; indeed, they may be considerably less legible! Forms are available[5] (Fig. 26.1), but few clinics or practices use techniques for formating the patient information for efficient review or even attempt to standardize the terminology.

Furthermore, with the large amount of patient information for even those patients requiring only primary care, we are far beyond the ability to process patient data efficiently from hand-written records, especially when we are dealing with large numbers of patients. Computers have been available for some time. (Dr Barness was one of the earliest pediatricians to try to utilize their analytic power.) Only a few clinics and inpatient services utilize them for recording and

PRESENT ILLNESS

Time Patient Seen by Provider:

General: ☐ Fever ______ duration ______ ☐ antipyretic ______

☐ Decreased activity ☐ somnolence ☐ irritability

☐ Decreased appetite ☐ intake last 24 hrs. ______

Usual formula/dilution (< 1 yr. old) ______ wght loss ______

☐ On antibiotic ______ ☐ On other meds ______

☐ Previous medical care for this episode ______

Skin: ☐ rash ______

HEENT: ☐ headache ______

☐ visual abnormality ______

☐ otalgia ___ ☐ hearing loss ___ ☐ otorrhea ___ duration ___

☐ rhinorrhea ______ ☐ sore throat ______ duration ______

Chest: ☐ cough ______ duration ______

☐ wheezing ______ ☐ SOB ______ ☐ stridor ______

☐ chest pain ______ ☐ cyanosis ______ ☐ apnea ______

GI: ☐ vomiting ______ ☐ nausea ☐ constipation

☐ abdominal pain ______

☐ diarrhea ______ ☐ blood ______

GU: ☐ dysuria ☐ frequency ☐ urgency ☐ hematuria

☐ enuresis ☐ oliguria/anuria ☐ polyuria

☐ other ______

sexually active ______ last intercourse ______

contraception method ______ GC contact ______

♀ LMP ______ Gr ______ Pa ______ If pregnant, duration ______

☐ vaginal discharge ______ ☐ itching ______ ☐ soreness/rash

♂ ☐ penile discharge ______

Musculoskeletal ______

CNS: ☐ LOC/Amnesia ______

☐ seizure ☐ focality ______ ☐ duration ______ ☐ No. in 24 hrs. ______

describe ______

☐ **Trauma** ______

Other symptoms ______

FIGURE 26.1. An example of part of a structured form for recording patient information. (*Source*: Cook and Heidt.[5] Reprinted with permission of authors and Oxford University Press.)

processing patient information. Even fewer use them for the actual evaluation of patient care.

Do these techniques for quality assurance actually contribute to improving patient care and to making ambulatory pediatrics more cost-efficient? Dealing with so many self-limited diseases in pediatrics, this is not always easy to prove. In our own application of some of this methodology at Kings County Hospital we were able to observe some improvements. For example, we were able to show

TABLE 26.5. Effect of guidelines on the use of antibiotics in patients discharged with diagnosis of pneumonia.

	Preguideline	Guideline
Probable bacterial pneumonia treated	75% (6/8)	80% (4/5)
Probable viral pneumonia treated	88% (15/17)	23% (2/9)
Unclassified pneumonia treated	20% (1/5)	29% (2/7)
All pneumonia treated	73% (22/30)	38% (8/21)
Correct[a] use of antibiotics	32%	79%

[a]Correct according to the guidelines.
Source: Reprinted from Cook CD and Heidt J,[5] with permission of authors and Oxford University Press.

that the management of patients with pneumonia became more appropriate (Table 26.5). We were also able to show that costs were reduced and, in our opinion, appropriately so, when the guidelines were applied (Table 26.6). We were also able to show that the outcomes for asthmatic patients improved with the use of guidelines.[5]

An additional factor that affects the quality of care emerges from the data of Duff et al, indicating that the quality of care improves as one progresses from solo, to two- and three-person practices and finally to larger group practices (Table 26.7). An appealing interpretation is that larger practices have more opportunities for self- and cross-examination, resulting in more critically evaluated, better care being given. The converse is that intellectual/professional isolation may not be conducive to optimal care.

TABLE 26.6. X-ray and laboratory charges.

	Adherent visits	Nonadherent visits
Asthma	$2.32	$6.17
Otitis media	0.21	0.99
Gastroenteritis	0.11	2.47

Source: Reprinted from Cook CD and Heidt J,[5] with permission of authors and Oxford University Press.

TABLE 26.7. Physician performance scores.

Type of practice	Mean score
Solo	3.82
Two members	4.00
Three to five members	7.27
Health plans	9.25

Source: Duff et al.[9] Used with permission.

Summary

I have pointed out (1) that serious and costly gaps exist between what we believe, in the light of present information, is best for pediatric patients and what we actually do; (2) that a critical challenge is to develop and implement standards of optimal care for children; (3) that to meet this challenge we need to use the modern technology provided by computers for data processing and information analysis and, therefore, for quality assurance; and (4) that the most critical challenge of all is to persuade all those who provide care to children that it is intellectually exciting and satisfying to examine continuously what is being done for children with the purpose of improving it. Socrates put it well: "The unexamined life is not worth living."[11]

If we and practitioners succeed, we will have more time to give to the humanistic components of patient care and to meet the challenge of the emotional needs of children, which Duff's study[9] showed are frequently neglected. We need time to take a careful history. We need time to understand our patients' and their families' psychosocial problems. A quality assurance system using new technology is an essential basis for achieving such goals.

References

1. Duff RS, Cook CD, et al: Use of utilization review to assess the quality of pediatric in-patient care. *Pediatrics* 49:169–176, 1972.
2. Duff RS, Cook CD, et al: A review of pediatric in-patient care. *Am J Dis Child* 129:1422–1424, 1975.
3. Kemper KJ: Medically inappropriate hospital use in a pediatric population. *N Engl J Med* 318:1033, 1988.
4. Phillipp JT, Rao M, Cook CD, et al: Impact of policy changes on in-patient care. *Pediatr Res* 12:447, 1978 (abstract).
5. Cook CD, Heidt J: *Assuring Quality Out-Patient Care for Children*. New York: Oxford University Press, 1988.
6. Cook CD, Cook CC: Unpublished data.
7. Paradise JL: Tonsillectomy and adenoidectomy: In Bluestone CD, Stool SE (eds): *Pediatric Otolaryngology*. Philadelphia: Saunders, 1983, p 998.
8. LoGerfo JP, Dynes IM, et al: Tonsillectomies, adenoidectomies, audits: Have surgical indications been met? *Med Care* 16:950–955, 1978.
9. Duff RS, Meyers A, et al: A critical study of pediatric practice: Strengths and weaknesses. Ann Arbor: Health Administration Press (in press).
10. Machiavelli: *The Prince*, 1513.
11. Plato: *The Apology* (38a), 5th–4th BC.

Index

MIX
Papier aus verantwortungsvollen Quellen
Paper from responsible sources
FSC® C105338

If you have any concerns about our products,
you can contact us on
ProductSafety@springernature.com

In case Publisher is established outside the EU,
the EU authorized representative is:
Springer Nature Customer Service Center GmbH
Europaplatz 3, 69115 Heidelberg, Germany

Printed by Libri Plureos GmbH
in Hamburg, Germany